Honest Aging

A Johns Hopkins Press Health Book

Honest Aging

An Insider's Guide
to the Second Half of Life

ROSANNE M. LEIPZIG, MD, PhD

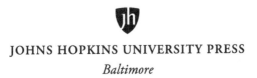

JOHNS HOPKINS UNIVERSITY PRESS

Baltimore

Note to the Reader: This book is not meant to substitute for medical care, and treatment should not be based solely on its contents. Instead, treatment must be developed in a dialogue between the individual and their physician. The book has been written to help with that dialogue.

Drug dosage: The author and publisher have made reasonable efforts to determine that the selection of drugs discussed in this text conform to the practices of the general medical community. In view of ongoing research, changes in governmental regulation, and the constant flow of information relating to drug therapy and drug reactions, the reader is urged to check the package insert of each drug for any change in indications and dosage and for warnings and precautions. This is particularly important when the recommended agent is a new and/or an infrequently used drug.

© 2023 Rosanne M. Leipzig
All rights reserved. Published 2023
Printed in the United States of America on acid-free paper
9 8 7 6 5 4 3 2

Johns Hopkins University Press
2715 North Charles Street
Baltimore, Maryland 21218
www.press.jhu.edu

Library of Congress Cataloging-in-Publication Data

Names: Leipzig, Rosanne M., 1951– author.
Title: Honest aging : an insider's guide to the second half of life / Rosanne M. Leipzig, MD, PhD.
Description: Baltimore : Johns Hopkins University Press, 2022. | Series: A Johns Hopkins Press health book | Includes bibliographical references and index.
Identifiers: LCCN 2021062978 | ISBN 9781421444697 (hardcover) | ISBN 9781421444703 (paperback) | ISBN 9781421444710 (ebook)
Subjects: LCSH: Aging. | Older people. | Geriatrics. | Popular works.
Classification: LCC HQ1061 .L4556 2022 | DDC 305.26– dc23/eng/20220104
LC record available at https://lccn.loc.gov/2021062978

A catalog record for this book is available from the British Library.

The illustrations in this book, including modifications and adaptations, were created by Jane Whitney unless otherwise noted.

Special discounts are available for bulk purchases of this book. For more information, please contact Special Sales at specialsales@jh.edu.

To my grandmother, Gussie Gordon, and my wife, Ora Chaikin—
my role models for how to adapt to one's new normal

Contents

Preface

I am a geriatrician, a specialist in the care of older adults. In my 40 years of practice, the number one question that I'm asked by patients, families, at parties, or when sitting next to someone on an airplane is "Is *this* normal for aging?" *This* can be a change in physical appearance, a new symptom or behavior, or difficulty doing something that's never been a problem before. There's a world of subtext in these questions: Is *this* a sign of a serious chronic illness? Is *this* the start of dementia? Will *this* kill me? Will *this* make it impossible for me to live independently? Can anything be done about *this*?

What is normal? Dictionary definitions include usual or typical. Normal doesn't mean there's never a cause for concern, or that there's nothing that can be done to make things better. Normal age-related changes can affect what you do day-to-day and how you feel, both physically and emotionally. We're lucky to live at a time when so many adaptive devices and technologies are available. When you turn 40 or so, you develop blurred vision while doing close-up work, reading, using the computer, or sewing, for example. This is called presbyopia. It is "normal," and hopefully you will respond by getting glasses to correct your vision. Without glasses, you wouldn't be able to live a normal life, and your new visual impairment would become a disability. We don't usually think of glasses as assistive devices, yet they are, just like canes or hearing aids. These devices can make an enormous difference in the quality of our lives as we age; however, this will happen only if we recognize how they improve our function and ability to engage with the world when using them.

How you react to age-related change determines how you will live. People age in different ways. Some fight it tooth and nail, denying that any changes are happening. Some are scared and anxious about every change they perceive. Some cave in, and some just keep living, looking at the changes as new and interesting challenges. The same holds for family and friends who have their own fears and concerns about the safety and quality of life of their loved ones as well as the effects this process may have on their own lives. Both worry about how changes related to aging will affect their relationships with each other. It is my hope that the answers, ideas, and suggestions you find in this book will help you and those you love to be creative, resilient, and engaged in this, the second half of your life.

Birth is a beginning and
death a destination;

But life is a journey.

A going, a growing from
stage to stage:

From childhood to maturity
and youth to old age.

FROM "LIFE IS A JOURNEY,"
BY ALVIN FINE

How to Use this Book

Honest Aging is a guide for you and your loved ones as you begin the next stage of your life. What should you expect as you age? Every person ages differently, yet there are common changes and challenges that all of us experience.

This book is not a prescription for aging backward or making 80 the new 60. It doesn't delve into DNA, telomeres, or other aspects of the basic science of aging. It is not a guide to self-diagnosis, nor should it substitute for regular visits with your medical provider. But it may come in handy when you and your practitioners are trying to figure out whether something is normal or if there are ways to help you function better.

This book is for older adults, their loved ones, and those who are curious about what to expect and who they can be as they age. Each chapter is written with an awareness and sensitivity relevant to each of these readers. For example, those concerned about their memory may not want to tell others, afraid that they will lose their autonomy and independence, but they still want information as to whether a loss of cognitive function is actually happening, and what they might do to limit it. Loved ones may not know how to discuss concerns about memory or make suggestions without engendering conflict. The curious run the risk of becoming "worried well," focusing on potential problems rather than being proactive.

Part I of the book, *Aging 101*, focuses on five spheres that are uniquely important to the health and well-being of older adults. Chapter 1 addresses personal and psychological responses to aging,

both for older adults and those who care about them. Chapter 2 provides an approach to medical care for older adults, comparing and contrasting 80-year-olds and 60-year-olds in the ways medical illness presents and should be treated, and introduces the focus of part II, geriatric syndromes and the Geriatrics 5M's. Chapter 3 discusses medication use and management in older adults. Chapter 4 presents a framework for deciding what care makes sense for you and how to discuss this with your providers, while chapter 5 addresses what should constitute "preventive medicine" when you're 65 and older.

Part II, *What Really Matters as You Grow Older*, focuses on the symptoms that cause my patients and their families to worry the most. There are chapters on memory, energy, moods, mobility, balance and falls, sleep, urination, vision and hearing, aches and pains, gastrointestinal concerns, weight and nutrition, and sex. These chapters cover the gamut of where things can and do go awry as we grow older. The chapters are structured similarly, beginning with questions and answers about *what's normal with aging* and *adapting to your new normal*. They also discuss *what isn't normal aging*, with *red flags* to alert you to serious symptoms that need prompt evaluation and *yellow alerts* that describe medications and common treatable conditions that may be causing or exacerbating the problem. Deeper dives into the science and age-related changes are contained within boxes in each chapter. The chapters in part II also discuss whether to get an evaluation, *when to see a specialist*, and *how to prepare for the visit*, including a *pre-visit checklist* (found in Appendix 3) for you to complete beforehand and bring to your visit.

Part III, *Difficult Decisions*, addresses some of the life concerns about which individuals and their families worry the most. Chapter 17 (along with chapter 4) discusses the overall process of decision-making. Chapters 18, 19, and 20 consider the options for, respectively, where you should live, if you should continue driving, and how to decide who should speak for you if you're unable to speak for yourself.

Loved ones is the term I use for those people who care about and for a person who is growing old. Recognizing how sensitive conversations can be between older adults and their loved ones, especially when contentious issues need to be discussed, I offer *advice for loved ones*, prudent ways to frame and have discussions, toward the end of most chapters in parts II and III.

In my experience, the key to aging well is having a sense of what to expect, what's normal and what's not, and what options there are for you and your loved ones when adapting to whatever is in your future. This is the purpose of this book. It's also to help you keep your eye on the prize—having an old age filled with contentment, meaning, well-being, and connection by being open and flexible as you experience the rewards and the challenges of aging.

Aging 101

CHAPTER 1

It's Only Aging, Get a Grip!

The key to aging well lies within you, the attitudes and responses you have to growing older and entering old age.

"Aging—it's better than the alternative" is a familiar quip. It's not often said with a lot of enthusiasm, and it's hardly a rousing recommendation for what may be up to a third of one's life. Yes, there will be inevitable physical declines and losses that can transform your life, but as long as you're alive, there will be new options for improving your well-being, happiness, and sense of purpose. Being resilient, facing challenges, and establishing a new normal can allow you to have a positive outlook about the future, to think outside the box you may find yourself in, and to appreciate the possibilities, humor, and joy that can be part of your life.

Old age is a new stage of life. It is *not* the same as middle age. Your abilities, your desires, and your circumstances are likely to change. What counts is how you deal with these changes. Not all change will be welcomed, but I bet this isn't the first time in your life you've needed to adjust to uninvited change. In my many years of practice as a geriatrician, I've seen different responses to aging, from head-in-the-sand ostriches, to obsessive worry warts, to wise old owls. These are *choices*. Facing reality head-on, using this book to discover what's likely to happen, what to expect, and what you can do will help you to turn this stage of your life into a time of growth, meaning, and happiness. But if you buy into the stereotypes and myths, you'll be at the mercy of the naysayers, including at times your health care providers. Be proactive, creative, and resilient in response to the new situations you will undoubtedly face.

Self-Fulfilling Prophecies

We develop stereotypes of aging when we are children. Some stereotypes are positive, and some are negative. These are often reinforced throughout our lifetimes, and they can become self-fulfilling prophecies, affecting our health and well-being in old age. Dr. Becca Levy and her colleagues conducted a series of studies and found that older adults with negative perceptions of aging performed worse on memory tasks and standardized hearing tests, and their hearing declined more rapidly, than those with positive perceptions of aging. In contrast, in a study with an eighteen-year follow-up, older adults with positive perceptions of aging lived 7.5 years longer and maintained more independence, including the ability to do heavy work and climb stairs, than those with negative perceptions of aging. This wasn't true only for those in old age. Over thirty-eight years, young and middle-aged adults, 18 to 49 years old, with negative perceptions of aging had more cardiovascular disease, and those aged 18 to 39 had more heart attacks after age 60.

At this point you're probably wondering how this could be. These health conditions are generally considered to be caused by diseases and age-related physiologic changes, not by one's attitude. Yet attitude can influence one's effort, expectations, adherence to medical advice, and use of adaptive strategies. For example, older adults with negative perceptions are less likely to seek preventive medical care.

The good news is that these self-perceptions are not immutable. In other studies, Dr. Levy's group randomly divided older study subjects into two groups. Each group had stereotypes of aging subliminally flashed on their screens while performing a task on a computer. The subjects were unaware that stereotypes were flashing on their screens. Stereotypes were negative for one group and positive for the other. Those exposed to positive stereotypes showed improved memory, handwriting legibility, and, in an exercise study, better strength, gait, and balance. They also had fewer negative self-perceptions of aging. Negative stereotypes, even subconscious ones, activate negative self-perceptions, which become self-fulfilling prophecies.

Your job, and that of those who love you, is to recognize that these stereotypes are not reality, to improve your own perceptions of aging by speaking up when you hear or see negative stereotypes, and to surround yourself with positive images of aging and empowered older people. Professionally run arts workshops, often called Creative Aging programs, engage older adults in opportunities for meaningful creative expression and have been found to improve their health, wellness, and connectedness. See the Creative Aging section of the Resources at the end of this chapter for ways to find programs.

What Is Old Age?

I'm often asked at what age "old age" begins. The great statesman Bernard Baruch said that "old age is 15 years older than I am." That works for me. But when do we *feel* that we've reached old age? That varies. Many of us are a bit surprised when we look in a mirror or at a photograph of ourselves—Who is that person staring back at me?

Individuals have lived into old age

throughout history, but never before have so many lived so long. For our society, old age now is a new phenomenon. Fifty percent of people born in 1900 died before they were 47. Infant mortality was high, and adults died from infections like pneumonia, tuberculosis, blood poisoning (bacteremia), accidents, and diseases like high blood pressure or diabetes. Today, many of these conditions can be prevented or cured, while the others are managed with behavioral change and medication.

This success has brought new challenges. Half of people born in 1965 will live into their eighties, and many will spend 20 to 30 years in retirement. With these additional years come age- and disease-related changes that can affect what you're able to do. In your eighties, you will not be the same as you were at 20 or even 50. Aging begins at birth. We reach our maximum abilities at different ages, but the reality is that many physical characteristics peak by our thirties, like muscle mass, bone density, and physical endurance.

But it's not all downhill. The truth is that most older adults, even the old-old (over age 85) are in good health and able to do much of what they want to do. For example:

- As many as 80 percent of people over 65, and 70 percent over 85, report that their health is good or excellent.

- Only 20 percent of people 65 and over, and 40 percent over 85, have significant limitations in vision, hearing, mobility, communication, cognition, or self-care.

- Only 4 percent of people over age 65, and 13 percent over 85, live in nursing homes.

There are real advantages to having lived longer. Older people are less insecure than their younger selves. They're more likely to say exactly what they're thinking and to do what they want. Societal norms and peer pressure become less compelling, allowing older people to better see the big picture. Yes, death is closer. But coming to terms with this fact and recognizing your time is limited often results in a greater focus on the present and what's really important, instead of dwelling on the past or the future. Older adults can have intense negative emotions, but studies show that, compared with younger people, these happen less often and are better controlled. Wisdom grows, including having a larger store of coping mechanisms and problem-solving strategies. For additional information, see the discussion of the paradox of aging in chapter 8.

Make Peace with Aging

For more people, old age will become their new normal. Normal doesn't mean there's never a cause for concern or that there's nothing you can do to make things better. The changes that come with aging can affect function and well-being. This book addresses what to expect as you age and what you can do about it. But none of this information will help if you still view aging as the enemy.

A great recipe for aging well is a passage from the familiar serenity prayer by Reinhold Niebuhr:

> *grant me the serenity to accept*
> *the things I cannot change,*
>
> *courage to change the things I can,*
> *and wisdom to know the difference.*

To benefit from this book, you need to accept the changes and limitations that come with aging and be open to novel ways of adapting and meeting these challenges. Think of these extra years as a gift.

Oftentimes it's how you react, not what's actually happening, that makes life difficult. The loss of loved ones, functional abilities, long-standing roles and responsibilities, and even of familiar environments are inevitable parts of aging. It's normal to respond with some sadness, grief, or even anger. But becoming resentful, isolating yourself, or refusing help doesn't help you cope with the loss. These reactions are not going to reverse time. In fact, they're likely to make you more miserable. See what new doors are opening. Try to see the humor in some of these situations. Don't view later life as a glass half empty because you're not able to do everything you were once able to; envision it as a glass half full of as yet unknown possibilities.

I know it's a lot easier to say this than to do it. And it's hardest to do it when the losses come as a total surprise. But no one knows what the future will bring, so it's never too soon to think about your future and make some plans. Reflect on what really matters to you, what's no longer so important, and what you might do in response to life's future challenges. What will you do if you retire, have difficulty walking, or lose loved ones? What resources do you have? Financial resources help, but equally if not more important are family, friends, and spiritual or other affinity communities that provide emotional support, not to mention your own inner life, ideas, and values.

Practices for a Happier Old Age, Regardless of Your Current Age

Resist Ageism

Older adults are commonly portrayed in the media as unattractive, childlike, confused, grumpy, and selfish. Has this been your experience? I find it so strange that we disparage and are prejudiced against our future selves, since most of us (the lucky ones) will eventually be members of this group. No wonder we're in denial. Become a role model for aging. You can do this simply by being yourself and telling people your age—you'll love the look of surprise on their faces. I see it often when medical students meet my patients.

Right-Size Your Expectations

Age doesn't need to change your passions. You can still be a daily walker or a competitive runner. But if you expect that by working out you will reclaim the speed and strength that you had when you were 40, you're wrong. Even those in the best shape will walk or run slower as they age. After all, there are Boston Marathon winners of all ages, but the winning time for 20- and 30-year-olds is about two hours, while it's twice that for 70- to 80-year-olds. Run marathons, walk daily, and work out to slow your age-related loss of speed and strength; just remember to adjust your goals and expectations.

Be Resilient, Adaptable, and Flexible

With aging, we lose people, roles, and abilities that have been central to our lives. How we react and respond influences our happiness, contentment, and sense of well-being. Being grateful for what you've had—and what you still have—can help your mood and bring your focus more to the present. Compassion, humor, and finding new meaning and purpose can help reestablish a positive outlook. How do you spend your days? Are you doing things that you find meaningful? Getting out daily? Helping other people? Consider volunteering. It's associated with longer life, better moods, and improved health, and it's a good way to meet new people and become more engaged in your community. Be proactive, and explore what you might do to reinvigorate your life.

Redefine the Term "Independent"

Independence is an important word to teenagers. It means they can do what they want, on their own. As we age, independence continues to mean being able to do what you want, but you may not be able to do this by yourself, and it can be difficult to accept help. Yet what's most important to many older adults is to be able to continue meaningful social and spiritual connections, important activities, and living arrangements. Needing assistance in these areas may feel like a threat to your independence, but accepting help can actually allow you to be more independent and do what you want to do. Help can come from a person, a device, by learning new skills, or by adjusting your perspective and doing things differently.

Never Say Never

It's easy to dig in your heels and proclaim you'll never use a hearing aid, move out of your home, have an aide, or take an antidepressant. What you're really saying is that change is scary, and the alternatives have downsides. Which is true. But they also have upsides. Any time you face a new change, make a list of the pros and the cons. If possible, do a trial to see what happens. For example, commit to using a walker for three months. Track your activities, your mood, how often you go outside and socialize, and whether you fall. Don't decide whether you'll keep using it until the end of the trial. Remember, making a change can be the key to having a more fulfilling and independent life.

Advocate for Yourself, and Allow Others to Advocate for You

Pain, shortness of breath, nausea, insomnia, sadness, and other symptoms affect your daily life. It's important to identify and treat the underlying cause of these symptoms, but some symptoms may persist. These symptoms are not benign (without consequences). They can start a spiral where you become less active, get deconditioned and weaker, more tired, depressed . . . the list goes on. Do not accept decline as a part of normal aging. Use this book as a guide, and get help to figure out what's causing the symptoms and what can be done to become as symptom-free as possible. Commit to trying the treatments, including therapy (physical, occupational, psychotherapy), medication trials, and behavioral modifications. Let others help you when you need it.

Select, Optimize, and Compensate

When you can't do everything you once did, for whatever reason, remember SOC: **select** what really matters to you, **optimize** by practicing and rehearsing what you are able to do ("use it or lose it"), and **compensate** by using alternative mechanisms and equipment. For example, if there is an evening show you really want to attend but don't feel you have the energy or stamina, do all you can to get a good night's sleep the night before: exercise, eat right, and schedule a nap for that afternoon. Consider using an assistive device to get to the event, like a cane, walker, or even a wheelchair, to conserve your energy. Remember, never say never. Don't let vanity and pride get in the way of your having a good time!

Laugh More

Cultivate your sense of humor, especially about those things that scare you or you can't control.

We all take ourselves seriously, sometimes a bit too seriously. Have you ever noticed how many comedians live and continue performing well into old age, and that they are often the butts of their own jokes? Think about George Burns, Bob Hope, Moms Mabley, and Lily Tomlin. Having a sense of humor can help you face the unknown.

Choose the Right Doctor

Get a doctor who knows the difference between caring for 80-year-olds and 60-year-olds, as we discuss in the preface and chapter 2.

Advice for Loved Ones: Adapting to Your Older Adult's New Normal

There is a section like this in almost every chapter of this book. It is intended to help loved ones with their own feelings as well as to offer some insight into what aging is like. It also provides older adults with some sense of what their loved ones may be experiencing.

Aging can be a time of positive change and growth for you and the older person you care about, but it can also be tough. Even if your previous relationship was perfect, there's lots of potential for conflict. At times the roles become reversed, and you begin to act like a parent and the older adult a child who is angry, resentful, or depressed that you are telling them what to do. Most older adults want to be independent, make their own decisions, and not become a burden. But their families can be burdened by fear that the older adult could get worse or be injured by refusing to adapt to their new normal. This is an understandable concern, and it requires patience and thoughtfulness to see both sides and negotiate solutions everyone can live with. This is especially true when the older adult has experienced cognitive or functional decline. Reframing what independence means, and how getting help can make one more independent, is important.

Older adults are more likely to try something you suggest if they're told the benefits rather than if they feel threatened with the negative consequences. To encourage walking, for example, emphasize that walking will improve their mood, memory, and mobility while decreasing the chance that they will have a heart attack or a stroke. Don't start by telling them that if they continue to be a couch potato they'll become fatter, weaker, or frailer, or that eventually they will only be able to walk using a walker or a wheelchair.

These can be difficult conversations, and the issues are rarely resolved in one sitting. From my experience I've developed what I call the "six-month rule," meaning it often takes about six months before any suggested significant life change, like using a walker or having an aide in the house, is accepted. I suggest you explore options together, without mandates, and make sure the person you care about knows their views have been heard. Consider using a third party—a therapist, doctor, or counselor at a senior or religious center—as a mediator. If you have serious concerns that your loved one may lack the mental ability to make a certain decision, speak with their health care provider (and see the Advice for Loved Ones section in chapter 17).

Caregiver Stress and Burnout

Caregiver stress can result in your becoming ill or depressed and cause your relationship with the person you're caring for to deteriorate. Signs and symptoms include irritability, overreacting, resentment, anxiety, difficulty sleeping, and neglecting your own needs. It's critical that you take care of yourself by participating in relationships and activities that give you pleasure, spending time outdoors, and maintaining your health. You cannot be a caregiver 24/7—you need time to nourish and care for yourself. Estimates put the chance of developing depressive symptoms at anywhere from 40 to 70 percent for primary caregivers, many of whom will neglect their own health and needs while caring for someone else's. Ask for help from other members of your family, friends, and religious or social organizations, and accept it when offered. See if your loved one could benefit from a respite program, where they can socialize and you can get a break. Your local Department of Aging can direct you to these and other community resources, including local and online support groups. Caregivers may find it helpful to connect, either in person on virtually, with others who are in the same position and at the same time receive support, discuss concerns, and exchange ideas with those who have had similar experiences. You may even make new friends who understand what you're going through.

Bottom Line

At some point, aging will be a new stage of life for all of us. The best approach is to take control of your aging. Have a sense of what to expect, and maintain an open and flexible attitude, actively embracing change. Work on enhancing your positive perceptions of aging, and don't let old stereotypes define you. If a symptom or physical condition con-cerns you or interferes with your daily routine, find out if it's normal or not, and in either case be willing to accept and adapt to your new normal. How you react to challenges is a choice—it is not preordained. Use this book to inform your decisions and to empower you and your loved ones to be advocates for an active and meaningful old age.

RESOURCES

Reframing Aging

Let's End Ageism
(https://www.ted.com/talks/ashton_apple
white_let_s_end_ageism?language=en)
TED talk by Ashton Applewhite.

Aronson, Louise. *Elderhood: Redefining Aging, Transforming Medicine, Reimagining Life*. New York: Bloomsbury Press, 2019.

Levy, Becca. *Breaking the Age Code: How Your Beliefs about Aging Determine How Long and Well You Live*. New York: William Morrow, 2022.

Aging for Life
(https://www.agingforlife.org/anti-ageism
-activism.html)
List of advocacy groups working to combat ageism.

New Opportunities

Coming of Age
(www.Comingofage.org/resources)
Resources for personal development, lifelong learning, volunteering, civic engagement/advocacy, employment, self-expression, e-newsletters, and more.

Where to Volunteer
(Volunteermatch.org)
The web's largest volunteer engagement network makes it easier for good people and good causes to connect.

Senior Citizen Guide for College
(https://tinyurl.com/28np8zaj)
States that provide tuition waivers or dis-counts for older adults to attend public colleges and universities.

AARP Free Online Classes
(https://www.aarp.org/personal-growth
/life-long-learning/info-01-2011/free
_online_learning.html)
The AARP offers classes on a variety of
subjects.

Creative Aging Programs

Ruth's Table
(https://creativeagingresource.org
/resource/ruths-table-virtual-drop-in-art
-workshops/)
Ruth's Table offers free, weekly online arts
workshops.

TimeSlips
(https://timeslips.org/services/family-friend)
An international network of artists and
caregivers committed to bringing joy to
late life by helping family and friends discover new and creative ways to meaning-
fully engage.

State Arts Councils
Arizona: https://azarts.gov/programs
/azcreativeaging/
Maine: https://mainearts.maine.gov/Pages
/Programs/CreativeAging

Caregiving

Gillick, Muriel. *The Caregiver's Encyclope-
dia: A Compassionate Guide to Caring for
Older Adults.* Baltimore: Johns Hopkins
University Press, 2020.

Houle, Marcy Cottrell, and Elizabeth
Eckstrom. *The Gift of Caring: Saving Our
Parents from the Perils of Modern Health-
care.* Lanham, MD: Taylor Trade, 2015.

AARP Caregiving Resource Center
(https://www.aarp.org/caregiving)
Provides information on medical, financial,
and legal matters, as well as on types of
long-term care, self-care issues, and caregiver support.

Family Caregiver Alliance
(https://www.caregiver.org/)
The online tool CareNav allows caregivers
to ask questions and receive follow-up
from the organization's staff. It also has a
Services by State portal to locate support
services wherever you are in the United
States.

National Alliance for Caregiving:
(https://www.caregiving.org/resources/)
This organization provides many resources, including support programs,
eldercare locator, and links to specific dis-
ease/condition caregiving sites.

Aging Life Care Association
(www.Aginglifecare.org)
Professional organization for geriatric care
managers. The Aging Life Care Association
explains the role of a geriatric care manager and provides a portal for locating a
geriatric care manager in your area. Certified geriatric care managers have varied
educational and professional backgrounds,
with a specialized focus on issues associated with aging and disabilities.

Eldercare Locator
(eldercare.acl.gov)
This service of the US Administration on
Aging gives information on resources for
the aging, including contact information
for your local Agency on Aging.

Administration for Community Living. "Profile of Older Americans." Last modified May 27, 2021. https://acl.gov/aging-and -disability-in-america/data-and-research /profile-older-americans.

All-Party Parliamentary Group on Arts, Health and Wellbeing. *Creative Health: The Arts for Health and Wellbeing*, 2nd ed. Lundwood, UK: All-Party Parliamentary Group on Arts, Health and Wellbeing, 2017. https://www.culturehealthandwell being.org.uk/appg-inquiry/.

Freund, A. M., and P. B. Baltes. "Selection, Optimization, and Compensation as Strat- egies of Life-Management: Correlations with Subjective Indicators of Successful Aging." *Psychology and Aging* 13 (1998): 531–43.

Levy, B. R. "Stereotype Embodiment: A Psychosocial Approach to Aging." *Current Directions in Psychological Science* 18, no. 6 (2009): 332–36.

Noice, T., H . Noice, and A. F. Kramer. "Par- ticipatory Arts for Older Adults: A Review of Benefits and Challenges." *Gerontologist* 54 (2014): 741–53.

Samuel, L. R. "Creative Aging." *Psychology Today*. September 29, 2017.

CHAPTER 2

What's Normal Aging?
Or, 80 Isn't 60

As you age, your body and your mental and physical abilities change. Some changes are apparent: hair turns gray, print seems a lot smaller, a potbelly appears, we recognize but can't name the actor on TV, and we're walking slower than we used to. Other changes are more subtle, like our response to medications, the steady increase in our blood pressure, how easily we become dehydrated or feel unsteady and worried about falling.

I consider these changes to be "normal," since they are what happens physiologically, psychologically, and functionally to most people as they get older. It's what to expect. But these changes don't occur in lock-step fashion or to the same degree in everyone. You won't age in exactly the same way that your peers do. The effects of aging manifest themselves in different ways and at different times in people of the same chronological age. Geriatricians have a saying: "If you've seen one 80-year-old, you've seen one 80-year-old." There is no group of people who differ more one from one another than older adults. After 85 or even 65 years, your choices have had an impact. Smokers, for example, are more likely to develop wrinkles, cancer, and osteoporosis than nonsmokers. What's normal also changes by generation, since each generation is exposed to different environments, diets, health care, and education.

This chapter provides an overview of how aging modifies the way medical conditions present. Aging also may affect one's ability to respond to physical and psychological stress, may change our options for treatments as well as their risks and benefits, and may impact what we want for and from our medical care. The chapter also discusses why diagnosis and treatment in older adults can differ from that for most middle-aged adults. Many medical providers have had limited training in the care of older adults even though they care for many older patients. You may find the approaches described in this chapter helpful as you discuss your health and care with your provider.

How 80-Year-Olds Differ from Most 60-Year-Olds

Note: I often compare 80-year-olds to 60-year-olds when I'm trying to explain how aging influences the medical care older people should and do get. I do not choose these ages based on scientific evidence, but rather from my experience of when age-related changes begin to influence a person's symptoms, illnesses, and their response to treatment. As discussed previously, aging progresses at different rates in different people.

Physiological Changes Happen to Everyone in Their 70s and Beyond

Physiological changes can affect your health and well-being, so it is critical that both you and your medical providers take note of them. Symptoms of an illness may differ from those in middle-aged people. For example, chest pain is the cardinal symptom of having a heart attack, but an older person having a heart attack may instead be short of breath or confused. Some of the most bothersome conditions, like incontinence or falls, are considered geriatric syndromes (see page 17). These aren't due to a single cause but to multiple contributing factors, and by addressing these factors you can have fewer accidents. The same dose of a medication you've been taking for years may cause new side effects as you age. Laboratory values considered normal for younger people may be abnormal for an older person, and vice versa. All of these are examples of "normal" aging. For some, these changes are evident before age 70.

Older Adults Are More Vulnerable to Serious Illnesses, Medication Adverse Effects, Trauma, and Environmental Extremes

Have you ever wondered why it's primarily very old people (and very young ones) who die during a heat wave? During a heat wave, people become dehydrated. Middle-aged people compensate by increasing their fluid intake and retention. They feel thirsty, so they drink more fluids, and because their kidneys concentrate their urine, they eliminate less fluid. Their heart rates also increase to maintain their blood pressure. Older people are physiologically less able to compensate for dehydration. They don't feel thirsty, so they don't increase their fluid intake, and they're less able to concentrate their urine, further increasing their dehydration. In addition, their heart rates don't increase, resulting in low blood pressure that can lead to shock or even death.

The result of these types of differences is called *homeostenosis*, a play on the term *homeostasis*, which is a basic concept in physiology that explains how the body uses its *physiologic reserves* to compensate for physical and environmental stressors. Homeostenosis refers to the narrowing of physiologic reserves. It's part of normal aging for everyone, but it often is not appreciated by patients or their doctors. A person's physiological and psychological reserves can be substantial. In general, we have more reserves than we need. After all, people have two kidneys, and most can donate one without it ever affecting their health. As shown in the figure below, as you age, you need to call upon more of these reserves just to do your daily activities. This results in a narrowing (stenosis) of the body's capacity to deal with stressors of all kinds, resulting in even further loss of physiologic reserves and resilience. Illness, disease, poor nutrition, lack of exercise, and many other factors can accelerate a loss of reserve that is not part of normal aging. Homeostenosis can leave a person on a precipice where they're unable to compensate for stressors, resulting in serious illness, organ failure, and possibly death.

Few Older Adults Participate in Clinical Trials

Clinical trials are critical to determine the benefits and safety of new treatments. Most medications and treatments are approved without being tested in lots of older adults. This is true even for diseases that mainly affect the older population, like arthritis and heart failure. If and when older adults are studied, the benefits and risks may differ from those found in younger people. For example, recent studies showed that an aspirin a day to prevent heart disease in people 70 and older without a history of heart disease didn't prevent heart disease but did increase the risk of death and major bleeding (see the Preventative Aspirin section in chapter 5). In younger adults, aspirin lowers the risk of heart disease, and their risk of bleeding is much lower.

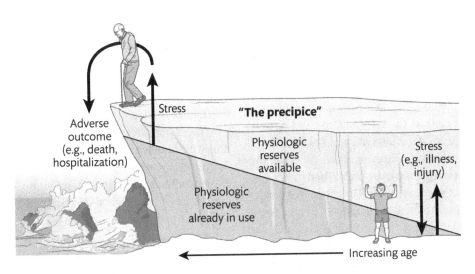

Homeostenosis: what happens to the body's reserves with aging. Adapted from A. Pelleg and R. Ramaswamy, "Differential Diagnoses in the Setting of Advanced Age and Multiple Conditions in Geriatric Practice," in *Geriatric Practice: A Competency Based Approach to Caring for Older Adults*, edited by Audrey Chun (New York: Springer, 2020), fig. 7.1

There are two major reasons why older adults are not included in clinical trials. One is that they may be excluded from the trial because of their age or the presence of certain medical conditions. The other is that they're not interested in participating. A clinical trial can be a hassle—it takes a lot of time and effort, including multiple visits, tests, keeping records, and so on. The good news is that many clinical trials soon will be unable to exclude people because of age. The National Institutes of Health, which funds much medical research, recently began requiring an explanation of proposed age limits, and why people with certain conditions are excluded, before granting funding. Studies will also have to track the number of older adults being enrolled. Discussion is also occurring on how to make study participation more appealing to older adults, including having study visits done at home or paying for transportation.

For now, however, most existing treatments and interventions have only been tested in younger adults before approval. Even when older people are included in trials, they are usually much healthier than my patients, so I don't know if the benefits and risks will be the same. Once approved, however, the treatment can be prescribed to people of all ages, races, ethnicities, genders, and abilities. As discussed in chapter 3, *the longer a treatment is available, the more will be known about its effects on older people.* For this reason, it usually makes sense to wait when a newly approved treatment is recommended for you (see chapter 3 for times when it may make sense not to wait).

Illness Scripts May Differ

Illness scripts detail the most common symptoms, physical examination findings, laboratory results, and prognostic course for a given disease. They are generally developed for a "textbook" middle-aged patient and are used by medical practitioners to learn the typical characteristics of a disease in order to make a diagnosis. The illness presentations of older adults can and do differ from the standard disease scripts and are thus called "atypical," but they're only atypical for younger people. They are quite typical for many older adults. Older adults who are ill may have vague symptoms that aren't representative of the disease or organ that is causing the illness. For example, those with pneumonia may have decreased appetite, fall, or become confused but not have a fever, cough, or sputum production. Hyperthyroidism, which causes tremor, heat intolerance, rapid heart rates, and frequent bowel movements in younger people, can present as depression, lethargy, weight loss and constipation in older people. So, the script for a given illness often needs to be different for 60- and 80-year-olds.

The importance of recognizing these differences cannot be overstated. I recently spent the greater part of a Sunday afternoon on the phone bumping heads with a surgical resident and fellow who were seeing my 86-year-old patient in the emergency room. She was there because she didn't "feel right," was nauseated, and had belly pain. They argued that because she didn't have a fever, her abdominal exam was normal, and her white blood cell count was not elevated enough to indicate an infection nothing "major" was going on, she probably had a gastroenteritis and should recover at home. I insisted on an imaging study, and when it was finally done, it showed that she had a perforated appendix with a raging infection. She was whisked off to surgery. Her symptoms were atypical for a young person, but totally typical for an older one. Sending her home and waiting until she became more severely ill (higher white count, lower blood pressure, or increasingly confused) would have increased her chances of further complications or death. Thankfully, she had surgery and recovered well.

A Symptom May Be Caused by a Combination of Disorders

When a person is ill or has a new medical concern, health care providers seek to find one diagnosis that will account for all the symptoms, physical findings, and laboratory results. As my neurology professor used to say, "No matter how you pinch and squeeze, it's [the symptoms and findings] got to fit just one disease." You may have heard of Occam's Razor. It states that causes (of a phenomenon) should not be multiplied beyond what is necessary. When applied to medicine, this principle encourages physicians to come up with one unifying diagnosis to account for all of a patient's symptoms, implying that the simplest diagnosis is often the right one. As explained below, however, this may not be the case for older adults.

In a younger person, feeling short of breath when walking is usually due to asthma, or possibly a pneumonia or a new anemia, but it is rarely all three. If you're 80 years old, however, you've

had a lifetime to accumulate a number of physiological changes and medical conditions that can contribute to both chronic and acute symptoms. In an older person, shortness of breath when walking could be due to an acute pneumonia, but it also may be the end result of a combination of effects from underlying heart disease, chronic anemia, smoker's lung disease, and muscle weakness from having stayed indoors throughout the winter (or during the COVID-19 pandemic). A pill won't necessarily fix the problem, but addressing each of these with a combination of behavioral changes (physical therapy, exercise program, stopping smoking) and medications will likely make the person feel better by decreasing the shortness of breath and increasing the distance they can walk.

Geriatric Syndromes Are Common in Older Adults

There is no perfect definition of a geriatric syndrome, but the term is used to differentiate diseases like pneumonia or appendicitis from disorders like cognitive impairment (dementia and delirium, or acute confusion), abnormal weight loss or malnutrition, falls and fractures, sleeping problems, loss of energy, urinary incontinence, depression, and frailty. In general, diseases have a single etiology, such as a bacterium or an anatomical obstruction, that interferes with normal physiology to cause symptoms. Geriatric syndromes are usually multifactorial, meaning they are caused by impairments in the physiology of several organ systems. These impairments interact to cause the syndrome. Often, the organ one would expect to be responsible for the syndrome isn't even involved. For example, delirium is rarely due to a new problem with the brain, and weight loss usually occurs in a person with a normal gastrointestinal system (specific syndromes are discussed in Part II of this book).

Understanding the underlying causes of geriatric syndromes provides a way to prevent or treat these disorders that can cause severe disability in older adults. Syndromes occur as a result of the interaction of a person's vulnerabilities and the challenges to which they are exposed. *Predisposing factors* increase a person's vulnerability to developing the syndrome, and *precipitating*

factors are responsible for triggering an episode of the syndrome. For example, a healthy 70-year-old who takes medications for high blood pressure is at low risk for falling after tripping on a crack in the sidewalk, but under the same circumstances, a 70-year-old with poor vision and balance problems who takes antidepressants and antihypertensives would be at high risk. A younger person without predisposing factors can also fall, but generally it requires a much stronger precipitating factor, like losing one's balance while on a ladder. These concepts as they apply to the geriatric syndrome of falls are demonstrated in the figure below.

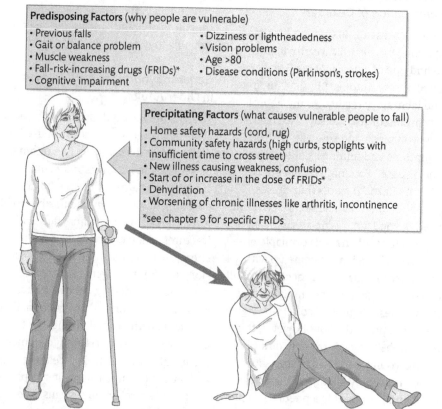

Predisposing Factors (why people are vulnerable)
- Previous falls
- Gait or balance problem
- Muscle weakness
- Fall-risk-increasing drugs (FRIDs)*
- Cognitive impairment
- Dizziness or lightheadedness
- Vision problems
- Age >80
- Disease conditions (Parkinson's, strokes)

Precipitating Factors (what causes vulnerable people to fall)
- Home safety hazards (cord, rug)
- Community safety hazards (high curbs, stoplights with insufficient time to cross street)
- New illness causing weakness, confusion
- Start of or increase in the dose of FRIDs*
- Dehydration
- Worsening of chronic illnesses like arthritis, incontinence

*see chapter 9 for specific FRIDs

Risk factors for falling (a geriatric syndrome)

Each geriatric syndrome has its own predisposing and precipitating factors. There can be overlap in predisposing factors, however, and geriatric syndromes can predispose a person to other geriatric syndromes. For example, pain can increase the risk of delirium, insomnia, falls, and depression. Delirium can predispose a person to falls, insomnia, malnutrition, and incontinence.

There are two pieces of good news. First, the more risk factors you can address, the less likely you are to develop the syndrome. Some risk factors can't be eliminated, but others will respond to interventions like exercise or physical therapy, medication changes, or hydration. Second, when you address a predisposing factor, you will decrease your likelihood of developing not just the syndrome you're concerned about, but several others. For example, when you commit to an exercise regimen, you not only decrease your risk of falls and fractures, but also your risk of cognitive impairment, urinary incontinence, sleep disorders, frailty, and depression. Similarly, drinking more fluids and avoiding dehydration will decrease your risk of cognitive impairment, malnutrition, and falls and fractures. Other common predisposing factors, in addition to the syndromes themselves, are medications, pain, hearing and vision impairment, deconditioning, and severe illness.

Competence in the Medical Care of Older Adults

Question: What are the most important domains for health care providers, patients, and families to focus on when older adults are receiving medical care?

Answer: The **Geriatrics 5M's**:

1. Mind
2. Mobility
3. Medications
4. Multi-complexity
5. what Matters most

Individual diseases and disorders are still relevant, but for most older adults, these five domains address what's most needed to have the best quality of life possible.

The importance of most of the 5M's is obvious. Many older adults and their loved ones are particularly concerned that they may develop dementia or become depressed (**mind**), or that they will become dependent because they can't walk without assistance (**mobility**). These concerns are further addressed in chapters 6, 8, and 9. Chapter 3 discusses how the risks and benefits of **medications** can change with age, and how important a regular medication review with your primary care provider is to ensure that you still need each medication at the dose you're taking and that none of your medications are responsible for symptoms that are bothering you.

Multi-complexity acknowledges that health depends on psychological and social concerns, as well as the ways in which the different disorders you may have accumulated through your lifetime interact with each other. As we said before, if you've seen one 80-year-old, you've seen one 80-year-old. For this reason, care must be individualized. This includes modifying medical guidelines (which almost always assume the only disease you have is the one being addressed) based on your other disorders, your life expectancy, and what's most important to you.

What **matters most** will drive discussions and decisions about what medical interventions you want to accept. As discussed in chapters 4 and 17, this can include relationships or connections with others, activities that provide enjoyment and satisfaction, and the ability to maintain your independence. When you're younger and get sick, your goal is usually to be cured and live as long as possible. When you're older, cure may not be an option, and the quality of your life may be more critical to you than the quantity. For this reason, when considering whether to have a medical intervention, it's essential for you and your medical team to consider the potential risks as well as the potential benefits. As one of my colleague's states, you don't want to win the battle but lose the war.

What Isn't Normal Aging?

If you notice or feel something new—particularly if it's affecting your function or making you worry—get it checked out. Many of us, even health care providers, accept stereotypical symptoms of aging as inevitable: memory impairment, incontinence, sleep disturbances, pain, difficulty walking, and more. Each of these can be age related, but they also can be due to treatable conditions or be amenable to therapy. Don't sell yourself short. Part II of this book discusses these symptoms, including what's normal and what's not. Even if a change is normal, specific underlying medical conditions or medications may be making the problem worse. Some symptoms can be modified or improved, resulting in your feeling and doing better.

Importantly, make sure you're working with a health care provider who isn't ageist. If you're questioning what that means, listen to my patient Ralph, who at age 90 went to see an orthopedist because of pain in his left knee. The doctor said, "What do you expect? You're 90 years old." Ralph's reply? "My right knee is also 90 years old, and it feels great!"

Advocate for yourself, and allow your loved ones to advocate for you as well. It can take a village to navigate our health care system!

Bottom Line

There are major differences between being 80 years old and 60 years old, especially when it comes to your health. Some of these are normal, some are not. Medical conditions may present differently, and there may be shifts in the balance of risks and benefits for treatments, many of which are unknown at the time the treatments first become available. Vulnerability to geriatric syndromes can be decreased to some extent by attending to relatively simple things, such as hearing, vision, fluid intake, and exercise. What you want for your life and medical care may differ. There is no one-size-fits-all approach. Be proactive—make sure you get appropriate advice and care for maintaining the quality of your life, using your own definition of quality.

RESOURCES

Finding Reliable Medical Information Online

National Institute on Aging. "Online Health Information: Is It Reliable?" Reviewed October 31, 2018. https://www.nia.nih.gov health/online-health-information-it -reliable.

US National Library of Medicine. "Evaluating Internet Health Information: A Tutorial." Last updated March 6, 2020. https:// medlineplus.gov/webeval/webeval.html.

 Health on the Net. "HONcode Certification." Last reviewed March 2020. https://www.hon.ch/en /certification.html. Look for the HONcode standard for trustworthy health information.

Finding Geriatric Health Care Providers

Health in Aging
(www.Healthinaging.org)
Service for locating geriatrics health care professionals in your area.

American Geriatrics Society
(www.AmericanGeriatrics.org;
212-308-1414)
Professional society for geriatricians that provides information on locating a geriatrician in your area.

Web-Based Resources for Geriatric Medical Information

American Geriatrics Society Health in Aging
(https://www.healthinaging.org/)
Provides up-to-date health and aging information to older adults and caregivers.

McMaster Optimal Aging Portal
(https://www.mcmasteroptimalaging.org/)
From the originators of evidence-based medicine, this portal gives access to high-quality information on healthy aging in topic form, on blogs, through video, and via e-learning.

MedlinePlus
(https://medlineplus.gov/olderadults.html)
Part of the National Library of Medicine, MedlinePlus gives access to trusted health information.

National Institute of Aging
(https://www.nia.nih.gov/)
A division of the National Institutes of
Health that studies aging in an effort to
extend life span.

Better Health while Aging
(https://betterhealthwhileaging.net/)
Dr. Leslie Kernisan's website contains practical information on aging to older adults and their children, including podcasts and a blog.

Focus on Health Aging
(https://universityhealthnews.com
/subscription-offers/mount-sinai-school
-medicine-focus-healthy-aging/)
Dr. Rosanne Leipzig is editor-in-chief of this monthly newsletter from the Mount Sinai School of Medicine that contains the latest news and practical advice on aging, to help you take charge of your health and well-being.

BIBLIOGRAPHY

Flacker, J. M. "What Is a Geriatric Syndrome Anyway?" *Journal of the American Geriatrics Society* 51, no. 4 (2003): 574–56.

Sharon, K., S. K. Inouye, S. Studenski, M. E. Tinetti, and G. A. Kuchel. "Geriatric Syndromes: Clinical, Research and Policy Implications of a Core Geriatric Concept." *Journal of the American Geriatrics Society* 55, no. 5 (2007): 780–91.

Tinetti, M. E., A. Huang, and F. Molnar. "The Geriatrics 5M's: A New Way of Communicating What We Do." *Journal of the American Geriatrics Society* 65, no. 9 (2017): 2115.

Tinetti, M. E., S. K. Inouye, T. M. Gill, and J. T. Doucette. "Shared Risk Factors for Falls, Incontinence, and Functional Dependence: Unifying the Approach to Geriatric Syndromes." *JAMA* 273, no. 3 (1995): 1348–53.

CHAPTER 3

Better Living through Chemistry?

Medications can be miracles, but they can also be toxic. Studies have shown that the more medications you take, the more likely you are to develop an *adverse drug event* (ADE), an injury resulting from the use of a drug, and older adults lead the pack when it comes to the numbers of medications taken. An ADE can be an exaggeration of the response expected from a medication, like having difficulty awakening or feeling hungover after taking a sleeping pill. Or it can be a completely different reaction, like stomach bleeding from certain over-the-counter (OTC) pain medications.

What counts as a medication? Your prescriber needs to know all nonfood substances you put into your body: prescription and OTC drugs, vitamins, herbal medicines, dietary supplements, and recreational drugs such as alcohol, marijuana, or cocaine. Your body reacts to each according to the principles described in box 3.1, and all have the potential to cause ADEs or interfere with the other medications you're taking. In this book, I'll use the words *medications* and *drugs* interchangeably to describe all of these substances.

This chapter is designed to empower readers to take a more active role in ensuring that the medications they take improve their health and quality of life. It describes age-related changes in how the body handles medications and in how the mind and body are affected by medications. It spells out high-risk medications for older adults and explains how the right medications and the right dosages for you may change as you age. Besides the medications mentioned here, each chapter in Part II of this book contains lists of drugs that may cause or worsen the conditions and symptoms discussed in that chapter.

What's Normal with Aging?

For a deeper dive into age-related changes in how the body processes and responds to drugs, see box 3.2.

Are ADEs the same in older people as in younger?

Few older adults participate in drug trials, and those who do tend to be healthier than most (see chapter 2). For this reason, ADEs in older adults may differ from those described in a drug package insert. These ADEs may be vague, like fatigue, dizziness, unsteadiness, or poor appetite. Often, they mimic conditions people think are normal with aging, like confusion, falling, constipation, or incontinence. For this reason, it's important to *consider that a medication may be the cause whenever you have a new symptom.* If an ADE is not recognized, a *prescribing cascade* may start, where one medication is prescribed to combat the adverse effects of another, when what's really needed is for the original drug to be stopped.

A common example is for an older adult with pain to start taking an over-the-counter nonsteroidal anti-inflammatory drug (NSAID) like ibuprofen (Motrin) or naproxen (Aleve). NSAIDs can cause fluid retention, resulting in an increase in blood pressure or a worsening of heart failure. If the medical provider doesn't know that you're taking the NSAID, they may prescribe additional drugs to treat these conditions instead of stopping the NSAID and discussing with you alternate methods of controlling your pain. This is another reason why it's important for you to inform your provider of all the medicines you're taking

I'm 83, and for decades I've had a glass or two of wine in the evening. But in recent years, I've been getting quite high after only one drink. Over the past month, I've fallen twice, both times after having a few glasses of wine while out with friends. What's wrong? Why can't I hold my liquor anymore?

With aging, increased sensitivity to alcohol and many other medications is not unusual. Older adults often get a

BOX 3.1

Medications and You

How you respond to a medication depends on the concentration, or *drug level*, it attains in your body and the sensitivity of your body's organs to the drug. The drug level, the organs affected by the drug, and how the drug is eliminated from the body are to some extent based on the dose of the drug and its solubility in body water and in body fat. Water-soluble drugs are eliminated unchanged by passing through the kidneys into the urine, while others are deactivated first in the liver or gut and then eliminated in the urine or stool. As a result, impairments in kidney, liver, or gut function can decrease elimination of drugs from the body and increase their levels. High drug levels can also be caused by drug–drug interactions.

In general, the larger the dose or the higher the drug level, the greater your response, including the possibility of developing an adverse drug event, or ADE. Drugs taken daily accumulate, resulting in a higher drug level than when only a single dose is taken. This is the reason why ADEs from a new medication may not occur until several weeks after you started it.

BOX 3.2

What Happens with Aging: A Deeper Dive

When it comes to medications, older adults often get more bang for the buck.
Older adults often get a greater response than younger people to a given dose
of a drug. Even medications taken at the same dose for many years may begin to
cause problems because of age- and disease-related changes in the way the body
processes them. Why?

*Drug levels are often higher for older than younger people taking the same dose
of the same drug.*
With age, body composition changes, resulting in increased body fat and decreased body water and muscle. Drugs like alcohol dissolve mainly in the water
compartments of the body, not in the fat. As we age, the same amount of alcohol
distributes into a smaller space, resulting in a higher concentration, and higher
blood levels. It also takes longer for alcohol to be deactivated by the liver. Remember, inside an 80-year-old person are an 80-year-old liver and 80-year-old
kidneys. Kidney function often decreases with normal aging, so blood levels are
often higher for drugs eliminated by the kidneys.

*The body organs of older adults may react more strongly to a given level of drug
than those of younger adults.*
Many body organs lose reserve with age, becoming more vulnerable to drug
effects. The older brain can be more sensitive to numerous drugs, including antihistamines like diphenhydramine (Benadryl) or muscle relaxants like cycloben-
zaprine (Flexeril), causing greater sedation, confusion, and falls.

greater response from a given dose of a drug. Even medications taken at the same dose for years may begin to cause problems because of age- and disease-related changes in the way the body processes them. The same dose of in-sulin can produce more episodes of low blood sugar, a sleeping pill now causes confusion or falls, or thyroid medica-tion may precipitate atrial fibrillation or a poor appetite.

Older adults often need a lower dose of a drug to get the same effect as younger adults because their drug blood level is higher (see box 3.2). When it comes to alcohol, this causes an in-crease in both the positive outcomes hoped to be achieved from the drug—feeling calmer and more sociable—and, unfortunately, outcomes you'd rather not have—feeling off-balance, having slurred speech, blurred vision, slowed reaction times, impaired judgment and self-control, and even at times a per-sonality change.

Another reason for new problems with drug dosages that were previously tolerated is that many body organs become more vulnerable to drug effects as one ages. The older brain, for ex-ample, is more sensitive to alcohol and sleeping pills.

The good news is that these changes are often predictable, so you can decrease the number or size of your drinks to avoid getting intoxicated. For other medications, your medical provider can help you minimize bad effects by prescribing a lower dosage or substituting a different drug. Lowering the dose may also save money.

The Goldilocks Approach, Step I

Remember the fairy tale "Goldilocks and the Three Bears"? Goldilocks entered the cabin and found one bowl with too much oatmeal, one with too little, and one that was just right. When it comes to your medications, it's important that you're taking what's just right for you. *The goal is to be sure that you need every medication you're taking, you're taking every medication you need, and that you're taking the right medication at the right dose for you.*

Too Much Medication?

Polypharmacy, the use of multiple medications by one person, is common in older adults. Just how many medications constitutes polypharmacy is a topic of debate. Some say it is taking five drugs, others say nine or even more. To me, it's not the number, it's whether each drug being taken is clinically appropriate for the person at that time. I try to minimize the number because as the number of drugs taken increases, so does the likelihood of having an ADE.

So, do you truly need each of the medications you're taking? Medications for disorders like infections or insomnia should be taken only for a limited time. Medications taken for chronic conditions, however, such as high blood pressure or diabetes, need to be taken throughout one's life, although if you lose weight or stop smoking, they may no longer be necessary, or you may need a different dose.

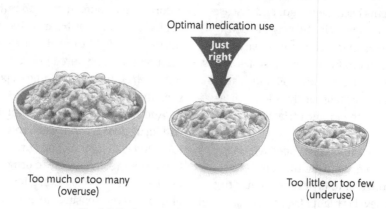

Optimal medication use

Just right

Too much or too many
(overuse)

Too little or too few
(underuse)

The Goldilocks approach to medication management

To determine whether you have polypharmacy, fill out the worksheet in table 3.1 with your medications and your medical conditions. Then note why you're taking each drug, and review the list with your health care provider. If your table looks like the example in table 3.1, you would ask your provider why you're taking atenolol and omeprazole, and whether you need to keep taking them.

If I think I'm taking too many medications, can I just stop them on my own?

No! Stopping a medication cold turkey can lead to withdrawal symptoms that can be uncomfortable or even life-threatening. Discontinuing a drug suddenly can also lead to a rebound situation where the condition being treated comes back with a vengeance, like developing extremely high blood pressure when certain antihypertensives are abruptly stopped.

Is there anything I can do to limit the number of medications I take?

Take an active role at the time when medications are being prescribed. Ask if there's something else you could try other than a new medication, like a heating pad, physical therapy, or a dietary change. You can also ask your health care provider whether you still need to be taking each of your medications, or whether any could be *de-prescribed*. This term means just what it says—stopping the prescription of a medication. Deprescribing usually involves slowly tapering the dose down to zero, while monitoring for recurrence of symptoms or improvement in how you

feel, although there are some drugs that can just be stopped. One of the main reasons health care providers are reluctant to deprescribe is a belief that patients will be resistant, so your request can open the door to streamlining your medication regimen.

When it's unclear whether you need a medication, or if you suspect that one of your medications is causing a symptom, discuss these concerns with your health care provider. She may be able to simplify your regimen, stop some drugs or decrease the number of daily doses, give you suggestions on how to help reduce those side effects, or switch you to another medication.

Too Little Medication?

You should be concerned not only with whether you need each of the medications you're taking, but whether you are taking all the medications you need. Your need for any medication is relative and depends on your priorities. There are some medications that are not prescribed as often as they should be for older adults, however. Examples include medications to treat osteoporosis if you've suffered a hip fracture (to decrease chances of a second fracture) and laxatives to prevent the constipation you're bound to develop if you're taking opioid medications.

Underdosing is not usually a problem for older adults. Because older adults are more sensitive to medications, health care providers "start low, and go slow" when prescribing for them. This is the right thing to do. Still, there are medications where the effective dose, even for older adults, is larger than the starting dose. Antidepressants

TABLE 3.1

Personal Medication List (Example and Worksheet)

Generic Name	Brand Name	Dose	Frequency	Reason	Who Initially Prescribed It and When?
Levothyroxine	Synthroid	100 µg	Daily	Low thyroid	H. Lutz, GNP 5/1999
Simvastatin	Zocor	20 mg	Before bed	High cholesterol	Dr. R. Kaplan 7/2010
Atenolol	Tenormin	25 mg	Daily	?	Dr. R. Kaplan 10/2015
Vitamin D		800 IU	Daily	Prevent osteoporosis and falls	H. Lutz, GNP 8/2005
Coenzyme Q		100 mg	Two times a day	Memory	Self 10/2013
Omeprazole	Prilosec	20 mg	Daily	?	Hospital 7/2019
Generic Name	**Brand Name**	**Dose**	**Frequency**	**Reason**	**Who Initially Prescribed It and When?**

Note: Complete as much of the worksheet as you can; you may not know the answer to every question.

and pain medications, in particular, are often underdosed for older adults.

Just-Right Medications?

As discussed above, you should only be taking medications that you currently need. Certain medications should be used with special caution in older adults. These fall into the following four categories.

Higher-Risk Medications

Anticholinergic drugs include muscle relaxants, antispasmodics, and some antihistamines, antidepressants, antipsychotics, and Parkinson's disease medications. The strongly anticholinergic drugs listed in table 3.2 should generally be avoided by older adults. These drugs can cause a variety of ADEs, including confusion, sedation, falls, and worsening dementia. Taking a high dose or more than one anticholinergic drug has been associated with increased emergency visits, hospitalizations, fractures, and possibly the development of dementia.

The Beers criteria lists medications to avoid and use with caution in older adults, including anticholinergics (see table 3.2). It is regularly updated by the American Geriatrics Society. Drugs like benzodiazepines—for example, lorazepam (Ativan), alprazolam (Xanax), and their cousin zolpidem (Ambien)—are used for sleep and anxiety and are considered drugs to avoid owing to the increased risk of cognitive impairment, delirium, falls, fractures, and car accidents in older adults taking them. They are also examples of medications that could have been taken safely for years, but whose risk increases significantly as you get older.

Blood thinners, digoxin, opioids, and the medications that cause low blood sugar are the medications most often associated with emergency hospitalization in older adults. These drugs often can't be avoided, as they can prevent serious medical events or improve one's quality of life. Discuss the pros, cons, and alternatives with your health care provider, including ways to decrease the chance of having a serious ADE.

TABLE 3.2

Medications to Avoid or Use with Caution in Older Adults

Medication Class	Examples	Adverse Drug Events
Drugs to avoid*		
Strong anticholinergics ⟶		Confusion, constipation, dry mouth, hallucinations, blurred vision, nausea, urinary retention, impaired sweating (hyperthermia), sedation, worsening dementia, falls, low blood pressure (hypotension).
First-generation antihistamines	Diphenhydramine (Benadryl); chlorpheniramine (Aller-Chlor); doxylamine (Unisom); hydroxyzine (Atarax)	

(continued)

TABLE 3.2 *(continued)*

Medication Class	Examples	Adverse Drug Events
Strong anticholinergics (cont.) ⟶		Confusion, constipation, dry mouth, hallucinations, blurred vision, nausea, urinary retention, impaired sweating (hyperthermia), sedation, worsening dementia, falls, low blood pressure (hypotension).
Some antipsychotics[‡]	Chlorpromazine (Thorazine); olanzapine (Zyprexa); thioridazine (Mellaril)	
Tertiary tricyclic antidepressants	Amitriptyline (Elavil); doxepin (Sinequan), doses over 6 mg; imipramine (Tofranil)	
Anti-Parkinsonian medications	Benztropine (Cogentin); trihexyphenidyl (Artane)	
Antispasmodics	Dicyclomine (Bentyl); hyoscyamine (Levsin, Anaspaz, NuLev, Levbid); propantheline	
Skeletal muscle relaxants	Baclofen (Lioresal); carisoprodol (Soma); cyclobenzaprine (Flexeril); methocarbamol (Robaxin)	
Antianxiety/sedative/ hypnotics	Alprazolam (Xanax); clonazepam (Klonopin); diazepam (Valium); lorazepam (Ativan); zolpidem (Ambien); eszopiclone (Lunesta)	Increased risk of cognitive impairment, delirium, falls, fractures, motor vehicle accidents.
Barbiturates	Butalbital (in Fiorinal); phenobarbital; secobarbital (Seconal)	Sedation, risk of overdose at relatively low doses.
Diabetic medications: long-acting sulfonylureas	Glyburide (Micronase); chlorpropamide (Diabinase)	Low blood sugar (confusion, loss of consciousness, sweating, palpitations).
NSAIDs	Indomethacin (Indocin); ketorolac (Toradol)	Indomethacin and ketorolac produce more ADEs than the other NSAIDs, including more confusion, GI bleeding, ulcers, and acute kidney injury.

TABLE 3.2 (*continued*)

Medication Class	Examples	Adverse Drug Events
Antipsychotics†	Prochlorperazine maleate (Compazine); haloperidol (Haldol); aripiprazole (Abilify); risperidone (Risperdal); ziprasidone (Geodon); quetiapine (Seroquel)	Increase risk of stroke and cognitive decline in people with dementia. Cause unsteadiness and slowed reaction time.

Drugs to use with caution†

Moderate anticholinergics ⟶		Same as serious anti-cholinergics, but occur less often.
Bladder relaxants	Tolteradine (Detrol); oxybutinin (Ditropan)	
Anti-dizziness	Meclizine (Antivert); dimenhydrinate (Dramamine); scopolamine (Trans-scop)	
Other antidepressants	Desipramine (Norpramin); nortriptyline (Pamelor); paroxetine (Paxil)	
NSAIDs	Aspirin >325 mg; ibuprofen (Motrin, Advil); naproxen (Naprosyn, Aleve); sulindac (Clinoril)	All NSAIDs cause increased risk of intestinal bleeding and ulcer disease in those age >75 or who take corticosteroids, anticoagulants, or antiplatelet agents.

Note: The information in this table, known as the Beers criteria, is from American Geriatrics Society (2019). Abbreviations are as follows: ADE, adverse drug effect; GI, gastrointestinal; NSAID, nonsteroidal anti-inflammatory drug.

Drugs to avoid: These drugs are likely to cause more harm than benefit to older adults and should be used sparingly, if at all.

†*Drugs to use with caution:* These drugs have a higher risk of causing harm in older adults. People taking them should be closely monitored for ADEs.

†Antipsychotics may be appropriate for treating schizophrenia or bipolar disorder or for short-term use for nausea during chemotherapy.

Newly Approved Medications

You're likely to be aware of new medications. They're the ones advertised on television and in newspapers and magazines telling you to "ask your doctor" whether they're right for you. Think twice before taking a newly approved drug. There may be a good reason for you to take it, but make sure there's not an already established medication that works just as well. *The longer a medication is on the market, the more will be known about its effects on older people.* When drugs are first approved, there are little data on the benefits or risks to older people (chapter 2). You can look in the package insert under "Geriatric Use" to see how many older adults participated in the trials. Once approved, the drug can be prescribed to anyone, including older adults excluded from the trials, and new, different, and serious ADEs are often identified.

Dietary Supplements

These include minerals, vitamins, herbals, amino acids, and enzymes. How do you know if they're right for you? Are they effective, what are the risks, and what's in the bottle? Even if not effective, supplements can cause an ADE or interact with medications you're taking. This is why you need to be sure to tell your health care provider if you take them. Recent investigations have found that many supplements contain little if any of the ingredients listed. Check out the Resources section at the end of this chapter for where to find trustworthy information about the effectiveness and risk of specific compounds, and for sites that have analyzed the composition of the product you're considering. See chapter 15 for a discussion of the dietary supplements you might need.

Medications That Have Caused You to Have a Previous ADE

Make sure your health care provider knows if you've had an ADE in the past. Many ADEs are due to genetic differences in drug processing pathways or to low organ reserve. If you've previously had an ADE and take another drug that is processed similarly to the one that caused the ADE or that affects the same organ, you may be at higher risk of another ADE. Make sure that you note these in the list of medications that you carry with you, and when you're asked if you have any drug allergies. Although you may not have had a true allergic reaction in the past (swelling, itching, low blood pressure), your prescribers need to know about any previous bad reaction to a medication in order to avoid prescribing it or a similar medication to you.

The Goldilocks Approach, Step 2

Getting the right medications—not too many, too little, or too likely to cause harm—is the first step. The second step is making sure you're taking the right dosage at the right times.

The Right Dosage

The "right" dosage for older adults is often less than the standard adult dosage. You can find recommended doses and concerns for older adults in most package inserts under "Indications and Usage," "Dosage and Administration," or "Geriatric Use."

As discussed in box 3.2, the dose or frequency with which a medication is taken may need to be adjusted for older adults because they may have higher blood drug levels or body organs that are more sensitive to drug effects. This increased sensitivity can come from age-related changes, disease, lifestyle effects, or genetics. The two major reasons for high drug levels are drug–drug interactions, which are more common in those taking multiple medications, and changes in kidney function.

Kidney function decreases over time in about two-thirds of older people. It is reported in blood work as *eGFR* (estimated glomerular filtration rate). Many medications depend on kidney function for elimination. When the eGFR is low, these medications will build up to higher levels and can cause ADEs. You can find your eGFR on your blood work reports, or you can ask your medical professional. If your eGFR is less than 50 ml/min, be sure your prescribers are aware, and ask whether they are adjusting your medication doses for your kidney function.

The Right Times

It can be hard to remember which medications to take and when, and to get refills before you run out, especially when you're taking several medications. For tips on taking your medications at the right time, see box 3.3.

Advice for Loved Ones

Taking medications correctly is a complex task that requires several steps. Some of my patients keep medications in their original bottles and often aren't sure if they've taken a particular medication that day.

Speak with the older person in your life about how they manage their medications. If they can't tell or show you what they're taking, or how they know which pills to take when, discuss how they may not be getting all the benefits they could from the medication, and that it can be risky to not be taking medications as prescribed. Look at box 3.3 together, and see if there are some easy fixes. If these suggestions don't work, see if your loved one will let you fill the pillbox for them every week or two, or discuss whether they would be open to using a pharmacy or mail-order service that provides daily packets of medications for the month. These packets, often called blister packs, include all medications that are to be taken at a particular time. If the drug regimen is too complex, ask prescribers if they can change the medications or their frequency so they only need to be taken a few times daily.

BOX 3.3

Tips for Taking the Right Medication at the Right Time

KNOW WHAT MEDICATIONS AND DOSAGES YOU'RE TAKING.

Keep a medication list, and review it regularly with your health care providers.
Fill out a medication list like the one in table 3.1. Include *all* medications, prescription and nonprescription, as well as herbal and dietary supplements. Keep it up-to-date and with you in your wallet or purse, and show it to each health care provider you see. Once a year, bring all the actual medication bottles to your primary care provider to be sure you're both aware of what you're taking.

Reconcile your medications with your health care providers whenever you're discharged from the hospital or rehabilitation.
Have some of the medications you were taking at home been stopped? New ones added?

Get all your medications from the same pharmacy.
By filling all of your prescriptions at the same pharmacy, you will ensure there is a complete record of your medications. In addition, the pharmacist can help identify potential problem interactions or adverse drug effects (ADEs).

Know your medications by name, not by color or shape.
Prescription and over-the-counter (OTC) drugs have both a brand name and a generic name. The company that develops a drug receives a patent to be the sole manufacturer for many years. The patent covers the drug ingredients, the pill's shape and color, and the brand name. Once the patent has expired, other manufacturers can make generic versions that are essentially equivalent to the brand name but have a different shape and color, and are often less expensive. Because they look different and have different names, it is easy to mistakenly take both. Make sure you know both the generic and brand names of your medications.

> Most of Jethro's medications are generic, and each time he refills a prescription, the pills he gets differ in color and/or shape from the last ones he got. He deals with this by putting a different-colored sticker next to each medication on his list and the same color on the medication bottle's top. He uses red for atorvastatin, so his atorvastatin is always in the red-topped bottle, regardless of the color or shape of the pill.

HAVE A ROUTINE

For knowing which pills to take:
- Make a list of the pills you take and the days and times you should take them.
- Each day check off each dose after it is taken. This will help to avoid missed or double doses. If you do this on a whiteboard or chalkboard, you can erase your checkmarks and start again the next day.

BOX 3.3 (*continued*)

- Get a pillbox with sections for each day and, if needed, different times of the day. These can be found at drugstores or online. If the box is empty, you've taken your pills!
- Set a regular time each week to refill your pillbox; for example, after dinner every Friday night.
- Ask your pharmacist for help if you need larger-print drug labels or bottles that are easier to open.

For remembering to take your medications:

- Take your medications at the same time every day, and link taking your pills to an activity. If the medication should be taken with food, place it on the table where you eat. I've found it helpful to link my nighttime medications to brushing my teeth before sleep and keep them in the medicine chest next to my toothbrush.
- Leave yourself reminder notes where you're likely to see them: on the bathroom mirror or the refrigerator, for example.
- If needed, use alarms to remember when to take your medications. There are an array of devices to help you, including pill containers that beep, smartphone apps, wristwatch alarms, and even voice reminders. Ask your pharmacist about these.

For making sure you have enough pills when you need them:

- Make a note on your calendar to call in for your refills a week before you're going to run out. Some pharmacies have automated systems that call or text you when it's time for a refill. In some states, you can get a three-month supply at your local pharmacy or through a mail-order pharmacy. Keep in mind that mail-order pharmacies may take a little longer to send the prescription, so plan accordingly.
- Plan ahead for traveling; you may need to get an early refill. Don't pack your medications in your luggage. Instead, keep them with you in case your luggage goes astray.
- Keep a few doses of your key medications in your purse or wallet, or at work, so you have them in case you forget to take them at home.

IF COST INTERFERES WITH GETTING YOUR MEDICATIONS

- Speak with your pharmacist.
- Ask if there is a generic medication that you can take instead.
- Revisit your Medicare D plan during open enrollment to see if there is another plan that better covers your current medications. The Medicare.gov website can help you find a pharmaceutical assistance program for the drugs you take.
- Check to see whether you are eligible for drug assistance programs in your state or from the companies that manufacture your medicines.
- Go to the medication's website. Oftentimes manufacturers offer coupons that can help lower the cost.
- See the Resources section at the end of this chapter for other programs.

Bottom Line

Medications can be a blessing and improve your life, but only if you are thoughtful about what you are taking. As you age, some medications may not provide you with the same benefits as when you started them, or they may cause new symptoms or conditions. Work with your health care providers to determine which medications are necessary and whether you might be able to take a lower dose. See chapter 4 if you need some guidance on how to have these conversations. Talk to your health care provider or pharmacist if you have questions or concerns about whether you're taking the right medications at the right dosages or need help taking them at the right time.

RESOURCES

Taking and Deprescribing Medications

Credible Meds
(www.crediblemeds.org)
Provides guides for safe medication use and tips for avoiding certain drug interactions.

Script Your Future
(www.ScriptYourFuture.org)
Gives guidance to help you take your medications as prescribed. This website offers a downloadable wallet card where you can keep track of the medications you take.

Safe Medicine Newsletter
(https://consumermedsafety.org/tools-and -resources/safe-medicine-newsletter)
Subscription newsletter that focuses on avoiding medication errors.

Deprescribing
(https://deprescribing.org/)
This website was developed by Canadian researchers who work with older people and are concerned about the risks associated with medications in this population. The advice on this site helps patients and prescribers participate in deprescribing.

National Institute on Alcohol Abuse and Alcoholism. *Harmful Interactions: Mixing Alcohol with Medicines.* Washington, DC: National Institutes of Health, revised 2020. https://tinyurl.com/7kcxsbvy.

Dietary Supplements and Complementary and Alternative Medicine

Office of Dietary Supplements
(https://ods.od.nih.gov/)
A division of the National Institutes of Health (NIH) that provides up-to-date information on dietary supplements.

National Center for Complementary and Integrative Health
(https://nccih.nih.gov/)
Also part of the National Institutes of Health, the NCCIH conducts scientific research on complementary and alternative approaches to medicine, and has reports on what works and what doesn't for specific symptoms and diseases.

MedlinePlus
(https://www.nlm.nih.gov/medlineplus/)
Part of the National Library of Medicine, MedlinePlus gives access to trusted information about drugs, herbs, and supplements.

US Pharmacopeia–Verified Products
(https://www.quality-supplements.org
/verified-products)
These products have been tested to ensure
that they contain the ingredients listed
on the label, in the declared potency and
amounts.

NSF International–Certified Products
(http://info.nsf.org/Certified/Dietary
/Listings.asp?StandardExt=FP&)
NSF tests products to ensure that they
meet standard requirements and that
labeling and claims are correct.

Help with Medication Costs

NeedyMeds
(needymeds.org)
Nonprofit organization that offers a free
prescription drug discount card for use in
most major pharmacies.

GoodRx
(goodrx.com)
This website provides coupons for lower-
cost prescription medications that can be
used at most US pharmacies.

WeRx
(werx.com)
WeRx compares the self-pay prices for
medications at your local pharmacies.
You'll be surprised at the variability in
pricing and how much you can save by
comparison shopping.

The Senior List
(theseniorlist.org)
This website lists discounts for prescriptions, groceries, restaurants, and travel for
seniors.

National Council on Aging
(ncoa.org)
Provides information on state pharmaceutical assistance programs and Medicare
Part D's Low-Income Subsidy (also known
as "Extra Help").

Medicare Interactive
(medicareinteractive.org)
Site that provides a national listing of state
pharmacy assistance programs, among
other information about Medicare.

BIBLIOGRAPHY

American Geriatrics Society. "Updated AGS
Beers Criteria for Potentially Inappropriate
Medication Use in Older Adults." *Journal
of the American Geriatrics Society* 67, no. 4
(2019): 674–94.

Steinman, M. A., and J. T. Hanlon. "Managing Medications in Clinically Complex Elders: 'There's Got to Be a Happy
Medium.'"*JAMA* 304, no. 14 (2010):
1592–601.

CHAPTER 4

More or Less

What's Right for You When It Comes to Health Care

I often joke that appropriate medical care for older adults can be an *evidence-free zone*, making it even more important that the medical care you get benefits you. As discussed in chapter 2, relatively few older adults participate in clinical trials, and those who do are fairly healthy, so a study's findings of benefit or risk may not apply to you. Neither might the outcomes be those you consider important. For example, stroke prevention trials are often focused on the numbers of deaths from stroke, whereas many of my patients are less concerned about dying than they are about how disabled they may be if they live. You're also not going to benefit from tests and treatments for conditions that are unlikely to ever cause you harm, such as screening for prediabetes or cervical cancer after you've reached a certain age or time of life (see chapter 5).

As the preeminent physician Sir William Osler (1849–1919) famously said, "The good physician treats the disease; the great physician treats the patient who has the disease." Have you ever wondered if you need all the tests, treatments, or types of care your health care providers order for you? Providers generally assume that you want to do everything possible to prevent an illness from developing or progressing, whether it be an infection, heart disease, or cancer. This may work for you, but at times, depending on how you feel, your age, and your priorities, you may wonder if all these measures are necessary.

Remember the maxim "Too many cooks spoil the broth"? This can also be true for health care providers, especially as you age. It's not uncommon for my new patients to have 15 or more doctors they see yearly to address specific concerns, including bladders, prostates, breasts and uteri, eyes, hearts, lungs, skin, gastrointestinal problems, and more. Do you need to see these providers every year? When decisions need to be made, do your doctors touch base with your primary care provider (PCP) or, if needed, other specialists? Specialists can be critical to diagnosing certain conditions, performing procedures, and managing certain treatments. After diagnosis, your PCP often can monitor your symptoms and treatments, referring you back to see the specialist if there is a specific need. Review your list of doctors with your PCP to see if she can help you decide when or whether you need to see a specialist again.

So, who should decide which treatment and tests you should have? What's your role in this decision? If you give your providers some key information about who you are and what matters most to you, they can suggest options that are tailored to you.

This chapter is designed to help you think through your medical care priorities and goals, and to empower you to share these with your providers and family so that you find your medical care to be more helpful, less burdensome, and better aligned with your personal definition of health.

What's the Right Medical Care for You?

I'm not a doctor or an expert in medicine. How should I know what's important, or whether a test or treatment will benefit me?

Everything that your health care providers suggest is in service of one primary outcome: your ability to live a life that's meaningful to you. You're the expert in this area. Take the time to figure out *what matters to you* so that your medical care reflects your wishes. Identify your *health priorities*—the goals and activities you want your medical care to help you with—taking into account what you are willing and able to do. Identifying your priorities, and sharing them with your providers, focuses your medical care on what is important to you.

This sounds complicated. How do I identify my health priorities and what matters most to me? Where do I start?

The information I'm about to summarize comes from the Patient Priorities Care Initiative (PPCI; see https://myhealthpriorities.org/). It is a user-friendly, self-directed online program that you can complete by yourself or with a loved one. The program takes about 20 minutes and guides you through the process of developing a personalized Health Priorities Document to share with your health care providers and family. The website contains tips on how to communicate these priorities to your providers. These tips are also included in last section of this chapter.

Five Steps to Identifying Health Priorities and Goals

Step One: Determine What Matters Most to You

To develop their model, the PPCI interviewed many patients, family members, and health care providers, and asked what issues were most important to them when they needed to make a medical decision. Their responses fell into four categories: maintaining the ability to connect with others, enjoying life, preserving or improving function, and managing health.

What do each of these categories really mean?

Connecting refers to your relationships with others and includes personal, professional, and spiritual connections. It includes time spent with friends and those with whom you share common interests, access to family gatherings, and helping others. Connecting is as simple as the feeling of belonging with others in a space where you are welcomed and wanted.

Enjoying life is anything you do that results in feelings of self-satisfaction, well-being, and a sense of purpose. It encompasses a wide variety of activities, from reading to playing sports or games to learning new things, fixing up your house or garden, creating art, or using your life experiences to mentor or teach.

Functioning includes physical, cognitive, and psychosocial functioning. Changes in any of these areas can impact one's sense of self, dignity, and independence. How would you feel if you couldn't be as physically active as you are now? What if you needed some help to be able to live at home? How much is your identity dependent on what you're able to do?

Managing health can overwhelm one's life. It can be time-consuming, or your symptoms may interfere with your ability to connect, enjoy life, or function. Some medical decisions force us to choose which is more important to us: how well we function (quality of life) or how long we live (quantity of life). The balance that's acceptable to you may change as you age.

Do any of these capture your health priorities, or is something else most important to you? Identify what really matters to you given your values and your experiences.

Step Two: Use Your Priorities to Develop Your Health Goals

Health goals are not numbers like blood pressure readings, cholesterol levels, or pounds on the scale. They're the activities that are most important to you, the ones that you want your medical care to facilitate, not constrain. One of the best ways to develop a health goal is to ask yourself, *How would I want to be spending my time and energy if I weren't feeling this symptom or dealing with this medical care activity?*

Be specific. Exactly what do you want to do, and how often do you want to do it? Make sure you're being realistic, that this is something that is possible given your current state of health. Be flexible. Try to understand why this activity is so important to you, and identify what else might replace it if you weren't able do it anymore (see chapter 17 for guidance).

My patient Sam provides a good example of this process. Sam's current stated health goal is *I want to be able to attend my nephew's graduation in June and celebrate with my family.* What's interfering with Sam's ability to go to the graduation? For one, he can't walk around the block even once without becoming so winded he needs to rest. He's also concerned because one of his blood pressure medicines increases his need to urinate, and he finds it difficult to get to the bathroom on time, especially when in public.

So, Sam's realistic health goal is: *I want to be able to attend my nephew's graduation. My poor breathing and frequent urination are barriers to this goal.* By modifying his health goal to include limitations brought on by his current state of health, Sam clarifies his priorities and identifies what he and his health care provider need to focus on if he is to achieve his goal.

Step Three: Review Your Health Care Tasks and Medications, and Decide Which You Find Helpful and Which Are Burdensome

Some people are willing to do anything to help them achieve their health goals, but others find some things just not worth the trouble. One way to think about this is to identify what medical care you consider helpful and what feels burdensome. *Helpful care* is that which you can do without too much difficulty *and* helps you with your health goals. For example, taking an antidepressant may increase your desire to spend time with friends, or a pain medication may improve your knee pain so that you can go golfing or take a walk with your grandchild. *Burdensome care* includes health tasks that you feel are too difficult, uncomfortable, time-consuming, unhelpful, or likely to just create a new problem you're not going to want to deal with. This could include following a restricted diet, having a colonoscopy, or going to the clinic for a weekly treatment.

You may not have strong feelings about whether a test or treatment is helpful or burdensome until you actually experience it. Sometimes you can try out a treatment or a type of care by working with your medical provider and setting a time limit for determining whether your treatment response is good enough or if the dose or treatment should be changed or even stopped all together. For every set of tests or treatments, you may start or continue care when it is consistent with your priorities and not too burdensome. You may choose to stop when the burdens outweigh the benefits or the care becomes inconsistent with your priorities. Make discussing the pros and cons of any medical treatment a regular part of your discussions with your health care provider.

Step Four: Identify Whether the Tests and Procedures Your Health Care Provider Is Suggesting Match Your Health Goals

Let's return to my patient Sam.

Sam and his provider decide that he needs to accomplish two shorter-term goals in service of getting to his nephew's graduation.

The first goal is that he be able to get around the block three times a week without needing to rest. To reach this goal, Sam needs to:

1. Regularly attend pulmonary rehabilitation (a program of exercise, education, and support to those with lung disease).
2. Learn to correctly use his breathing inhaler so that he gets the full dose of medication.

The second goal is to decrease and better control his urinary incontinence. To reach this goal:

1. Sam's diuretic dose is decreased by half to see if his incontinence improves.

2. He takes his blood pressure daily to see if he will need another medication to control his pressure now that he's taking a lower dose of diuretic.

Sam agrees and enrolls in pulmonary rehabilitation, decreases his diuretic dose, and checks his blood pressure daily. His incontinence is better, but he's still concerned about having an accident in public. Two months before the graduation, he is still unable to get around the block twice without stopping to rest.

His provider then suggests that Sam:

1. Use a wheelchair to attend the graduation.

2. Use a nebulizer machine, which uses mist rather than liquid to administer his breathing medications, since he never really was able to get a full dose of medication using a hand-held inhaler.

3. Learn to do daily pelvic floor and urge suppression exercises (see chapter 11) to help control his incontinence.

This is where Sam starts to draw the line between what's helpful and what's burdensome. He needs to decide if following his health care provider's advice will help or interfere with achieving his goal of getting to the graduation. He has always said he would never use a walker, let alone a wheelchair, and that he didn't want to be "chained by machines" for his health.

Step Five: Determine What Trade-Offs You're Willing to Accept to Meet Your Health Goals

Trade-offs are what you're willing or unwilling to do to find, diagnose, or treat a medical problem based on your feelings of what's helpful and what's too burdensome. Trade-offs aren't written in stone and can change as your circumstances change. They can also be temporary, like Sam using a wheelchair just for getting to and around the graduation. If Sam understood that the nebulizer isn't a "chain" but is only used for five minutes a few times a day, he might be willing to try it and see if it helps.

You and your health care provider can make decisions that align with your goals by basing them on your priorities, your understanding of your options, and a sense of your likely future health status, and then determining what trade-offs you're willing to accept.

There is other important information you and your provider need to discuss before making a decision. For example, if you're considering a diagnostic or screening test, what are the next steps if the test is abnormal? Are these steps you would want to take? If you're considering a treatment, what is the likelihood that you'll benefit from the treatment, and what are its risks? What are your other options? If you're discussing surgery, what are the best-, worst-, and usual-case scenarios for outcomes and recovery if you have the surgery? What if you don't have surgery?

Envisioning what it would be like to live in different states of health and function can help you decide on trade-offs when you're making a medical decision. For example, if you have terrible pain from an incurable cancer and have a remaining life expectancy of three to six months, radiation might provide pain relief but could cause you to be severely fatigued for a few weeks. Is this acceptable to you? Would you rather try pain medication? What if the pain medication makes you confused or increases your daytime sleeping? Would you be willing to take a lower dose of medication and live with some pain to be more awake and mentally clearer? Thinking through these trade-offs will help you make a decision that is more in line with your health priorities and goals.

Communicating and Discussing Your Priorities with Your Health Care Providers

I'm afraid my provider will think I am pushy or demanding if I question or refuse to take some medications or have a test done. How can I avoid this situation?

Working collaboratively with your health care provider is vital to making the right decisions for you. What kind of relationship do you have? All relationships, whether professional or personal, are built on trust, clear communication, and mutual respect. If you don't feel that these basic factors are in place, it will be important to see if you can improve things by being honest about how you feel. If not, you might do better with a different provider.

My appointments already feel so rushed. My provider seems to have so much to cover. Could sharing my priorities make matters worse?

There is only one way to find out if sharing your priorities is helpful: you have to try. If you have specific questions you want to address during the visit, write them down and tell your provider at the start of the visit. If you have lots of questions or medical concerns, it may help to first identify your health priorities by completing the PPCI process or by filling in the form in the figure on page 44 and bringing it to your visit. Having a clear, well-stated priority to anchor your visit can help you avoid wasting time on burdensome medical care that is meaningless to you.

For each of your visits, especially with your PCP, try to concentrate on one or two health goals. Before the visit, complete the following:

"The thing I most want to focus on today is [*symptom or problem*] so that I can do [*health outcome goal*] more easily or more often. I think [*health problem or medical care activity such as a medication, self-management task, health visits, etc.*] is [*helping or worsening the symptom or problem*]."

You may be surprised to find that asking your provider to focus on what matters the most to you improves the flow of the visit and optimizes everyone's time.

Name _____ **Date** _____

■■■ What Matters Most ■■■■■■■■■■■■■■■■■■■■■■■■■■■■■■■■■■■
Examples: Spend time with family, volunteering, reading books
_____
_____
_____

■■■ Most Important Health Goal ■■■■■■■■■■■■■■■■■■■■■■■■■
Examples: Watch grandchildren after school 2-3 times weekly, volunteer in library twice weekly
_____
_____
_____

■■■ Current Health Care Tasks and Medications ■■■■■■■■■■■

Most bothersome symptoms or health problems
1. _____
2. _____

Helpful health care tasks: *The medications, self-management tasks, clinical visits, tests, or procedures, that I think are helping me most with my health goals and I can do them without too much difficulty*
Examples: Exercise, physical therapy, bloodwork and imaging, acetaminophen for arthritis pain
1. _____
2. _____

Helpful Medications:
1. _____
2. _____

Burdensome health care tasks: *The medications, self-management tasks, clinical visits, tests, or procedures that don't think are helping my goals and are bothersome or too difficult for me. I would like to talk with my doctor about whether these are helping my goals. If not, can I stop them or cut back? If they are helping, is there a way to make them less bothersome or less difficult?*
Examples: using CPAP, being hospitalized
1. _____
2. _____

Burdensome medications
1. _____
2. _____

■■■ The One Thing to Focus On ■■■■■■■■■■■■■■■■■■■■■■■■■■
The one thing about my medical care I most want to focus on is
(fill in a health problem that you think is keeping you from achieving your health outcome goal OR the medical care task that is most bothersome or difficult) so that I can do (desired activity) more often or more easily.

I want to focus on _____
_____
_____
_____

Health priorities template. Modified from https://myhealthpriorities.org

Do you have any tips on how to discuss my medical care goals and preferences with my providers?

The way in which you start these discussions matters. You want to be heard, but you don't want to be accusatory or have your health care provider get defensive.

Start with a general statement that puts your thoughts in context, like *I've been thinking about how my health and medical care affect my ability to do the things that are important to me. I've been reading about patient-centered medical care priorities and have been trying to identify my medical care priorities, goals, tasks, and symptoms. I'd like to review it with you and start working with you on these.*

Frame your questions and concerns in terms of asking for help and clarification given your health goals. If your provider is interested in learning more about patient-centered care, refer them to the Patient Priorities Care Initiative at www.patientprioritiescare.org. Tips from the PPC website suggest that you ask questions such as, *Is there something that will help me walk around my house without being so short of breath?* or *Will this medicine affect my energy in the morning, making it more difficult for me to walk my dog?*

Be specific. Instead of saying "I don't like this medicine," say "This medicine makes me feel weak and dizzy, and I can't get out to visit friends or see my family." Voice your preferences. Tell them what you are able to do and what you think is helping in addition to what is not helping or is bothersome.

The PPCI website also provides certain words and phrases that can help open up a topic, such as:

- The one thing I want to focus on is _____. What do you think will help with that?
- I really don't like _____ because _____.
- What concerns me most is _____.
- My main health goal is making sure I can _____.
- I want help with _____.
- I'm willing to _____ if it helps me meet my goals.

Advice for Loved Ones

Working through these five steps with the person you're concerned about, or for whom you may be health care proxy (HCP) and called on to make decisions in their name, gives you insights into what's important to them and what they would want for themselves. Knowing what's helpful and what's burdensome can provide a touchstone, especially when there are so many options for care. Shining a laser focus on what really matters, what makes life worth living, can bring a new sense of clarity to these discussions.

In this arena, I'm a loved one.

My spouse has a complex illness that involves several specialists and frequent decision-making. We completed the

PPCI online and were able to identify what she felt was most burdensome to her at that time. This provided us with a clear goal to work toward when making decisions with her doctors and other health care providers.

Bottom Line

At the risk of repeating myself, the real bottom line is that everything your health care providers suggest is in service of one primary outcome: your ability to live a life that's meaningful to you. You need to decide what really matters and how you can best achieve it. At times, identifying health priorities requires making some hard decisions, but this may be easier if you use the PPCI website or the five steps described in this chapter. If possible, do this with your family or special friends so that they get the chance to understand your thoughts and feelings, and be sure to discuss your conclusions with your health care providers.

RESOURCES

Patient Priorities Care Initiative (https://myhealthpriorities.org/) The PPCI website contains its self-directed online health priorities guide; a summary of the health priorities you decide on (https://patientprioritiescare.org/wp -content/uploads/2018/11/Patient -Summary-of-Health-Priorities.pdf); a conversation guide (https://patient prioritiescare.org/wp-content/uploads /2018/11/Conversation-Guide-for -Patients-and-Caregivers-for-Identifying -their-Health-Priorities.pdf); and informa- tion for medical providers (https:www .patientprioritiescare.org).

National Institute on Aging. *Talking with Your Doctor: A Guide for Older People.* Washington, DC: National Institutes of Health, 2016. https://order.nia.nih.gov /sites/default/files/2017-07/TWYD_508 .pdf.

BIBLIOGRAPHY

Boyd, C. M., J. Darer, and C. Boult. "Clinical Practice Guidelines and Quality of Care for Older Patients with Multiple Comorbid Diseases: Implications for Pay for Perfor- mance." *JAMA* 294, no. 6 (2005): 716–24.

CHAPTER 5

An Ounce of Prevention

As Ben Franklin said, an ounce of prevention is worth a pound of cure. Prevention takes several forms. It includes vaccinations that decrease your chances of contracting an infectious disease; early detection to avoid the serious consequences of a disease, like diagnosing and starting treatment for glaucoma before it affects your vision; and behavioral changes such as exercising regularly to decrease one's chances of developing dementia or heart disease. The differences between screening and prevention, what disorders screening may prevent, and why recommendations for screening and prevention can change over time are described in box 5.1.

Deciding what preventive measures to do becomes more complicated as we age. Recommendations developed by medical societies and national task forces often differ from each other, change over time, and don't usually consider whether there's a point where the risks of the measures outweigh the benefits. This point could be an age, but it could also be the presence of other medical conditions and disabilities that make it less likely that you will benefit or more likely that you will be harmed. These recommendations are evidence based, but all too often older adults are poorly represented in the studies that produce the evidence. Lack of evidence is not evidence that something doesn't work. It just means we're more uncertain of the benefits and risks.

What prevention or screening should you do? I spent five years as a member of the US Preventive Services Task Force (USPSTF), evaluating the evidence and making recommendations to primary care practitioners for what screening and prevention should be done, and when to stop screening.

In this chapter, I'll put the various approaches to prevention into context. I will also give you a framework to help you decide what you should do every year, and when you should consider screening and preventive measures to prevent infections, cardiovascular disease, other diseases, and cancer.

When all is said and done, you should discuss the benefits and risks with your health care provider and decide what makes sense for you.

Note: The recommendations in this chapter are current as of June 2022. These may change as new high-quality studies are published. See the Resources section at the end of the chapter for websites that publish updated recommendations.

BOX 5.1

Screening and Prevention 101

Screening for a medical problem and preventing a medical problem are two different things. Screening is actually early detection, as it refers to detecting conditions or diseases before they cause symptoms, then intervening to decrease suffering or death. Prevention is changing behaviors or taking vaccines or medications to prevent the development of a condition. Concerns with screening include *false positive* screens, where people are falsely identified as having a condition they don't actually have, and *false negative* screens, where people are told they don't have a condition that they actually do have.

Screening often involves more than the initial testing. Occasionally there can be harms. Abnormal tests may lead to further diagnostic tests, such as radiological scans or biopsies, or to treatment recommendations such as medication, chemotherapy, surgery, or radiation. Before you get screened, make sure you know what the next diagnostic and therapeutic steps would be. If you would not want to follow through with these, you shouldn't get screened. Discuss the options in advance with your health care provider.

Why don't we try to detect all diseases as early as possible?
There are many diseases where early treatment doesn't result in better outcomes than if you wait until after you develop signs or symptoms. If treated early for these diseases, you're at risk of suffering the harms of treatment years before you might benefit from it. For other diseases where there's no effective treatment, early detection only increases the amount of time you're aware that you have an illness, but it doesn't delay suffering or help you live longer.

A screening test needs to accurately differentiate what's normal from what's not. For example, if the prostate-specific antigen (PSA) test for prostate cancer is abnormal, biopsies are done to look for cancer cells. Unfortunately, it's hard to tell which of these cells will develop into symptomatic prostate cancer. Autopsies detect prostate cancer cells in 60 to 80 percent of men 80 years and older who didn't have symptomatic prostate cancer during their lives. If these men had been biopsied and treated as a result of an abnormal PSA, they would have run the risk of immediate complications like erectile dysfunction, incontinence, and diarrhea even though they would never have developed full-blown prostate cancer. That's why there's so much controversy about PSA screening. Other screen-detected cancers don't become symptomatic until 10 years after detection. If you're unlikely to live this long, the risks clearly outweigh the benefits.

Why aren't the screening recommendations from the medical community all the same? Am I supposed to be doing breast self-examination, getting a yearly eye exam, things like that?
It's not unusual for recommendations for screening to differ depending on the group that wrote them. Specialty society recommendations are often written by

BOX 5.1 (*continued*)

doctors who primarily see people who are already diagnosed with a disease, and so they see mainly the benefits of treatment, often making recommendations that are biased toward screening. Primary care recommendations are written by clinicians who refer many people for screening, few of whom are diagnosed with the disease, but they also see patients who are harmed without any benefit, so they tend to be more conservative in their recommendations. The US Preventive Services Task Force (USPSTF) is an independent body that consists of primary care physicians, nurses, and other experts like statisticians, public health professionals, and epidemiologists. The USPSTF tends to be the most conservative, only making recommendations when there is high-quality evidence showing that screening or prevention results in a greater benefit than risk to the well-being and survival of most people, not just an improvement in their laboratory tests. Using these criteria, breast self-examination doesn't improve cancer survival, and yearly tests of your visual acuity (your ability to read) by your primary care provider doesn't improve your vision, except in people with diabetes, so these screens are not recommended by the USPSTF.

How can recommendations for screening change so drastically over time, from "you must do this" to "don't even think about it"?
These changes are actually a good thing. Recommendations are based on the preponderance of evidence from high-quality studies, and new ones are constantly being published and added to the mix. For example, low-dose aspirin was a mainstay of prevention of heart attacks for people without cardiac disease. Several years ago, the USPSTF evaluated studies and found that the risk of bleeding from low-dose aspirin increased to the point where, for those over age 79, the benefits didn't necessarily outweigh the risks. Then, in 2018, new high-quality studies were published that showed not only that the risk of bleeding increased with age, but also, because so many people were using other preventive measures for heart disease like blood pressure and cholesterol-lowering medications, there was no additional benefit of prophylactic aspirin in people 60 years and over without a history of heart disease. In 2022, the USPSTF began recommending against starting low-dose aspirin for primary prevention of CVD in adults 60 years or older. See the Resources section at the end of this chapter for websites that contain up-to-date recommendations.

Annual Wellness

The lists of recommended screenings and shots seems to get longer and longer each year. What really makes a difference as I get older?

I had a friend, Mark, who weighed over 300 pounds, smoked like a chimney, and always wanted my opinion on whether or not he should get screened for prostate cancer. My advice to him, and to you, is to prioritize what matters to you. Getting screened for prostate cancer may decrease your chances of dying from prostate cancer, but it won't affect overall health and well-being. Yet there are many other things that you can do that will positively affect longevity and quality of life. My list doesn't start with screenings—it highlights behaviors and habits that when incorporated into your daily life are likely to improve your health, function, mood, and longevity. The reasons why are described in the chapters noted below.

- Stop smoking. Within weeks of quitting smoking, you decrease your risk of having a heart attack, improve lung function, decrease shortness of breath and coughing (although initially you will cough more because your lungs will begin to get rid of the mucus that has accumulated). By the end of a year, your risk of a heart attack will be cut in half.
- Limit your alcohol consumption to no more than one drink a day (chapter 3).
- Exercise regularly (chapter 7).
- Monitor your weight and eat nutritiously (chapter 15).
- Use seatbelts in all vehicles, including taxicabs. (You can tell I live in New York City!)
- Socialize regularly (chapter 8).
- Do everything you can to prevent falls and fractures (chapter 9).
- Avoid extreme heat or cold. Although not discussed in a specific chapter, older adults are more likely to develop severe dehydration in the heat, even developing *heat exhaustion* (severe fatigue, sweating, muscle cramps) or *heat stroke* (high fever, confusion, inability to drink), which is a medical emergency that can lead to organ failure and death. Cold weather is responsible for twice as many deaths as hot weather, possibly due to thickening of the blood, causing clots, which can cause heart attacks and strokes. If you must go out, stay hydrated and dress appropriately.

What health screenings should be on my yearly checklist?

I think of a yearly health checklist like a mechanic thinks of a car tune-up. It's helpful to identify where the problems are, what's starting to go, and what needs to be repaired or replaced to ensure that you get the most out of your car, or in this case, your mind and body. My suggestions for your yearly tune-up are found in box 5.2.

BOX 5.2

Yearly Tune-Up for Older Adults

Eye Care
See an eye care specialist to monitor you for glaucoma, macular degeneration, and cataracts every one to two years (chapter 12).

Oral Health
See the dentist once or twice yearly to prevent tooth loss and gum disease, which can interfere with your ability to eat well and enjoy food.

Primary Care
- Get your blood pressure and weight measured.
- Review medications, including supplements, and ask if there any medications you can stop taking (chapter 3).
- Review and update your advance directives (chapter 20).
- Get your flu shot in the fall, and check if you're due for any other immunizations (chapter 5).
- Review your history of smoking, drinking alcohol, use of recreational drugs, exercise, and how you spend your time, and discuss ways to change your lifestyle, if needed.
- Review your current living situation. Are you able to get healthy meals? Do you need help organizing or paying your bills? Are you feeling lonely or isolated?
- Review and update your list of primary care and specialist doctors—dentist, podiatrist, and so on—yearly.
- Let your health care provider know if you:*
    - leak urine (chapter 11)
    - are having difficulty walking, have fallen, or are afraid of falling (chapter 9)
    - are worried about your memory or your thinking (chapter 6)
    - feel sad or unmotivated a lot of the time (chapter 8)
    - drive a motor vehicle (chapter 19)
    - are concerned about your hearing, or if someone else is (chapter 12)
    - are concerned about sex or your sexual function (chapter 16)

*Each of these chapters has a pre-visit checklist you can find in Appendix 3. Complete the checklist before your visit to give your provider additional information that will help them better understand your concerns and determine what next steps should be considered.

Does Medicare cover my yearly tune-up?

To an extent. Medicare covers the Welcome to Medicare visit, an initial preventive physical exam that can only be completed within the first 12 months of enrollment, and an annual wellness visit (AWV) for those who have had Part B coverage for more than 12 months. The Medicare AWV is a time for you and your health care provider to discuss what you might need to improve your health now and in the future. It is a good start at identifying what screens and preventive measures you may need, what risk factors you have for chronic diseases, and what may be interfering with your ability to function at your best in your daily life.

At the end of these visits, your provider should give you a list of risk factors and a personalized screening and prevention schedule for the next five to ten years, as well as advice or referral to health education or preventive counseling on weight loss, physical activity, tobacco cessation, fall prevention, or nutrition, should you need them.

Not all primary care providers offer Medicare AWVs, but you can still make an appointment with them to go through the items in box 5.2. Remember, the Medical AWV is not a substitute for regular medical follow-up. The AWV is an appointment specifically to review your individual risks and identify ways to improve your health and function.

Recommendations for Prevention and Screening

Vaccines

Among the recommendations your health care provider will make is that you get up to date on any needed vaccinations (see table 5.1). Immunizations are one of best ways to help you avoid serious illness from a variety of diseases.

I got the pneumonia shots and still got pneumonia. I got the flu shot and still got the flu. Why should I keep getting vaccines?

Vaccines can make it less likely you'll get an infection, but they're not infallible; they don't protect you from all flu- or pneumonia-causing organisms. But they can decrease infection from specific strains, and if you do get infected with that strain, your illness will be less serious.

There are other reasons that older adults should still get vaccines. Some vaccines like tetanus are only protective for a certain period, so you will need a booster to be fully immunized again. Others, like the flu, are reformulated yearly because the strains that are most likely to cause disease change. As you age, you may lose some of your immunity and need certain revaccinations. New and more effective vaccines may also become available, like Shingrix for shingles. Also, it's important to consider the people you spend time with when deciding on your prevention plan. Older adults can easily transmit flu and pneumonia to friends and family, children can give you whooping cough and measles, and shingles can transmit chicken pox to those who never had the disease or the chicken pox vaccine, which became available in 1995.

TABLE 5.1
Summary of Immunization Recommendations for Older Adults

Conditions	Frequency	Provisos for Older Adults
Pneumococcal pneumonia	Depends on previous vaccination status and age at vaccination	• If never vaccinated: one dose of PCV20. • If vaccinated with PPSV23: PCV20 or PCV15 at least one year later. • If vaccinated with PCV13: one dose of PPSV23 at least one year later. • Many older adults have already received both PCV13 and PPSV23. It is not known whether PCV20 provides significant additional protection. • If vaccinated with PPSV23 before age 65, you will need another dose after age 65 (at least five years after your first dose).
Influenza	Early in the fall of each year	• Tell provider if you have egg allergy. • Get a quadrivalent vaccine, which provides a "higher dose," if possible (Fluzone High-Dose, Flublok Quadrivalent, or Fluad Quadrivalent). The standard-dose trivalent or quadrivalent vaccine may not provide adequate coverage for older adults. • The intranasal vaccine FluMist does not provide protection for older adults.
Tetanus/diphtheria (± pertussis)	Booster every 10 years	• If you never completed a three-shot initial series, or don't know if you did, get it now. • If you've never had a pertussis booster, get a Tdap shot, especially if you spend time around young children.
Shingrix: shingles (H Zoster)	Two doses six months apart Need for booster dose not yet known	• 90% effective at reducing shingles • Recommended to get Shingrix even if you had Zostavax, the first shingles vaccine. • You are at risk for shingles and should get the vaccine if you had chicken pox. If you are not sure if you had it, get tested for immunity to varicella zoster virus. • In a small percentage of people, the vaccine causes fever and aches for a few days.
Measles		• Check immunity, particularly if you spend time around children. You may need boosters.

(continued)

TABLE 5.1 (continued)

Conditions	Frequency	Provisos for Older Adults
COVID-19	Two doses of Pfizer or Moderna (three and four weeks apart, respectively). First booster five months later, second booster at least four months after first.	• Older people are at greatest risk for hospitalization and death. • Available vaccines are effective in older adults. • Up-to-date information is constantly changing and is available at www.cdc.gov/vaccines/covid-19; www.coronavirus.gov; and www.who.int.

Influenza

Influenza causes more than 7,500 deaths and 150,000 hospitalizations a year in those 65 and older. People with chronic diseases like diabetes, asthma, or a heart condition, or who live in a nursing home or are in the hospital, are at the most risk of having serious complications from the flu. We learned during the COVID-19 pandemic that wearing a mask, social distancing, and handwashing are the best protections against getting the flu. As a result, in the 2020 and 2021 seasons, the number of influenza deaths decreased dramatically. The next best way to prevent influenza is to get a yearly flu shot. The flu season is from late October to May, and it takes about two weeks after vaccination for you to achieve immunity, so you should try to get vaccinated in the early fall if possible. Although there is an advertising push to get your flu vaccine in the summer, wait until fall, as you will want it to last throughout the whole flu season.

Getting a flu shot is not an absolute guarantee against getting the flu. There are many different influenza viruses, and the yearly vaccine contains protection against only the three or four strains judged by experts to most likely cause illness during the upcoming flu season. I have had many patients say to me, "I have never had a flu shot and I have never had the flu, so I don't need the shot." There is no science behind this belief, especially because both the flu shot and the flu strains that cause illness each year are different. In my opinion, these people have been lucky. I have cared for too many people who have died from the flu. One of my patients who died got it from his wife, who will never forgive herself that they hadn't been vaccinated. Influenza is a serious illness, and vaccination is the best prevention, other than continuing to follow the COVID-19 precautions.

The immune response to vaccination for older adults is often less than for younger people, so the standard dose vaccine isn't as protective. Influenza consists of two different types of viruses, influenza A and B, and there are many different strains of each. Influenza A is responsible for most of the illness in older adults. All trivalent flu vaccines contain the same two influenza A antigens and one influenza B. Quadrivalent vaccines contain two influenza B antigens. *Higher-dose, recombinant, and adjuvanted vaccines produce greater immunity in older adults than standard vaccines.* The intranasal vaccine, FluMist, is not as effective for older adults, so it is not recommended.

Side effects from the flu shot can include soreness, tenderness, redness, or swelling around where the shot was given. You may also get some flulike symptoms such as headache, muscle aches, fever, nausea, or fatigue, but not nearly as much as if you actually contracted the flu. The high-dose, recombinant, and adjuvanted flu vaccines may have more of these side effects. *But you cannot get the flu from the vaccine.* If you get sick after your flu shot, it's because you were exposed to it one to four days before your shot and now you've developed the flu.

Pneumonia

There is no vaccine that prevents all pneumonia because there is no single cause of pneumonia. Many different organisms can cause pneumonia, and the current pneumonia vaccines only prevent disease caused by some of the 90 different strains of the *Streptococcus pneumoniae* bacteria, also called pneumococcus. Pneumococci cause about one-third of community-acquired pneumonias. This bacterium can also cause *invasive disease*, infecting joints, heart valves, and the coverings of the brain (meningitis) after entering the blood or spinal fluid. Pneumococcal pneumonia also may occur after flu in older people. As with flu, older

adults are more likely to die from these infections.

Currently there are four pneumococcal vaccines. Pneumococcal polysaccharide vaccine, or PPSV23, covers 23 strains, while the pneumococcal conjugate vaccines (PCV or Prevnar) cover 13 (PCV13), 15 (PCV15), and 20 (PCV20). Children began to receive PCV13 in 2010, while adults 65 years or older began receiving it in 2014. PCV13 use in children reduced the transmission of the disease to older adults and over time is expected to even further decrease it.

New recommendations for pneumococcal vaccination were released in 2022 by the Centers for Disease Control and Prevention (CDC). Older adults who have never been vaccinated or whose vaccination status is unknown should be vaccinated with PCV20 (see table 5.1 for additional information). It is not yet known if PCV20 provides additional protection against pneumonia in those previously fully vaccinated with both PPSV23 and PCV13. Some older adults are at higher risk for PCV-type invasive pneumococcal disease, particularly those who live in nursing homes, other long-term care facilities, or in places where PCV13 vaccination of children is low; those with chronic heart, lung, or liver disease, diabetes, or alcoholism; current smokers; and those who have more than one chronic medical condition. If this is you or someone you love, discuss whether PCV20 should be given with a medical provider.

Tetanus, Diphtheria, and Pertussis

These three bacterial infections have become much rarer since vaccines became available. Tetanus, also called lockjaw, causes painful muscle tightening that make it difficult or impossible for you to open your mouth, swallow, or even at times to breathe. Diphtheria causes a thick coating in the back of the throat and can lead to problems with breathing, heart failure, paralysis, and death. Pertussis, also called whooping cough, causes severe coughing spells, which can result in difficulty breathing, vomiting, and disturbed sleep. Although pertussis is usually considered a disease of children, there have been growing numbers of cases reported of in older adults.

Tetanus and diphtheria in the United States have decreased by 99 percent, and pertussis has decreased by 80 percent since vaccines became available. Most people receive a three-dose primary series in childhood. As a person ages, however, immunity lessens, so booster doses are needed. There are two different vaccines to prevent these diseases. One, called Td, protects against tetanus and diphtheria but not pertussis. A Td booster should be given every 10 years. If you've never received a booster pertussis shot, Tdap can be given in place of a Td booster. This is particularly important if you spend time around young children, as you can get pertussis from them (and then give it to other children). In general, tetanus boosters need to be given every ten years, but if you develop a deep and dirty puncture wound or laceration, you should get one if your last booster was more than five years ago. Side effects from this vaccine may include soreness, redness, or swelling at the injection site and a slight fever.

Shingles

Shingles, also known as herpes zoster, is a painful, blistering rash that comes from the reactivation of the chicken pox virus that lives within the nerves after a childhood infection. The rash usually develops on one side of the trunk or the face, following the path of a nerve. It can threaten vision when it appears on the forehead or nasal areas. Rarely, it presents as severe pain alone without any skin signs. The blisters scab over in 7–10 days. Although the skin manifestations are gone in two to four weeks, many people, particularly older adults, develop postherpetic neuralgia (PHN), a severe continuation of the pain that can last years and become debilitating. The risk of shingles and PHN increase with age. One out of every three people over age 60 will develop shingles, and one of six will develop PHN. People with shingles can give chicken pox to those who have never had it or the chicken pox vaccine; they remain contagious until all the lesions are scabbed over.

There is no medication that cures shingles or PHN. But there are two shingles vaccines. The newer vaccine, Shingrix, is 90 percent effective, compared to the 50 percent effectiveness of the previous vaccine, Zostavax. The vaccine is protective even if you've already had shingles (you can get another attack), if you have other chronic illnesses, or if you're immunocompromised (Zostavax is a treated live virus, so is contraindicated in immunocompromised people). Even if you've had Zostavax, you should get Shingrix because of its increased effectiveness. It requires two shots, two to six months apart. Side effects include pain, redness, and swelling at the injection site, and in a small number of people, a few days of headache, fever, shivering, or an upset stomach.

Preventing Cardiovascular Disease

Cardiovascular disease (CVD) includes many health problems and is one of the leading causes of death worldwide. Thankfully, cardiovascular disease can also be preventable. See table 5.2 for a list of recommended primary preventions.

⚠ CAUTION **If you have had a heart attack or a stroke, this section is NOT for you. Discuss with your doctor what you should do to prevent recurrences of these disorders.**

So far I've been lucky and haven't had any heart disease or strokes. I exercise and eat healthily, and I try to follow the other recommendations. But it seems that these recommendations are constantly changing, and often they have no suggestions for older people. What do you recommend to your patients?

Exercise, quitting smoking, eating healthily, and controlling your blood pressure are key to cardiovascular health. In younger adults, there are good data that support primary prevention (prevention for those who haven't had CVD) by lowering cholesterol, controlling blood glucose, and taking aspirin to prevent heart attacks and stroke. But these studies enrolled few older adults who haven't had previous heart disease or stroke, so the results may not apply to this population. In this section we'll discuss the evidence (or lack

thereof) and some provisos to consider when deciding what you should do.

Blood Pressure Screening

When I was in medical school, we were taught that systolic blood pressure (the top number) increases as part of normal aging (true—90% of those who live to 90 will have high systolic blood pressure), and that if we treated it, the patient could have a stroke (false—it's now evident that treatment of high blood pressure reduces the risk of stroke, coronary disease, and death). Blood pressure screening should occur at least yearly, and only if your pressure is high on two separate occasions a few weeks apart should it be treated. Be sure the right-size cuff is used to measure your blood pressure (if it's too small, your reading will be falsely high; if it's too large, it will be falsely low). If you're concerned that it's high because you're at the doctor's office and feel nervous (known as "white coat hypertension"), have it checked at your pharmacy, buy your own cuff and check it at home, or ask your doctor to order ambulatory blood pressure monitoring for you, which will record your blood pressure automatically over at least 24 hours.

What's the "right" blood pressure for older adults?

This is an area of controversy. Your systolic pressure should be 150 mmHg or less, and if you have chronic conditions like heart disease, diabetes, or kidney disease, it probably should be lower. A recent study showed that older adults, even those who were frail, lived longer and did better the closer their systolic pressure was to 120 mmHg. The concern is that getting one's systolic pressure to 120 mmHg usually requires several medications, and some people may get medication side effects or light-headedness from them. Blood pressure goals and treatments are not one-size-fits-all for older adults, and there are circumstances that will change a particular goal or medication decision. The safest approach is to discuss a blood pressure target with your doctor and slowly increase medication doses to reach that target—this way it's unlikely you'll have a bad side effect.

Diabetes Screening

A blood test to measure either fasting blood sugar (FBS) or glycosylated hemoglobin (HbA_{1c}) is recommended every three years for those between ages 35 and 70 who are overweight or obese. Identifying diabetes early through screening may prevent heart attacks, strokes, and eye, kidney, or nerve damage. Screening will tell you that you are either not diabetic, have diabetes, or have prediabetes. Diabetes is defined as an FBS of 126 mg/dl or greater, or an HbA_{1c} of 6.5 percent or greater.

TABLE 5.2

Summary of Recommendations for Primary Prevention of Cardiovascular Disease

 Primary prevention means preventing disease in individuals who do not already have the disease. The information in this table is not for those who already have cardiovascular disease.

Primary Prevention	Frequency	Provisos for Older Adults
BP screening	At least yearly; ideally at every doctor visit.	See the text for discussion of BP targets for older adults.
Diabetes screening (blood test for FBS or glycosolated hemoglobin, HbA1c)	Every three years for those between ages 35 and 70 *and* overweight or obese.	If you are over 70 years old or diagnosed with prediabetes, see the text for more information.
Cholesterol screening (blood test for total cholesterol, LDL, and HDL)	Every three to five years for those between the ages of 40 and 75.	If you are over 75 years old, see the text for more information.
Aspirin	Adults 60 and over without a history of CVD *should not* take aspirin to prevent CVD.	New USPSTF recommendation as of 2022.

Note: Abbreviations are as follows: BP, blood pressure; CVD, cardiovascular disease; FBS, fasting blood sugar; HDL, high-density lipoprotein; LDL, low-density lipoprotein; USPSTF, US Preventive Services Task Force.

What about diabetes screening if you are over 70?

The benefits and risks of screening aren't known, so discuss what is best for you with your health care provider. Screening only makes sense if you're at risk of developing the complications of diabetes. Complications can begin to develop early in the diagnosis of diabetes but generally take 10 or more years to affect your health or well-being. Knowing whether you are diabetic may influence your decision to take cholesterol-lowering agents to prevent cardiovascular disease (see below).

What is the target glucose goal for diabetics over age 70?

The American Geriatrics Society and the American Diabetes Association agree that target blood glucose goals for people over 70 should be higher than for younger people because of shorter life expectancy and greater risks from hypoglycemia. Older adults who are otherwise healthy with few other illnesses and intact cognitive and functional impairment status should have an HbA_{1c} that is less than 7.0 to 7.5 percent. Those with multiple illnesses, cognitive impairment, or greater risk from blood sugar becoming too low (such as falls, seizures, confusion, or functional dependence) should aim for an HbA_{1c} that is less than 8.0 to 9.0 percent. The goal for younger adults is an HbA_{1c} that is less than 7.0 percent.

What is prediabetes?

If you have prediabetes, it means you have a blood sugar level that is between normal and diabetic, usually an HbA_{1c} level between 5.7 and 6.4 percent. Prediabetes *does not* mean you will develop diabetes. Somewhere between 20 and 30 percent of people of all ages with prediabetes will develop diabetes within 10 years. In older adults, that risk appears to be lower, about 10 to 20 percent over 10 years. A major study done in middle-aged people (average age 51) found that lifestyle changes (losing weight and regular exercising) and a medication called metformin can decrease the likelihood of prediabetes progressing to diabetes.

The jury is still out on whether lowering HbA_{1c} to normal levels in older adults with prediabetes decreases the complications of diabetes. If there are benefits, for the most part they won't be seen until more than 15 years after screening. Discuss the pros and cons of lowering HbA_{1c} levels with your provider if you are prediabetic.

What should I consider if I decide to be treated for diabetes or prediabetes?

- Weight loss can be an effective way to improve your blood sugar.
- Treating high blood pressure and other cardiovascular risk factors is as important as blood sugar control in preventing the complications of diabetes.
- Don't let your blood sugar get too low. A low blood sugar can cause more problems—such as confusion, seizures, and blacking out—than having a slightly high blood sugar.

Cholesterol Screening

Having a low-density lipoprotein (LDL) cholesterol of >130 mg/dl or a high-density lipoprotein (HDL) cholesterol of <40 mg/dl are major risk factors for CVD. Others include male sex, diabetes, hypertension, and smoking. Cholesterol screening is done to determine whether you are at high risk of developing cardiovascular disease. If you are 40–75 years old, you should have your blood tested for total cholesterol, LDL, and HDL every three to five years.

⬦ CAUTION **CHOLESTEROL GUIDELINES**
The 2019 guidelines from the American College of Cardiology/American Heart Association (ACC/AHA) state that individuals who have a low-density lipoprotein (LDL) level of >190 mg/ml should be treated. The other guidelines are based on an age-adjusted risk calculator for CVD. Those in whom the calculator estimates that the risk of a cardiovascular event in the next 10 years is 20 percent or greater should be treated, and treatment should be considered in those whose risk is >7.5 to 19.99 percent. However, the calculator always estimates that those over 75 have a risk that exceeds 7.5 percent. For this reason, you need to discuss with your doctor what your risks are for developing cardiac disease independent of the calculator to decide if you should be treated for high cholesterol.

Should people over age 75 take statins for primary prevention?

The benefits and risks of taking statins if you're over age 75 and don't have cardiovascular disease aren't known, and as mentioned above, the calculator overestimates the risk of cardiac disease in this age group. If you are interested in being screened and starting a statin,

or if you're wondering whether to continue the statin you're taking, discuss the following with your doctor:

- Are you likely to live long enough to benefit (generally at least five years)?

- Would noninvasive tests, like the coronary artery calcium score, help determine whether you are at higher risk of developing CVD and therefore more likely to benefit from medication?

- What are the potential risks of the medication, and how will your doctor monitor for them? Risks from statins include muscle aches, drug interactions, weakness, and possibly diabetes.

- Is it more important for you to minimize the numbers of medications you take and possible adverse drug events, or are you more concerned about having a heart attack or stroke? This isn't a trick question— What really matters to you? (See chapter 4.)

Preventive Aspirin

Adults 60 and over without a history of CVD *should not take* low-dose (81-mg) aspirin. It doesn't prevent CVD, but there is a major risk of bleeding. Of note, enteric-coated or buffered aspirin formulations *do not* reduce the risk for serious bleeding.

The ACC/AHA guidelines also state that low-dose aspirin (75–100 mg orally daily) might be considered for the primary prevention of atherosclerotic CVD among select adults 40 to 70 years of age who are at higher risk of having a CVD event in the next 10 years but not at increased bleeding risk. Risk factors for bleeding include male sex, stomach or esophageal pain, gastrointestinal ulcers, taking other anticoagulants or using nonsteroidal anti-inflammatory drugs, and having diabetes or uncontrolled hypertension.

Cancer Screening

Cancer screening identifies cancers that, if treated early, result in less suffering and a reduced risk of death than if you waited until you had symptoms before being diagnosed and treated. For certain forms of extremely aggressive cancer, screening isn't warranted because early treatment rarely stops them.

To decide whether to be screened, you need to evaluate the process itself and the potential benefits and risks for you (see table 5.3). Screening may just be a blood test, but diagnosis can include additional scans or biopsies, while treatment may include chemotherapy, surgery, or radiation. If you would not be willing to undergo treatment, there's little reason to be screened.

Aging can change the balance of benefits and risks of screening. It's a fact that the older we are, the fewer years we have left. Will we live long enough for a screen-detected cancer, which is generally so small it's only seen under the microscope, to develop into one that will cause us suffering or death? For certain cancers we have a sense of how long this takes. For example, it's about 10 years for colon and breast cancer. Prostate cancer is variable, and at the moment it's hard to predict if prostate cancer cells will ever grow into a tumor that will cause illness. Do you have other health concerns that will be more likely to affect your quality of life and survival than what you're screening for?

For these reasons, recommendations for cancer screening have begun to give age ranges for stopping screening. This tends to be the point at which identifying cancer when it's asymptomatic is unlikely to produce benefits, or the harm from diagnostic tests and treatments would occur sooner than if treatment were delayed. Most clinical trials of screening benefit have not included people 75 and over, so to some extent this is another "evidence-free" zone. However, we can look at the biology of the cancer, the likelihood of adverse events from diagnosis or treatment, and a person's health, life expectancy, and previous screening to make suggestions for when to stop.

There are websites that have decision aids to help older adults decide whether to continue breast or colorectal cancer screening. (See the Resources section at the end of this chapter.)

Why should we ever stop cancer screening?

Breast cancer screening has been shown to be beneficial to age 74. There are no high-quality data for older women. Breast cancer screening is not recommended for women with less than 10 years remaining life expectancy because the harms are immediate, and the chance of benefit is low.

Cervical cancer screening should stop at age 65 for those with adequate prior screening.

Adequate prior screening means either three negative pap smears or two negative human papilloma virus (HPV) tests in the past 10 years, with the last

TABLE 5.3
Summary of Recommendations for Cancer Screening in Older Adults

Cancer (Test)	Frequency of Screening	Provisos for Older Adults
Breast cancer (mammography)	Every two years if <75; discuss pros and cons after that.	Stop if life expectancy is likely to be less than 10 years.
Cervical cancer (pap smear or HPV testing)	Pap smear every three years or HPV testing every five years.	*Stop after age 65 if you have had adequate prior screening.* See the text for the definition of adequate prior screening.
Prostate cancer (PSA)	The American Urological Association suggests every two years; other agencies decide frequency by PSA level. Discuss the pros/cons with your provider.	*Stop at age 70,* or if your life expectancy is likely to be less than 10 years. May continue to 75 in very healthy men. High false positive rates. Treatment harms can include incontinence, erectile dysfunction, and diarrhea that occur years before cancer may be evident to patient.
Colon cancer (stool-based tests)	Yearly from ages 45 to 75; individualize decisions from ages 76 to 85. Does not apply to those with previous adenomas.	*Stop at age 86,* or if your life expectancy is likely to be less than 10 years.
Colon cancer (direct visualization)	Colonoscopy every 10 years or CT colonography every 5 years to age 75. Individualize decisions from ages 76 to 85. Does not apply to those with previous adenomas.	*Stop at age 86,* or if your life expectancy is likely to be less than 10 years. Risk of bowel perforation and other complications increases with age. Flexible sigmoidoscopy every 5 years does not result in as many life-years gained as the other visualization tests.
Lung cancer (low-dose CT)	Consider annually in those 50–80 years old who have a 20 pack-year smoking history and are either current smokers or quit within the past 15 years.	*Stop at age 80,* if you have not smoked in 15 years, or if you have a condition that substantially decreases your life expectancy.

Note: Abbreviations are as follows: CT, computed tomography; HPV, human papilloma virus; PSA, prostate-specific antigen.

one being no more than 5 years before, and not being at high risk (such as previous high-grade precancerous lesion, diethylstilbestrol exposure, or immunocompromised). The reason is that the incidence of high-grade cervical lesions significantly declines after middle age, and the risk of false-positive screening tests increases.

Prostate cancer screening of men 70 and older rarely if ever decreases death from prostate cancer, although to some extent this will depend on life expectancy.

Colon cancer screening has been shown to be beneficial to age 75. Colon cancer is one of the most preventable cancers if screening is done regularly. Continuing to age 85 depends on how healthy the person is, whether they are likely to live another 10 years, and whether they want to undergo yearly stool tests, flexible sigmoidoscopy or computed tomography (CT) colonography twice, or one more colonoscopy. Screening should stop at age 85 because most people diagnosed at this age will not live long enough to have colon cancer be their cause of death. If someone has never had a colonoscopy, however, a colonoscopy even after age 85 may save their life. (Author's note: I've never had a patient get upset when I told them they were done with screening colonoscopies!)

Lung cancer screening has been shown to be beneficial to age 75. Three successive annual screens reduced death from lung cancer by about 20 percent. There was, however, a higher false-positive rate in people over the age of 65, resulting in more invasive procedures occurring in people who didn't have cancer. The US Preventative Services Taskforce recommends annual screening with low-dose CT in adults aged 50 to 80 years who have a 20-pack-year smoking history and currently smoke or have quit within the past 15 years. Screening should be discontinued 15 years after stopping smoking, if there is significant comorbidity that substantially limits life expectancy, or if you are unable or unwilling to have curative lung surgery.

Other Disease Detection

Disease detection diagnoses a disease while it is asymptomatic, before you're aware of it. Several diseases can be detected during your yearly evaluation or Medicare annual wellness visit. The conditions listed in table 5.4 should be tested for at least once in a lifetime. As with cancer screening, you should only get screened if you are willing to be treated, so discuss this with your doctor before you have the test.

TABLE 5.4

Screening for Other Disorders

Condition (Test)	Who Should Be Screened and How Often?	Provisos for Older Adults
Osteoporosis (bone mineral density/DEXA)*	Women: at least once after age 65, or at age 60 if high risk (patient age, BMI, parental fracture history, and tobacco and alcohol use)	Rate of fractures begins to decline 18–24 months after starting osteoporosis treatment. Screening for men is controversial. One in eight men will have a hip, wrist, or vertebral fracture after age 50. Recommendations include screening men over 65 who have had a previous fracture, and screening all men over 70 or 80.
Abdominal aortic aneurysm (ultrasound)	Once for men 65–75 who ever smoked, or anyone 65–75 with a family history of abdominal aortic aneurysm	Medicare pays for this screening once.
HIV (blood test)	Consider if at high risk (multiple sexual partners, intravenous drug use)	About 20% of people with HIV are over age 50.
Hepatitis C (blood test)	One time for those aged 18–79	Usually from a transfusion before 1992, when blood screening for hepatitis C began, or IV drug use.

Note: Abbreviations are as follows: BMI, body mass index; DEXA, dual-energy x-ray absorptiometry; HIV, human immunodeficiency virus.

*See chapter 9 for further discussion.

Advice for Loved Ones

Preventive measures are done primarily to delay death or to improve current quality of life. Screening for the latter, like eye or hearing exams, provide benefit right away, whereas the benefit of cancer screenings usually does not occur for many years. The results of screening and prevention should match the values of the person getting screened. I have patients who will do whatever it takes to avoid living with disability from a stroke but don't want to do anything that would require chemotherapy, surgery, or radiation to prolong their lives. Some have been told they're prediabetic and change their diets, only to lose the joy they had gotten from eating. If your loved one doesn't want to be screened for cancer or take statins for high cholesterol, it's their decision. Encourage them to do those things that will improve their lives now and in the near future.

Bottom Line

Even in old age, there are some effective measures that can prevent illness and disability, and certain disorders that, if identified early, can be treated to improve health and well-being. But the benefits and risks can change with age, so it's important to individualize which screens and preventive measures meet your goals. Many screening tests, particularly for cancer, don't benefit those who have a life expectancy less than 10 years, but the screening and treatment can cause immediate harm. Make sure you know what you would need to do after an abnormal screening test, and don't do the test if you would refuse the treatment for the disease. Ask your provider how long it would take for you to realize the potential benefit of a screening test or behavioral change.

RESOURCES

Up-to-Date Information on Prevention and Screening

My Healthfinder
(https://health.gov/myhealthfinder)
Provides easy access to current recommendations by age and sex. Maintained by the Office of Disease Prevention and Health Promotion (ODPHP) in collaboration with the Agency for Healthcare Research and Quality (AHRQ).

US Preventive Services Task Force
(www.uspreventativeservicestaskforce.org)
Current recommendations and in-depth explanations of reasoning for these recommendations.

American Cancer Society Guidelines for the Early Detection of Cancer
(https://www.cancer.org/healthy/find
-cancer-early/american-cancer-society
-guidelines-for-the-early-detection-of
-cancer.html)
Recommendations for screening tests for various types of cancer.

Medicare Wellness Visits
(https://www.medicareinteractive.org
/get-answers/medicare-covered-services
/preventive-services/annual-wellness-visit)
A detailed explanation of the eligibility, covered services, and costs of Medicare's annual wellness visit.

CDC Vaccine Recommendations and Explanations
(https://www.cdc.gov/vaccines/schedules
/hcp/imz/adult.html)
Recommended immunization schedule for adults, including COVID-19 vaccines. For more information on COVID-19, see https://www.coronavirus.gov/.

Cardiovascular Primary Prevention

For the latest information on preventing cardiovascular disease, do an Internet search for updated American College of Cardiology / American Heart Association guidelines on the primary prevention of cardiovascular disease. The information in this chapter is based on the 2019 guidelines.

Diabetes and Prediabetes Prevention and Screening

CDC Diabetes Website
(https://www.cdc.gov/diabetes/index.html)
Provides resources for preventing, treating, and living with diabetes.

National Institute of Diabetes and Digestive and Kidney Diseases
(https://www.niddk.nih.gov/health
-information)
The NIDDK provides health information that is reviewed by doctors to help you better understand and manage diabetes.

Community Preventive Services Task Force
(https://www.thecommunityguide.org
/findings/diabetes-combined-diet-and
-physical-activity-promotion-programs
-prevent-type-2-diabetes)
The Community Preventive Services Task Force recommends diet and physical activity promotion programs to prevent type 2 diabetes among persons at increased risk.

Cancer Screening

Decision Aids
(http://cancerscreening.eprognosis.org/)
Decision aids can help older adults decide whether to continue breast or colorectal cancer screening.

BIBLIOGRAPHY

American Diabetes Association. "Older Adults: *Standards of Medical Care in Diabetes—2021." Diabetes Care* 44, suppl. 1 (2021): S168-79.

Arnett, D. K., R. S. Blumenthal, M. A. Albert, et al. 2019. "ACC/AHA Guideline on the Primary Prevention of Cardiovascular Disease: A Report of the American College of Cardiology/American Heart Association Task Force on Clinical Practice Guidelines." *Journal of the American College of Cardiology* 74, no. 10 (2019): 1376–414.

Leipzig, R. M., E. P. Whitlock, T. A. Wolff, et al. "Reconsidering the Approach to Prevention Recommendations for Older Adults." Annals of Internal Medicine 153, no. 12 (2010): 809–14.

PART II

What Really Matters as You Grow Older

CHAPTER 6

Mind Matters

Geriatricians are asked questions about memory almost every day, whether from a patient concerned about themselves or from a spouse or relative concerned about a loved one. But memory is just one of the parts of the mind that change with aging. *Cognition*, a term that describes our ability to think, reason, and remember, includes the overall functions of the mind. Broader than memory, cognition also refers to how we interpret sensory input and react from an emotional per-spective. For an overview of cognition and its components, see box 6.1.

This chapter discusses differences between normal aging and dementia, presents suggestions for preserving and improving your cognitive abilities, and identifies conditions and medications that can mimic memory loss and dementia. It also describes changes that are not normal aging and what to expect when you have a medical evaluation for cogni-tive concerns.

What's Normal with Aging?

Just like physical abilities, cognition can change as a person ages. For a deeper dive into age-related changes in cogni-tive abilities, see box 6.2.

I'm having more "senior moments." Am I developing dementia?

Senior moments, when you might have a problem finding a specific word or name, are common with normal aging. Sometimes they are called the "tip of the tongue" phenomenon—you know what you want to say but just can't find the word. Oftentimes the word will pop into your brain when you stop trying so hard. Once you've gotten the word, it's usually retained, and rarely does that word give you a problem again. In con-trast, people with dementia are unable to remember the word even if they're given a cue or a list of possibilities to choose from. *The major memory problem in dementia is the inability to store new information.* If you identify the word with cues or choices, it means that the word has been stored in your brain, and the problem you're having is with retrieving it. This is not dementia.

It takes more effort for me to learn new things. Is this normal?

Yes. Like physical abilities, some cogni-tive abilities—remembering where you parked the car or calculating a tip in a restaurant, for example—peaked in your twenties and thirties. Only some of this decline is due to a true loss of memory. Much of the difficulty learning something new is due to other cognitive changes, particularly the ability to quickly process information (see box 6.2).

With aging you have to work harder, needing more focused attention, repetition, and strategies to learn new things and accomplish tasks. Multitasking is more difficult, and processing takes longer, so reaction times are slower (both mentally and physically). You also don't perform as well when there's time pressure. All of this is normal aging.

How about dementia? Is it normal aging? That is, does everyone develop dementia if they live long enough?

No. Dementia is a disease, not normal aging. A little more than a third of people who live into their nineties have dementia, and many people live to be over 100 with intact cognition.

BOX 6.1

Cognition 101

Cognition is defined in the *Oxford Dictionary* as "the mental action or process of acquiring knowledge and understanding through thought, experience, and the senses."

Cognitive functions include memory (remembering things seen, heard, or otherwise experienced), but also being able to learn new things, pay attention, speak and understand, and visualize objects in space, such as pieces of a jigsaw puzzle or the location of a parked car.

Executive functions are an extremely important part of cognitive function and include the ability to solve problems, make decisions, set goals, plan, and quickly process new information. They provide a structure for how we live our lives and organize our days, including things like time management, date planning, and organization. These skills include the mental processes that allow us to hold information in our minds as we are working through tasks. Executive function also has an emotional component that includes flexibility when situations change, self-control over emotion and actions, and perseverance when things become challenging.

Each cognitive function has a primary home in a specific area of the brain. As shown in the figure on page 71, executive functions live in the frontal lobe, memory in the temporal lobe, sensory perceptions in the parietal lobe, and vision in the occipital lobe. Pathways exist that allow these areas to communicate with each other and with other parts of the nervous system to allow these functions to be carried out. Intact cognitive functioning allows individuals to learn and remember new things, set and achieve goals, and communicate with others. Disruptions in these areas or pathways cause impairments in these functions.

BOX 6.1 (*continued*)

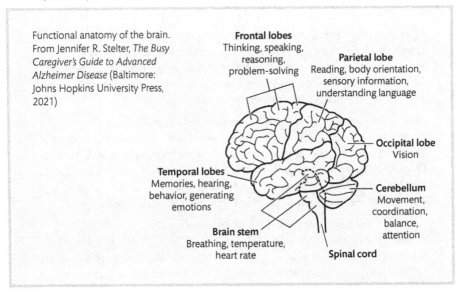

Functional anatomy of the brain. From Jennifer R. Stelter, *The Busy Caregiver's Guide to Advanced Alzheimer Disease* (Baltimore: Johns Hopkins University Press, 2021)

Frontal lobes
Thinking, speaking, reasoning, problem-solving

Parietal lobe
Reading, body orientation, sensory information, understanding language

Occipital lobe
Vision

Temporal lobes
Memories, hearing, behavior, generating emotions

Cerebellum
Movement, coordination, balance, attention

Brain stem
Breathing, temperature, heart rate

Spinal cord

BOX 6.2

What Happens with Aging: A Deeper Dive

Not all aspects of cognition decline with aging.
You keep the skills and knowledge that you've acquired throughout your life. Remote memory, language comprehension, and vocabulary remain largely intact with aging.

Reaction time increases with age both for cognitive processing and motor skills; that is, it takes longer to respond to stimuli.
These changes may be due to age-related declines in brain dopamine and some changes in the white matter around the ventricles of the brain. As a result, we're less able to quickly adapt to sudden changes or to solve problems as efficiently as we once could. Performance on tests that require speed declines, and reactions to stimuli usually take more time. This can affect one's ability to play sports or, more crucially, to drive (see chapter 19).

Executive function declines a bit.
The gradual decline in executive function probably occurs because of decreased processing speed. However, in general, it doesn't have a lot of impact on day-to-day activities.

It takes more time and effort to learn new information.
More repetition and focused attention are needed, for example, to learn a list of words. *Free recall* is the ability to recall the words you've tried to learn without

(*continued*)

BOX 6.2 (continued)

being given any clues. *Cued recall* is when you need to be prompted to recall a word in the list. Clues for the word "rose," for example, could be a category that the word fits in, like flower, or a written list containing the word "rose," allowing *recognition* to jog the memory. When older adults have repeated chances to practice, free recall increases, but not nearly as much as cued recall.

Finding the right words, particularly nouns, may be harder.
As noted above, sometimes we can't recall a word without a clue. But if you're able to retrieve it at all, that means the word (or the memory) was stored in your brain. Needing a clue shows that it's the ability to retrieve these from storage that gets weaker with age. This is the difference between a "senior moment," or a problem with retrieval, and dementia, which is a problem with storage.

For most older adults, memory is best in the morning.
Performance on many behaviors and tasks controlled by circadian rhythm is best one to two hours earlier than when we were younger (see chapter 10 for more information on age-related changes in circadian rhythm). For example, when older adults have their recognition memory tested in the early morning, they perform as well as younger adults, but when tested later in the afternoon, they perform significantly worse.

The ability to maintain attention persists, but multitasking becomes harder.
It's more difficult to divide your attention and concentrate on two or more things at once. As described above, processing speed also decreases, making it harder to pay attention to more than one thing at a time.

Some other abilities worsen with age.
Other functions, such as your ability to rotate an object or assemble objects in your mind, or to copy complex geometric designs, often decline with aging even when you're given unlimited time to do these things.

Adapting to Your New Normal

There is good news: you have been adapting and compensating for a change in cognition for years. My favorite study demonstrating this phenomenon looked at expert typists who used typewriters (it's an old study!). Older women were as fast and accurate as their younger colleagues when typing a manuscript, even though the younger women had faster reaction times; that is, they hit a typewriter key faster than older women in response to a stimulus. How did the older typists keep up their speed? They unconsciously read ahead when typing text, anticipated the next keystrokes, and moved their fingers toward the relevant keys much sooner than the younger typists. When the typists couldn't look ahead because the next part of the text was concealed, the older experts typed slower than the younger ones.

You say these changes are "normal," but they're annoying and frustrating to me. Is there anything I can do?

As shown in box 6.3, making a memory requires that your senses capture new information and events and store them in a way that you can retrieve them. You can often improve your memory by using the following strategies.

Pay More Attention

Anything that interferes with your sensory abilities or your ability to pay attention affects your ability to create a new memory. If you can't hear, you won't be able to remember what was said. Hearing impairments may mimic a true memory disorder. Hearing aids and related adaptations are a potentially easy fix in this circumstance (see chapter 12).

When you are distracted, you're unable to prioritize owing to the barrage of sensory input you encounter every hour. Think about what happens when someone speaks to you when you're reading a book. Do you really hear what's being said? When you need to concentrate, don't multitask, and work in a quiet environment with minimal distractions.

BOX 6.3

How Are Memories Made?

The schematic below combines features of different scientists' models of making a memory.

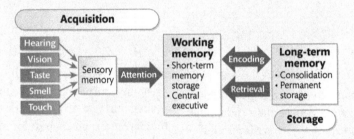

To create a memory, your senses must capture new information and events and then store them in your brain in a way that you can retrieve them.

New information is acquired through your senses—hearing, seeing, smelling, touching, or tasting. But more than your senses are needed. Since we're bombarded with input all day long, there's a limit to the amount of information we can absorb at one time. To really absorb new information, attention is key. You need to be alert and concentrating for the new information to be transferred into

(continued)

BOX 6.3 *(continued)*

working memory. *Anything that interferes with your sensory abilities or your ability to pay attention affects your ability to create a new memory.*

Working memory consists of short-term memory (STM) and the central executive (CE), which acts like the CEO (chief executive officer) of an organization. STM lets you remember recent events, like the question you've just been asked or the beginning of a sentence you're reading. It's also where information is rehearsed or manipulated prior to entering long-term memory. The CE is in charge of *executive functions*, such as planning or deciding what to prioritize and what to pay attention to when there is competing input—the television or the boarding announcement when you're at the airport, for example.

Long-term memory (LTM) is where our memories live, the parts of the brain where new information is *permanently* stored, and from which we can retrieve it as needed. Sleep is critical to memory storage, as this is when memories are strengthened and integrated into what we already know—a process called *memory consolidation*. Consolidation seems to occur during the last third of a night's sleep, when we are in stage N2 and REM (rapid eye movement) sleep (see box 10.1 in chapter 10).

Encoding is how new information or events are programmed for storage in and retrieval from LTM. The strength and methods of encoding influence our ability to remember, that is, retrieve a memory. This starts with how you acquire the memory in the first place. Have you ever pushed yourself to remember something by reconstructing where you were when you heard or saw it? Certain characteristics of the event make it more "sticky," or more likely to be robustly encoded. Information that elicits strong emotion, like when a grandchild is coming for a visit, is usually easier to remember than an appointment for a haircut, even if both are six months away.

Work at Your Own Pace

Studies show that when there is time pressure, older people make more mistakes than when they have unlimited time to complete a task. Make sure you have enough time to accomplish what you're trying to do.

Identify the Best Time of Day for You to Learn New Things

As discussed in chapter 10, morning is often the best time for many older people to learn new things. Figure out what's the best time of day for you. I read my journals and wrote this book mainly during morning hours. I find that late afternoon is best for me to delete emails and return phone calls.

Use Strategies to Help Your Memory

Make Stronger Memories

- Use as many senses as possible to reinforce a memory: repeat it aloud, write it down, visualize it (take a picture or imagine a movie in your mind if you can).

- Review what you want to remember before sleep. This exercise promotes memory retention.
- Test yourself by asking and answering questions about what you're trying to remember. This practice makes it easier to recall the information later.

Organize Material into Shorter Meaningful Groups

- *Chunking:* Break down large groups of words or numbers into three to five smaller chunks. For example, it's easier to learn a telephone number as three chunks—555, 671, and 9323—than as ten digits—5556719323.
- *Categorizing:* Group items by similarities. When making a grocery list, note which fruits, vegetables, meats, canned goods you need rather than just writing down whatever comes to mind.
- *Sequencing:* Provide a 1-2-3 order to things, events, or errands based on their time or location. An example is to write your grocery list based on the sections of the supermarket and how you make your way through the store.

Remember Names and Faces with These Tips

- Practice saying the person's name during the conversation, comment on it, use it at the end of the conversation. "Helen, like Helen of Troy?"
- Connect the name to something familiar and possibly meaningful. "Your name is Sara? That's my aunt's name." Or, "Do you spell Sarah with an h?"

- Picture the name. For example, if the person's name is Robin Brown, visualize a brown robin.
- Connect a facial feature to the person's name. Harry has a moustache, for example.

Keep Track of Things

- Identify a specific storage place for each item that is often lost, like your keys, glasses, or watch.
- Use an organizer, such as a calendar or a notebook, and make it a habit to jot down everything important in it: appointments, to-do lists, birthdays.
- Leave yourself a cue. If I want to order something online, I leave a note or a reminder near the computer.
- Don't panic if you happen to misplace something. Stay calm—it will show up!

I'm doing okay at the moment, but I'm worried about the future. What can I do to preserve my cognitive abilities?

There is no magic bullet to prevent age-related cognitive change or the development of dementia, but there are certain behaviors associated with better cognitive function. Engaging in these behaviors can benefit cognition, whether or not you have a cognitive problem. A recent Finnish study found that a two-year intervention (including diet, exercise, cognitive training, and vascular risk monitoring) improved cognition, particularly executive function and speed of processing, in people 60–77 years old at high risk of dementia.

Brain Health Is Heart Health

The risk factors for many types of dementia, including Alzheimer disease, are the same as those for heart attacks and strokes. Controlling blood pressure, cholesterol, and blood glucose; minimizing intake of trans fat (which is most common in fried or processed foods), red meat, and salt; being physically active; stopping smoking; and losing weight have contributed to a 25 percent decline in dementia, as well as a significant decline in heart attacks and strokes. It's never too early or too late to change habits that put you at increased risk for cognitive decline.

Reduce Exposure to Secondhand Smoke and Air Pollution

A study found that women 55–64 years old with secondhand smoke exposure had greater memory loss than women who were not exposed, and that the longer they were exposed, the worse their memory loss. Quitting smoking has been found to decrease the risk of dementia for older smokers, and likely for those exposed to secondhand smoke as well. In another study, older adults living in areas where pollution levels are the highest had a 40 percent greater risk of being diagnosed with dementia than people living in areas where pollution levels were low. Try to reduce exposure by avoiding outdoor exercise near busy roads and by using a high-efficiency particulate air (HEPA) filter in your home's furnace.

Limit Alcohol Use to No More Than One Drink Daily

Chronic alcohol overuse, binge drinking, and dependence are associated with an increased risk of dementia, especially early-onset dementia, which occurs in people under the age of 65.

Get Off the Couch

Any amount of exercise can be beneficial to people who are sedentary. You don't need to get out of breath or sweat profusely. Strength training, tai chi, gardening, dancing, and long, regular walks (30 minutes, five times a week) all count as exercise (chapter 7). Studies suggest that physical exercise improves executive function as well as global cognitive functions, such as learning, memory, language, and visuospatial abilities. Strength training improves cognitive function in those with mild cognitive impairment.

Get Adequate Sleep

Memory consolidation occurs during sleep, strengthening and integrating new memories into what we already know. Sleep disturbances and sleep medications can affect cognition and are associated with problems with attention and executive function. Don't medicate your sleeplessness or depression with alcohol, and stay away from sleeping medications, even those available without a prescription. See chapter 10 and your health care provider for help improving your sleep.

Sharpen Your Senses

Events, words, scents, and flavors must first enter your brain before they can be remembered. For more information on what you can do to improve your hearing, vision, and sense of smell and taste, see chapters 12 and 15.

Protect Your Head

Head trauma is associated with cognitive impairment. Wear a helmet when riding your bike or doing other sports that may result in head trauma.

Use It or Lose It

Participate in activities that make you think—crossword puzzles, reading, writing, board or card games, discussion groups—and use the computer or play a musical instrument. Studies suggest that people engaged in these activities in middle or late life are less likely to develop dementia. The jury is out on whether computer-based cognitive training improves cognitive functioning; in particular, it's not known whether these exercises translate to improvement in day-to-day tasks.

Engage Socially

Socializing with friends and families; being involved in clubs, religious services, travel, and cultural events; and learning new things will keep you intellectually stimulated and can help hold depression at bay.

Decrease Stress and Anxiety

Stress and anxiety can interfere with paying adequate attention and your ability to process new information. Physical activity, psychotherapy, particularly problem-solving types of therapy, and meditation have all been shown to reduce stress (chapter 8).

Do supplements help?

There is no evidence that any supplement enhances cognition unless you have vitamin B_{12} or thiamine deficiency. Many supplements have not been adequately tested, but among those that have, there has been no cognitive benefit associated with gingko biloba, multivitamins, vitamin E, vitamin C, beta-carotene, or B vitamins, including folic acid and vitamin B1.

What Isn't Normal Aging?

 Red Flags: Symptoms Needing Prompt Medical Attention

Any of the symptoms below may happen occasionally and be normal, but if they recur regularly, you should be evaluated, as they may indicate a cognitive problem that can be treated.

- Cloudy or foggy thinking.
- Nodding off to sleep during the day or an overwhelming feeling that you need to take a nap.
- Difficulty following and participating in conversations, often losing your train of thought.
- Feeling overwhelmed if you need to make a decision or a plan, or when following specific instructions.
- Losing objects and not being able to retrace your steps to find them.
- Personality and behavioral changes: you're irritable, withdrawn, anxious, depressed, impulsive, or have little interest or motivation.

- You frequently repeat questions or statements and forget recent events or conversations, which you still really don't remember even after being told about them by others.
- You miss important appointments or events.
- You've missed bill payments.
- You are having difficulty managing your medications.
- You've gotten lost when driving or walking in a familiar area.
- You lose your ability to communicate in a second language, even if you've been using it for many years.
- Your family and friends voice concern about any of the above.

⚠️ **Yellow Alerts: Common Conditions That Can Mimic or Worsen Cognitive Concerns**

When I see patients concerned about their cognition, I ask three questions.

The first is, "When and how did the problem start—was it abrupt or gradual?" If the symptom appeared abruptly, I'm concerned about delirium, a new confusion usually due to a new or worsening medical problem. Dementia, other than that due to a stroke, does not suddenly get worse. This is an important point to remember.

My second question is, "What medications are you taking, at what dose, for how long, and why?" I ask about prescription and nonprescription drugs, as well as supplements and vitamins obtained at the health food store. In older people, any new symptom may be caused by a medication or supplement.

Finally, I ask whether the person might be depressed, since depression can mimic cognitive impairment in some people. These are not the only treatable causes of cognitive impairment, but they are the most common.

Delirium

On Tuesday, Marsha, an independent 85-year-old woman with hearing impairment who lives with her daughter, went out with friends to dinner and a movie. On Wednesday afternoon, her daughter found her sleeping, not eating or drinking, and unable to remember that she'd seen a movie the day before. Although she wasn't coughing and didn't have a fever, her doctor diagnosed her with pneumonia. After a short course of antibiotics, she was back to her usual self.

Cognitive changes that come on abruptly, or that come and go over the course of the day, should receive prompt medical attention, as they may signal a serious underlying medical condition. Older brains are very sensitive to disease, medications, and environmental change. For example, a urinary tract infection rarely if ever causes confusion in a 50-year-old, yet it commonly does so in older adults, particularly those who are frail. Some medical conditions may present solely with confusion and not with the typical symptoms one might imagine. For example, the majority of people over age 80 having a heart attack don't have chest pain, but 10 percent of them have new or greater confusion as their main presenting symptom. As with Marsha, confusion may be the only sign of pneumonia; fever and cough can be absent.

Delirium is the medical term for this type of change. Delirium is *not* dementia, although people with dementia are more likely to become delirious. People with delirium may not know where they are or the time of day, they may sleep a lot, and their speech may not make sense or be understandable. Some become agitated, see things that aren't really there, or pick at things in the air. Delirium is rarely due to a new brain disease like a stroke, meningitis, or a brain tumor. It is a geriatric syndrome (see chapter 2) that occurs when a vulnerable person (one with difficulty caring for themselves, dementia, vision or hearing loss, depression, history of stroke, alcohol misuse, or over age 70) is exposed to certain medical or environmental triggers (see below). The more vulnerable one is, the less noxious the trigger needs to be to cause delirium. Delirium can be scary for family members and for the delirious person, but it usually clears once the underlying cause has been addressed. Even so, some studies suggest that the longer the delirium lasts, the less likely a person will return to their previous cognitive function, so it's extremely important that a person with delirium, or an acute change in their cognitive function, gets urgent medical attention.

What can cause delirium?

Many conditions can cause delirium, including:

- Worsening heart, liver, kidney, or lung function
- Nutritional deficiencies, such as thiamine or vitamin B_{12} deficiencies
- Fevers and infections (which don't always cause a fever in older adults)
- Dehydration or electrolyte abnormalities (low sodium, for example)
- Urine or stool retention
- Sensory impairments
- Sleep deprivation
- High or low levels of thyroid hormone, calcium, glucose, or cortisol
- Inadequately treated pain
- Medications, including abruptly stopping certain medications

Changes Caused by Medications

Fred is a 79-year-old man who recently experienced worsening angina (chest pain from the heart not getting enough oxygen) and was started on a new medication. His angina improved, but over the next few months, he became aware that his thinking had become fuzzy. The doctor checked the medical literature and found nothing suggesting that the new medicine could be the cause of his cognitive concerns. Nonetheless, she decreased the dose. Within a week, Fred's fuzzy thinking was a thing of the past, and his cardiac symptoms remained controlled.

Older people are more likely to develop medication-related changes in cognition, such as cloudy thinking, inattentiveness, sedation, confusion, and actual worsening of memory (see chapter 3). Additionally, there are three other situations that should be considered when evaluating the relationship of medications to cognition.

Over-the-Counter Medications

Every year, I see at least two patients for a dementia evaluation and discover they're regularly taking a product containing diphenhydramine, or Benadryl, such as Tylenol PM or Advil PM. When they stop these products, they return to their former selves. Dementia symptoms can also occur with the H₂ blockers sold for acid reflux, like Tagamet, Zantac, Axid, and Pepcid.

Specific Medication Effects on Elders

Some drugs that have not been reported to cause cognitive change may do so in older people (see table 6.1). There are several reasons why such side effects are not recognized before approval of a medication by the US Food and Drug Administration (chapter 3). If you suspect that a new medication may be causing your cognitive symptoms, speak with your health care provider like Fred did. You and your doctor can see if decreasing the dose over time causes the cognitive changes to improve. If so, you may be able to take a lower dose and still get the drug's benefits, or your provider may be able to prescribe a different medication altogether.

Abruptly Stopping Medication

Stopping certain medications cold turkey can result in withdrawal symptoms that include cognitive changes (see table 6.2). The dosage of these drugs should be slowly decreased over time under the supervision of your health care provider.

Depression

The cognitive impairment of depression in older adults is primarily a problem with executive function—that is, planning, problem-solving, paying attention, and maintaining self-control. Personality changes and apathy, or lack of interest, are also seen. Depressed people often complain of memory problems, yet when being evaluated, they may not even try to answer cognitive screening questions, instead saying, "I don't know." This differs from patients with dementia, who are often unaware of their own deficits and will guess and try to give an answer. See chapter 8 for additional discussion of depression in older adults.

Dementia

What is dementia?

Dementia is a brain disease that causes impairment in memory, executive function, language, and the performance of previously learned skills. To be diagnosed with dementia, these impairments must be severe enough to affect one's everyday life.

Are Alzheimer disease and dementia the same thing?

There are several types of dementia. Alzheimer disease (AD) is the most common type of dementia in the United States, followed by vascular dementia. Some patients have a *mixed dementia* and present with features of more than one type of dementia. The most common mixed dementia is that with features of both AD and vascular dementia. For information on the most common types of dementia, see box 6.4.

TABLE 6.1
Medications That Can Cause Cognitive Impairment

Examples of cognitive impairment include confusion, oversedation, increased forgetfulness, and occasionally hallucinations. If you're not sure whether a drug you're taking is in one of the drug classes listed, ask your pharmacist or health care provider.

Drug Classes	Examples
Blood pressure, cardiac, and diuretic medications	
Beta-blockers	Carvedilol (Coreg); metoprolol (Lopressor); propranolol (Inderal)
Diuretics	Hydrochlorothiazide; metolazone (Zaroxolyn); triamterene-hydrochlorothiazide (Dyazide); furosemide (Lasix)
Pain relief	
GABA-ergic neurogenic pain medications	Gabapentin (Neurontin); pregabalin (Lyrica)
NSAIDs	Ibuprofen (Motrin, Advil); naproxen (Naprosyn, Aleve); indomethacin (Indocin); ketorolac (Toradol)
Opioid analgesics	Morphine; oxycodone (in Percocet); hydromorphone (Dilaudid); hydrocodone (in Vicodin); tramadol (Ultram)
Muscle relaxants	Cyclobenzaprine (Flexeril); carisoprodol (Soma); metaxalone (Skelaxin)
Neurological, psychological, and sleeping medications	
Sleep and/or antianxiety drugs	Alprazolam (Xanax); lorazepam (Ativan); diazepam (Valium); triazolam (Halcion); eszopiclone (Lunesta); zolpidem (Ambien)
Melatonin receptor agonists	Ramelteon (Rozerem); tasimelteon (Hetlioz), melatonin
Anti-dizziness drugs	Meclizine (Antivert, Bonine); dimenhydrinate (Dramamine); scopolamine (Trans-scop)
Antidepressants	
SSRIs	Possibly paroxetine (Paxil)
Tricyclic anti-depressants and SNRIs	Amitriptyline (Elavil); doxepin (Silenor); nortriptyline (Pamelor); desipramine (Norpramin); venlafaxine (Effexor); duloxetine (Cymbalta)
Other antidepressants	Mirtazapine (Remeron); bupropion (Wellbutrin, Zyban); trazodone (Desyrel)

(continued)

TABLE 6.1 *(continued)*

Drug Classes	Examples
Antipsychotics	Thioridazine (Mellaril); haloperidol (Haldol); quetiapine (Seroquel); risperidone (Risperdal)
Anticonvulsant medications	Phenytoin (Dilantin); valproic acid (Depakote); lamotrigine (Lamictal); levetiracetam (Keppra)
Barbiturates	Butalbital (in Fiorinal and Fioricet); primidone (Mysoline); phenobarbital
Gastrointestinal medications	
Antispasmodics	Clidinium-chlordiazepoxide (Librax); dicyclomine (Bentyl); propantheline
Antidiarrheal	Hyoscyamine (Levsin, Levbid); atropine/diphenoxylate (Lomotil)
H₂ blockers	Famotidine (Pepcid); cimetidine (Tagamet)
Proton pump inhibitors	Omeprazole (Prilosec); lansoprazole (Prevacid); pantoprazole (Protonix)
Anti-Parkinsonian medications	
Decarboxylase inhibitor	Levodopa/carbidopa (Sinemet)
Dopamine agonist or potentiator	Pramipexole (Mirapex); amantadine (Symmetrel); bromocriptine (Parlodel)
Anticholinergic	Benztropine (Cogentin); trihexyphenidyl (Artane)
Other drugs	
First-generation antihistamines (used for itching, allergies, cold symptoms)*	Diphenhydramine (Benadryl); chlorpheniramine (Aller-Chlor, Chlor-Trimeton); hydroxyzine (Atarax)
Bladder relaxants	Tolteradine (Detrol); oxybutinin (Ditropan); solifenacin (Vesicare)
Fluoroquinolone antibiotics	Ciprofloxacin (Cipro); levofloxacin (Levaquin)
Corticosteroids	Prednisone; dexamethasone (Decadron); methylprednisolone (Solu-Medrol)

Note: Abbreviations are as follows: GABA, gamma amino butyric acid; NSAID, nonsteroidal anti-inflammatory drug; SNRI, serotonin-norepinephrine reuptake inhibitor; SSRI, selective serotonin reuptake inhibitor.

*Second-generation antihistamines do not cross the blood–brain barrier, so rarely cause cognitive symptoms. Examples include fexofenadine (Allegra), loratadine (Claritin), cetirizine (Zyrtec), desloratadine (Clarinex), and levocetirizine dihydrochloride (Xyzal).

TABLE 6.2
Medications That Can Cause Cognitive Symptoms When Abruptly Stopped

Drug Class	Examples	Withdrawal Symptoms
Alcohol		Confusion, anxiety, depression.
Benzodiazepines and benzodiazepine receptor antagonists (for sleep and anxiety)	Temazepam (Restoril); triazolam (Halcion); lorazepam (Ativan); zolpidem (Ambien); zaleplon (Sonata)	Apathy, confusion, dizziness, poor short-term memory, panic, anxiety.
SSRI antidepressants	Paroxetine (Paxil); escitalopram (Lexapro); citalopram (Celexa)	Irritability, anxiety, insomnia or vivid dreams, dizziness, tiredness.
SNRI antidepressants	Venlafaxine (Effexor); duloxetine (Cymbalta)	Anxiety, dizziness, tiredness.
Opioid analgesics	Morphine, oxycodone (in Percocet); hydromorphone (Dilaudid); hydrocodone (in Vicodin); tramadol (Ultram)	Confusion, clouding of mental function, drowsiness, tiredness.

Note: Abbreviations are as follows: SNRI, serotonin-norepinephrine reuptake inhibitor; SSRI, selective serotonin reuptake inhibitor.

My husband's doctor diagnosed him with mild cognitive impairment. Does this mean he's going to develop dementia?

Mild cognitive impairment (MCI) is diagnosed when neuropsychological testing finds that a person has cognitive changes that are worse than those expected with normal aging, but they don't interfere with the person's everyday life. MCI does not always progress to dementia. Some people with MCI improve; about 15 percent develop dementia within two years of diagnosis. Overall, about 33 percent of people diagnosed with MCI eventually develop some form of dementia.

What are some of the earliest signs of dementia?

Forgetting appointments, losing keys, and getting lost are usually *not* the first signs of dementia. Changes in *executive functioning skills* are, particularly the ability to perform complex tasks. These tasks are made up of several actions, each of which needs to be done correctly. Examples include paying household bills, filing taxes, and managing medications.

One of my cognitive screens is to ask patients if they are still paying the bills and managing their medications. If they are, I ask if they've made any errors recently. Sometimes a spouse will mention that she took over the bills six months ago. I always ask why. This is one way to find subtle (and not-so-subtle) signs of early disease.

BOX 6.4

Common Types of Dementia

Alzheimer disease (AD): Early features include difficulty with memory and performing tasks that require planning, like managing medications or paying bills (executive function). These difficulties worsen gradually over time. A person with AD may increasingly repeat themselves as the disease progresses. There are two forms of AD, an early-onset form that occurs in people under the age of 65, and the more common late-onset form seen in older adults. Both forms of AD begin in the hippocampus of the temporal lobe.

Vascular dementia (VD): Early features include problems with planning, con-centration, and processing speed. New learning and memory, although affected, are less impaired than in those with AD. VD is caused by strokes, blockages of blood vessels that occur mainly in people with long-standing high blood pressure and diabetes. Strokes can be obvious, causing loss of speech or the use of an arm or a leg, or they can be *ministrokes*, causing no symptoms or subtle changes in cognition or function. Cognitive deficits from a stroke appear as a sudden decline and then stabilize unless another stroke occurs. This is called a stepwise decline, as opposed to the gradual decline usually seen in Alzheimer disease. Strokes can occur in blood vessels in any area of the brain, although they happen most com-monly in the frontal lobe and the motor and sensory cortices.

Mixed dementia occurs in people with both AD and VD. Symptoms are a combination of what is seen in each disorder.

Parkinson's disease (PD) and Lewy body dementia (LBD): People with these disorders develop both dementia and the features of PD, including tremors, slow movement, stiffness, and a shuffling gait, but at different times. In people with PD who develop dementia, the dementia starts several years after the movement problems, while in LBD, both occur at the same time. Additionally, people with LBD have fluctuations in their alertness, vivid and realistic visual hallucinations, and may act out their dreams during sleep. This is called rapid eye movement (REM) sleep behavior disorder (see chapter 10). Dementia of PD and LBD are as-sociated with changes in neurons in both the brain stem and the cerebral cortex.

Frontotemporal dementia (FTD): FTD usually occurs at a younger age than AD. There are two forms of FTD. Personality changes and inappropriate behaviors are most prominent in one form, while difficulties with speech and language are most prominent in the other. Both worsen gradually over time. As implied in its name, both the frontal and temporal lobes are primarily affected.

Normal pressure hydrocephalus (NPH): People with NPH have a wide-based "magnetic gait," cognitive decline, and urinary incontinence. In a magnetic gait, the feet seem attached to the floor as if by a magnet, and one has to wrench each foot to get it off the ground to walk. NPH is not common, but the diagnosis should be considered since surgery may be able to stop or improve the demen-tia. NPH is caused by the buildup of fluid in the ventricles that are in the middle of the brain, causing pressure on and damage to nearby brain tissue.

Getting Evaluated for Cognitive Concerns

Many people are ambivalent about getting a cognitive evaluation. It totally makes sense if you are worried and want to know more, such as, "Is this normal or the start of dementia?" or "What can I do to improve my memory?" But if you feel there isn't a problem or refuse an evaluation and your loved ones think it's needed, this can become a real bone of contention. Your loved ones are concerned about your safety and well-being, and they may be worried about what the future will bring for both you and them. An evaluation may help both of you and result in ways to improve your day-to-day life and your relationship. Having an evaluation may identify treatable conditions or medications impairing your cognition, while cognitive testing can identify your strengths and weaknesses to help you develop compensatory strategies to improve your quality of life.

The biggest concern for most people is that the evaluation will result in a diagnosis of MCI or even dementia. It's important to recognize, however, that even with these diagnoses, there is a great deal of uncertainty as to how your future will unfold. With MCI, there's no way to know if or when dementia will eventually develop, and with dementia, the rate of progression is variable and can be quite slow for some.

The good news is that right now the vast majority of your brain is functioning well. There are things that you can do to help slow the progression of cognitive decline while continuing to do the things you enjoy and that give

purpose to your life. This is also a good time to review and make decisions about legal and financial affairs, as well as to designate a health care proxy who can make medical decisions if you're not able to do so yourself. Your proxy needs to know your wishes about medical treatment (see chapters 4 and 20).

Should I See a Specialist?

Most health care providers are not trained to do in-depth cognitive assessments. That's the reason they refer their patients to me and my colleagues in geriatrics, neurology, and psychiatry— to clarify the type and extent of the memory problems and to identify any conditions that may be interfering with cognitive functioning, such as medications, nutritional deficiencies, thyroid disease, infections, silent strokes, sleep apnea, depression, untreated pain, pulmonary issues, cardiac problems, or kidney disease. Another reason to see a specialist is that they often can provide resources for those with cognitive impairment and their loved ones. For example, many geriatricians work with social workers on-site and can link patients to helpful community-based programs, support groups, counseling, and home care.

Preparing for the Appointment

At your appointment, you'll need to discuss the specifics of your memory concerns and how things differ from before; for this reason, it's important that you prepare for the visit. Fill out this chapter's pre-visit checklist on page 369 in Appendix 3, bring it to the visit, and review it with your provider. Medications and supplements can cause problems with attention as well as memory itself, so the medical provider needs to know exactly what you're taking. You may be given a short test to assess your cognitive abilities and have blood work, brain imaging, and neuropsychological testing ordered. The latter is especially helpful when trying to detect cognitive impairment in high-functioning people, since even if they've lost some cognitive function, they can still ace the short tests typically administered in the office. For example, a 79-year-old woman with a PhD in English literature may need more in-depth testing to tease out a cognitive disturbance than the usual short screen. Even though I suggest you bring along someone else who is familiar with your cognitive concerns, *make sure you have time alone with your health care provider if there are private issues you wish to discuss.* Ideal times to ask others to leave are during the physical exam or cognitive testing.

Advice for Loved Ones

It's not uncommon for older adults, family, or friends to be concerned that senior moments, word-finding problems, or trouble taking medications indicate the start of dementia. One way to determine whether this is likely is to answer whether, over the past several years, there have been changes in any of the following that you think are due to cognitive problems:

- Problems with judgment (such as falling victim to online scams, making bad financial decisions, buying inappropriate gifts)
- Reduced interest in hobbies/activities
- Repeating questions, stories, or statements
- Trouble learning how to use a tool, appliance, or gadget (smartphone, computer, microwave, remote control)
- Forgetting the correct month or year
- Difficulty handling complicated financial affairs (such as balancing checkbook, filing income taxes, paying bills)
- Difficulty remembering appointments
- Having consistent problems with thinking or memory
- Problems with driving, accidents, or errors in calculating routes

An answer of yes to two or more of these is suspicious for a diagnosis of dementia, and an evaluation should be considered.

Other behaviors that may suggest dementia include personality changes, poor hygiene, weight loss, withdrawal from activities, missed appointments, unpaid bills, medication errors, and increased clutter in the home. There may be variability in abilities and behaviors at different times of the day. Memory is usually best in the morning for people living with dementia. Evenings may bring "sundowning"—that is, increased confusion and agitation.

You may worry that discussing your concerns about memory or offering suggestions like those in this chapter will cause conflict to arise between you and the older person in your life. Your preexisting relationship will play a major role in how these discussions go. It's important that you make sure the older adult knows that you're making suggestions because you care about them, and you want to help them remain independent and able as they age. Let them know that you use some of these strategies yourself to help with multitasking and remembering important things.

Some older people are afraid that if cognitive impairment is identified, they will be stigmatized or infantilized, losing autonomy or independence. Many people fear that a diagnosis of dementia will lead to placement in a nursing home. They may fear that this is the beginning of a process they'd rather not know about—one that will end up with their being unable to care for themselves or make their needs known, and becoming a "burden"—like friends or family they've seen in the end stages of dementia. Such fears are understandable. In this case, it helps if older adults and their loved ones strive to develop "radical empathy," putting themselves in the other's shoes and trying to understand the other's feelings, fears, and what might be gained or lost by an evaluation.

It can be difficult to diagnose cognitive impairment early on, especially in people who have been high-functioning. But going to a specialist may be more than an older adult wants to deal with. In this case, their primary care provider can be asked to evaluate whether the older adult has any of the medical concerns discussed above.

In the same way that I suggest making sure the patient has some alone time with the evaluating provider, it may also be helpful for concerned loved ones to have the opportunity to speak openly about their concerns during an evaluation. This can be difficult when the older adult resists the idea that they might have a memory problem. Asking your older adult if it is okay for you to speak with the health care provider, or writing down your observations for the provider to read, may be a helpful way around this difficult dynamic.

What if this is dementia?

If there *is* real cognitive decline, and particularly if you notice that it is progressing, don't argue over the small stuff, such as slight differences in recollections. Choose your battles carefully. Recognize that these cognitive changes are not volitional—the person doesn't remember that they've asked the same thing several times before; they have a condition that makes it difficult, sometimes impossible, to learn new things. You may find it hard to spend time with this person who looks the same as always but isn't. Conversations, personality, and behaviors may be different and at times upsetting to you. Some refer to this as an "ambiguous loss," not a death but still the loss of the essence of a person important in your life. It's a loss you need to acknowledge and perhaps mourn. You may wish to speak to a therapist or read more on this subject to help you cope with this loss while the person is still alive. Caregiver support groups can be helpful.

Even a person with moderate or severe dementia can still be involved in making choices about advanced medical care. Health care providers, in either the office or the hospital, can help to determine whether the patient has the required understanding to make these choices. There is good evidence that patients with this more advanced level of disease can still appoint a health care proxy and communicate that they trust a specific individual to serve in this role.

Bottom Line

Cognitive changes are part of normal aging. But these changes don't mean that you are losing your mind. There are strategies to help improve memory and thinking. Like many human organs, the brain needs exercise to stay in shape—and exercise is the best medicine we have for dementia prevention. But some people do develop more serious cognitive decline. The Red Flags section in this chapter lists a number of situations that should be discussed with a medical professional. If you or your family observe any these symptoms, it is time to see a geriatrician, neurologist, or psychiatrist for an evaluation. Remember that the sudden onset of confusion is more likely to be delirium, not dementia, and requires an urgent medical evaluation. Medications, underlying physical conditions, and depression can cause cognitive impairment that is short term and treatable. Most importantly, the majority of mental challenges you notice will *not* be first signs of dementia. Rather, they are a call to action.

RESOURCES

Maintaining and Improving Your Memory

Green, C. R. *Total Memory Workout: 8 Easy Steps to Maximum Memory Fitness.* New York: Bantam, 2001.

Lorayne, H., and J. Lucas. *The Memory Book: The Classic Guide to Improving Your Memory at Work, at School, and at Play.* New York: Random House, 1996.

Robledo, I. C. *Practical Memory: A Simple Guide to Help You Remember More and Forget Less in Your Everyday Life.* Seattle, WA: CreateSpace, 2017

For Those with Cognitive Impairment and Their Loved Ones

Alzheimer's Association (www.alz.org)
This organization provides resources, support groups, and educational seminars for those with memory loss and their families.

Boss, Pauline. *Ambiguous Loss: Learning to Live with Unresolved Grief.* Cambridge, MA: Harvard University Press, 2000.

Mace, Nancy, and Peter V. Rabins. *The 36-Hour Day: A Family Guide to Caring for*

People Who Have Alzheimer Disease, Other Dementias, and Memory Loss. 7th ed. Baltimore: Johns Hopkins University Press, 2021.

Family Caregiver Alliance. "Caring for Adults with Cognitive and Memory Impairment." Accessed November 29, 2021. https://caregiver.org/caring-adults -cognitive-and-memory-impairment.

National Institute on Aging. "Cognitive Health and Older Adults." Reviewed October 1, 2020. https://www.nia.nih.gov/health /featured/memory-cognitive-health.

Interest in Participating in Trials to Delay Dementia or Improve Cognition

Clinical Trials
(https://clinicaltrials.gov)
This search tool is part of the US National Library of Medicine. Use it to find clinical trials by entering terms like "memory," "dementia," "mild cognitive impairment," and the like.

Alzheimer Disease Resource Center
(https://www.adrcinc.org/ClinicalTrials.asp)
A division of the National Institute on Aging, the Alzheimer Disease Resource Center provides educational training, an assistance center, a list of medical professionals, safety products, and support groups.

BIBLIOGRAPHY

Baddeley, A. D., and G. Hitch. "Working Memory." In *The Psychology of Learning and Motivation: Advances in Research and Theory*, vol. 8, edited by G. H. Bower, 47–89. New York: Academic Press, 1974.

Croft, S., B. Cholerton, and M. Reger. "Cognitive Changes Associated with Normal and Pathological Aging." Chapter 62 in *Hazard's Principles of Geriatric Medicine and Gerontology*, 6th ed., 751–65. New York: McGraw-Hill, 2009.

Galvin, J. E., C. M. Roe, K. K. Powlishta, M. A. Coats, S. J. Muich, E. Grant, J. P. Miller, M. Storandt, and J. C. Morris. "The AD8: A Brief Informant Interview to Detect Dementia." *Neurology* 65, no. 4 (2005): 559–64.

Hall, C. B., R. B. Lipton, M. Sliwinski, M. J. Katz, C. A. Derby, and J. Verghese. "Cognitive Activities Delay Onset of Memory Decline in Persons Who Develop Dementia." *Neurology* 3, no. 5 (2009): 356–61.

Hood, C. N., and S. Amir. "The Aging Clock: Circadian Rhythms and Later Life." *Journal of Clinical Investigation* 127, no. 2 (2017): 437–46.

Inouye, S. K., S. T. Bogardus Jr., P. A. Charpentier, L. Leo-Summers, D. Acampora, T. R. Holford, and L. M. Cooney Jr. "A Multicomponent Intervention to Prevent Delirium in Hospitalized Older Patients." *New England Journal of Medicine* 340 (1999): 669–76.

Inouye, S. K., R. G. J. Westendorp, and J. S. Saczynski. "Delirium in Elderly People." *Lancet* 383 (2014): 911–22.

Institute of Medicine. *Cognitive Aging: Progress in Understanding and Opportunities for Action.* Washington, DC: National Academies Press, 2015. http://www.iom .edu/Reports/2015/Cognitive-Aging.aspx.

Livingston, G., J. Huntley, A. Sommerlad, et al. "Dementia Prevention, Intervention and Care: 2020 Report of the Lancet Commission." *Lancet* 396 (2020): 413–46.

Ngandu, T., J. Lehtisalo, A. Solomon, et al. "A 2 Year Multidomain Intervention of Diet, Exercise, Cognitive Training, and Vascular Risk Monitoring versus Control to Prevent Cognitive Decline in At-Risk Elderly People (FINGER): A Randomised

Controlled Trial." *Lancet* 385, no. 9984 (2015): 2255–63.

Salthouse, T. A. "Effects of Age and Skill in Typing." *Journal of Experimental Psychology: General* 13 (1984): 345–71.

Salthouse, T. A. "Expertise as the Circumvention of Human Processing Limitations." In *Toward a General Theory of Expertise: Prospects and Limits*, edited by K. A. Ericsson and J. Smith, 286–300. Cambridge: Cambridge University Press, 1991.

Wilson, R. S., P. A. Boyle, L. Yu, L. L. Barnes, J. Sytsma, A. S. Buchman, D. A. Bennett, and J. A. Schneider. "Temporal Course and Pathologic Basis of Unawareness of Memory Loss in Dementia." *Neurology* 85, no. 11 (2015): 984–91.

CHAPTER 7

Energy Cycles

Remember Pete Seeger singing "my get up and go has got up and went"? This is a real concern for many of my patients. What's "normal" for energy with aging is the second most common concern I'm asked about, after questions about memory. People become worried when doing their usual activities becomes too much for them. With aging, there are physical and psychological reasons why you may feel that you have less energy, and there are ways to adapt to these changes. .

Everyone's usual energy level is different: despite having metastatic cancer, my patient Annie ran rings around me at 85! Another of my patients, Nancy, stopped doing things she had loved 20 years before she died because she couldn't accept that she couldn't do them as she had at 40.

This chapter addresses low energy, loss of endurance, decreased exercise tolerance, and frailty. Sleepiness and drowsiness are discussed in chapter 10.

For an overview of energy production, heart function, and blood pressure, see box 7.1.

What's Normal with Aging?

For a deeper dive into age-related changes in energy production, requirements, and reserves, see box 7.2.

I've always been active. Now, at 80, I feel much more tired doing the same things I've always done. Is this normal?

Energy reserves and exercise tolerance (your ability to do physical activity) decrease with aging. Your muscles need fuel—predominantly food and oxygen—to generate energy. As you age, your food intake may decrease, especially the amount of protein you eat, and the lungs transfer less oxygen to the blood.

Additionally, the heart becomes less efficient with aging.

The result of all these changes is that muscle mass and strength decrease, and you generate less energy. As you age, accomplishing the same tasks at the same speed as when you were younger requires more energy. So, if less energy is generated and more is used to do usual activities, there won't be as much left for doing other things. Most people compensate by modifying their activities so they don't feel fatigued. If you don't compensate, you'll feel tired.

So, to some extent, feeling more tired is "normal." But if a major loss of energy is not addressed, it can set off the *cycle of frailty* (box 7.3), where the normal becomes abnormal. Age-related decreases in muscle mass and strength can be made worse by poor nutrition, inactivity, illnesses, and medications, resulting in further loss of strength, walking speed, and ability to do exercise, resulting in low energy, exercise intolerance, and a feeling of exhaustion. This results in *sarcopenia*, a loss of muscle mass and strength greater than expected from aging alone.

What is frailty?

Just like US Supreme Court Justice Potter Stewart's definition of pornography, frailty is hard to define but you know it when you see it. Frail people are vulnerable and have less physiologic reserve and resilience, so their ability to cope and bounce back from illness, stress (as a result of chemotherapy, surgery, hemodialysis, extremes of heat or cold, emotional difficulties), or trauma (including falls) is limited (see the homeostenosis figure on page 15). Their strength, performance, energy, activity, and sometimes weight are decreased, and they are at higher risk for becoming functionally impaired, dependent, hospitalized, and dying. Low energy does not necessarily progress to frailty, but it can set off the cycle of frailty. Prevention and intervention can interrupt the cycle.

I'm overweight, so I guess I don't have to worry about getting frail, right?

Wrong. You may think that sarcopenia and frailty only occur in those who are underweight. Not so—and the numbers with sarcopenic obesity have been skyrocketing with the increase in obesity we see in the United States. People who are both obese and sarcopenic are more functionally impaired than those who are only one or the other. Why? Their muscles are infiltrated with fat, so they are of poorer quality and strength. In general, obese people are less active. Obesity itself increases chronic inflammation, causing additional fatigue and exhaustion, more inactivity, and even more severe sarcopenia. Weight loss and resistance exercise can help to reverse this cycle.

Is frailty inevitable with aging?

Becoming frail is not inevitable; only about 25 percent of people 85 years or older are frail. Things you can do to make frailty less likely are described in the next section.

BOX 7.1

Energy 101

Energy is defined by the *Oxford Dictionary* as the capacity to do work, and the strength and vitality required for sustained physical or mental activity. Everything a person does uses energy. Metabolic equivalents, or METs, are a way to measure the energy needed to perform activities. One MET is defined as the energy it takes to sit quietly for a minute. Increasing exercise intensity requires an increase in METs. For example, sleep uses only 0.9 METs per minute, while jogging uses 7 METs per minute.

The body's energy is stored in a molecule called adenosine triphosphate (ATP) that can provide readily releasable energy. Little ATP is stored in the body, so it must be constantly regenerated using building blocks from food—particularly carbohydrates, fats, and protein—as the starting material. Although a small amount of ATP can be produced anaerobically (without oxygen), oxygen is required for the vast majority of ATP production. The maximum amount of energy a person can produce depends on the lungs' ability to oxygenate the blood, the heart's ability to pump the oxygenated blood to muscles and organs, and the muscles' and organs' ability to remove oxygen from the blood and use it to produce more ATP.

The heart plays a major role in energy generation, and understanding its normal anatomy and function will help explain how age-related changes affect both energy and blood pressure. An efficiently functioning heart is necessary for adequate energy production.

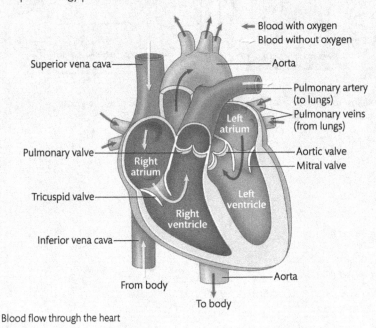

Blood flow through the heart

(continued)

BOX 7.1 (*continued*)

As shown in the figure on page 93, the heart has four chambers, two atria and two ventricles. Both ventricles are filled by blood flowing in from the atria during a period known as *diastole*. Toward the end of diastole, an electrical impulse causes the atria to contract, squeezing the remaining atrial blood into the ventricles. The ventricles contract forcefully during *systole*, pushing blood into arteries that take it to the lungs and the rest of the body. The amount of blood pumped out from the heart into the circulatory system is called the *cardiac output*. As shown in the schematic below, blood is oxygenated in the lungs and then goes out the heart's left ventricle to the body, the muscles, kidney, brain, and organs, returning to the right side of the heart with considerably less oxygen, where it again enters the lungs to get reoxygenated.

Blood pressure (BP) consists of two numbers. *Systolic BP* is the top number and reflects the pressure generated when the ventricles contract. *Diastolic BP* is the bottom number and reflects ventricular pressure during filling.

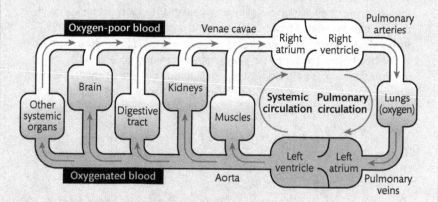

Blood flow through the body. Adapted by permission from Lauralee Sherwood, *Human Physiology* (Boston: Cengage, 2016), chap. 9

BOX 7.2

What Happens with Aging: A Deeper Dive

You generate less energy. Why?

- Hearts work harder and less efficiently. Ninety percent of Americans develop high systolic blood pressure (BP) by the time they're 90. This is caused by atherosclerosis, or hardening of the arteries, and as a result, the contracting heart needs to generate more pressure to maintain cardiac output. You may think high systolic BP is not a problem for older adults, since almost everyone has it. But treating systolic pressure in older adults protects against heart failure and stroke. The only question is how low to go (see Yellow Alerts below).
  - The left ventricle stiffens, decreasing the amount of blood that enters passively from the atria, and making ventricular filling more dependent on the atria that are actively contracting. This is why older people are more symptomatic if they develop rapid heart rates or disorders like atrial fibrillation, both of which cause inefficient atrial contractions, resulting in decreased cardiac output, lower BP, weakness, and shortness of breath.
  - Maximum heart rate decreases with age, limiting the amount of exercise we can do and energy we can generate.
  - The lungs transfer less oxygen to the blood.
- Appetite and food intake decrease (chapter 15).
- Muscle strength declines even more than muscle mass. In fact, the average person loses 0.5 to 1.2 percent of their current muscle mass and 3 percent of their strength every year after age 50.
  - Older people's dietary protein intake decreases. During exercise, protein ingestion stimulates muscle synthesis. It takes more protein for older people to stimulate muscle synthesis than it does for younger people.
  - Resistance (strengthening) exercise in particular can increase muscle mass and strength with aging.

You need more energy (more metabolic equivalents, or METs) to do the same activities at the same speed as when you're younger.

- The energy cost (the amount of energy needed) to walk at a given speed increases. Walking efficiency decreases from the loss of muscle mass, strength, coordination, and the change in our center of gravity.
- The energy cost of walking is even greater if one has heart, lung, or mobility impairments such as arthritis or other joint or muscular conditions.

Therefore, energy reserves decrease.

It's basic math: if less energy is generated and more is used doing usual activities, there won't be much left for doing other things. This is particularly true for tasks that require endurance, such as walking a long distance or vacuuming a larger room.

And we compensate by modifying our activities so we're able to do more.

Most healthy older people have a preferred walking speed that is slower than when they were young, allowing them to conserve energy and reduce fatigue.

BOX 7.3

Cycle of Frailty

Frailty occurs when *sarcopenia*, a loss of muscle mass and strength greater than expected from aging alone, combines with inadequate nutrition and age-related physiological changes to affect the body's ability to produce and use energy, causing further loss of strength, exercise ability, and endurance. Feelings of fatigue and exhaustion follow, gait slows, and physical activity further decreases, causing a cycle of increasing sarcopenia, weakness, and eventually frailty. Unhealthy environments, injury, disease, and inflammation can intensify this cycle. Without activity and proper nutrition, energy reserves and maximum exercise capacity decline further, so that everyday activities consume even more energy, decreasing the amount of physiological reserve available for other needs (see the homeostenosis figure on page 15).

Sarcopenia is usually the first sign of frailty. About 10 percent of 60-to-70-year-olds and 50 percent of those over age 80 are sarcopenic. Inactivity, undernutrition, chronic diseases (such as diabetes, lung or heart disease, cancer, and HIV), acute illness, and certain medications accelerate muscle and strength loss. Even short periods of inactivity, as often happens during a harsh winter, can worsen sarcopenia.

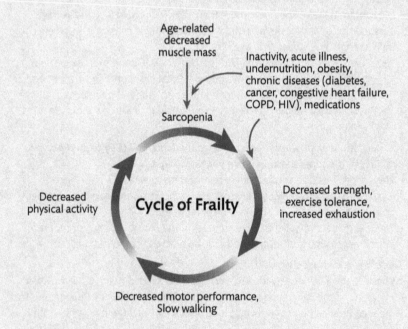

Cycle of frailty. Data from L. P. Fried, C. M. Tangen, J. Walston, et al., "Frailty in Older Adults: Evidence for a Phenotype," *Journals of Gerontology, Series A: Biological Sciences and Medical Sciences* 56, no. 3 (2001): M146–56

Adapting to Your New Normal

The two best things you can do to preserve or improve your energy are watching what you eat and developing a regular exercise program that works for you.

I'm a little overweight, but I try to eat a healthy diet. Will I have more energy if I lose weight or eat differently?

Being a little overweight is actually fine for most older adults. If you're considerably overweight or obese, or your weight is interfering with your activities, you can try to lose weight sensibly (see chapter 15).

To increase your energy, increase your protein intake. You need much more than the 58 grams (about 2 ounces) that is recommended by the US Department of Health and Human Services for a 160-pound older adult. This recommended amount is the *minimum* needed to stop lean muscle loss. More importantly, it is woefully inadequate to maximally stimulate muscle growth. To enhance muscle, about 0.5 grams per pound (or 0.8 grams per kilogram) of body weight are needed to stimulate muscle synthesis in conjunction with exercise. So, that 160-pound person would need to increase their daily protein to 80 grams. A little increase goes a long way. In a study of frail 80-year-olds, an increase to 3.5 ounces of daily protein caused a significant uptick in their physical performance compared to those who ate only 2.5 ounces.

Your protein goal depends on your weight and your activity level. The National Academies of Sciences, Engineering and Medicine's calculator can help you determine how much protein you should be getting. You should eat one-third of your protein goal at each meal.

The number of grams in an ounce of protein differs depending on the type of protein. For example, 30 grams of protein are found in about 3 ounces of skinless roasted turkey or chicken breast, 4 ounces of tuna or salmon, 4 cups of milk, and 1.5 to 2 cups of Greek yogurt (see the Resources section at the end of chapter 15 for websites that list the protein content of foods). It's always best to limit the fat that accompanies protein-rich foods, which can be done by eating lean meats and low-fat milk and cheese.

CAUTION If you have *liver or kidney disease*, you may need to limit your protein intake. Discuss what your daily protein intake should be with your doctor.

I know you're going to tell me to exercise. Why is it important, especially at this point in my life?

To have more energy, you need to exercise. *Exercise is the only "anti-aging drug" that works.* It can reverse some of the age-related declines in energy and physical work capacity by improving your strength, walking speed, stamina, and exercise tolerance. Exercise can improve your mobility and decrease falls and injury, as discussed in chapter 9.

It doesn't matter if you're out of shape or frail. Cardiorespiratory fitness improved 15 percent over two to three months for the average unfit older adult who followed the multicomponent regimen described in the American College of Sports Medicine's guidelines for older adults. The risk of developing frailty was cut almost in half when older sedentary adults at risk of mobility disability followed a similar exercise program for a year.

I've never exercised. How do I start?

Sit less. Older adults, even those without chronic diseases, spend an average of more than nine hours per day sitting (and during the COVID-19 pandemic, much more than that). Your aerobic capacity declines twice as fast if you're not physically active. The more fit you become, the more you will be able to do. Have an active lifestyle. Walk to the mailbox, park farther away from your destination, count your steps. Improved fitness can reduce the number of metabolic equivalents (METs) needed to perform an activity, while inactivity increases the number.

Consider using a fitness device or mobile app. Personally, I spend most of my day sitting in front of screens, reading, or having meetings. Time passes, and I have no idea when I last got out of the chair. Then I got a step tracker, which vibrates to let me know it's been almost an hour since I last stood or walked 250 steps. This woke me up! Now, whenever I feel that vibration, I try to take a 5- to 10-minute walking break. It's done wonders for my step count, and the exercise renews my ability to concentrate.

Okay, I'm getting up every few hours and walking for 5 to 10 minutes. What's next?

Check out the precautions for starting to exercise in box 7.4. Remember, any exercise, no matter how little, is a good starting point. The idea is to do something you like doing, at your own pace, and work up from there. Some of the things you may already be doing for fun are considered exercise, like walking, dancing, gardening, cycling, and tai chi.

Try to exercise with others. It's easier to be motivated to exercise if you do it as part of a group or in a physical therapy program. You can find community-based exercise programs at senior centers. Some malls and neighborhoods have walking programs. You can start with chair yoga if your balance or endurance are a concern.

What's the best kind of exercise for older adults?

There are different types of exercise that increase strength, endurance, flexibility, and balance. Multicomponent exercise programs address all of these areas. That being said, you don't have to start with a multicomponent program; each individual component has benefits and often increases your ability to do the others.

Strength Training

Strength training, also called *resistance exercise*, can counteract the loss of muscle and increase bone strength by increasing muscle mass, strength, and stability, and can decrease the energy cost of walking, that is, the amount of energy used. If you consume about

BOX 7.4

Exercise: Precautions when Getting Started

- If you've been sedentary or are functionally limited, start slow. You may need to get stronger or improve your balance before you can start endurance exercises.
- If you're just beginning to exercise, work with a physical therapist or a trainer to get the right form and routine for you. Make sure they're used to working with older adults who are just starting to exercise.
- Warm up before starting. To warm up, do some light exercise for two to five minutes to bring your body temperature up, loosen your muscles, and increase your heart rate to get the blood flowing before starting an exercise routine.
- Don't buy into the saying "no pain, no gain." You can get significant benefit from exercise without making yourself miserable for the rest of the day. If you have chest pain or pressure or shortness of breath, stop and notify your doctor.
- Give your body a chance to recover from workouts. Muscles need rest to strengthen and grow from exercise, and they need time to recover from any soreness that develops. You can still do less vigorous activities on your rest days, such as walking more leisurely, swimming, or doing yoga.

0.5 grams of protein per pound body weight over the course of a day (about one-third of the daily total at each meal), muscle mass and strength will increase by maximizing the protein synthesis that occurs after exercising. Building additional muscle mass and strength also helps to improve aerobic capacity and thus endurance, which is how long you can exercise. Some older people find elastic resistance bands easier to use than weights.

Aerobic Endurance Training

Aerobic activity improves cardiovascular conditioning and exercise tolerance, and decreases energy expenditure. Aerobic exercises include walking, playing a sport, dancing, or any other activity that utilizes large muscle groups. Alternatives for those who can't walk distances include water and/or stationary bike exercise.

Stretching and Balancing Exercises

These exercises improve flexibility, joint movements, and your awareness of where your body is in space and as you move, resulting in better balance and stability as well as a lower energy cost to walking. Do stretching and balancing exercises at least twice a week. Working to improve your balance can help prevent falls (see chapter 9).

How hard do I have to exercise to get these benefits?

Activity can be divided into three levels of intensity:

- *Mild activity* is any activity. When it comes to walking, a brisk walk is best, but there are benefits to strolls and slower walking as well.

- *Moderate activity* is something you can do while talking, but singing would take too much effort.

- *Vigorous activity* is intense enough that you can't say any more than a few words without pausing to take a breath.

You will get benefits from any regular exercise routine you choose, but the more aerobic exercise, strength training, and balance work you do, the lower your risk of developing age-related functional limitations. That said, type 2 diabetics who do some regular activities have much lower mortality than those who do none at all, and they benefit almost as much as if they did moderate activity 150 minutes a week. For older adults, doing moderate to intense activity at least 33 minutes a week reduces the risk of having an injurious fall. That's less than 5 minutes a day.

I'm worried I'm going to hurt myself using weights. How heavy do the weights need to be for me to get stronger?

Studies in young men show the same gain in muscle strength and size with fewer injuries when, instead of straining with heavy weights, they followed the program below.

- Start with a weight or resistance band that feels tolerable, and lift or stretch repeatedly until you've grown tired and the effort of your final repetition is at least an 8 on scale of 1 to 10.

- Do three sets of the above three times a week.

- Increase the number of repetitions or the weight if your effort is less than an 8.

I'm afraid to start exercising by myself because of my medical conditions. What can I do?

Discuss any exercise plan with your health care provider. You may qualify for one of the rehabilitation programs covered by Medicare that are listed below.

Physical Therapy

A physical therapist can teach you exercises and strategies to improve your walking and balance while decreasing the energy cost. You might want to try out an assistive device; it may help you increase your energy if you use it regularly (see Appendix 2).

Cardiac Rehabilitation

A cardiac rehabilitation program provides exercise, education, and counseling to those with functional limitations from heart disease. Speak with your cardiologist to see if you are a candidate.

Pulmonary Rehabilitation

If you have moderate to severe lung disease, pulmonary rehabilitation may help. It provides exercise, education (including how to best use your inhalers), and support. Ask your pulmonologist if you would benefit from this type of program.

What if I'm at a point where I really can't do what I want to be able to do day to day?

If you have low energy, you may find it hard to do everything you or others want you to do on a daily basis. You need to conserve your energy. A helpful strategy in this situation is SOC, as discussed in chapter 1: **select** what really matters to you, **optimize** yourself and your environment, and **compensate** by using alternative mechanisms and equipment. Don't let pride, or not wanting to appear "old," keep you from having a richer, fuller and more active life.

Select: Prioritize

- Focus on things you enjoy doing.
- Be realistic with yourself.

Optimize: Plan Your Time Based on What Works for You

- What's your best time of day? Plan events and work for these times.
- Alternate tasks that take lots of energy with those that take less.
- Give yourself more time to do tasks.
- Take rest breaks.

Compensate: Make Things Easier for Yourself

- Rearrange your household so that the things you use most often are near each other and within reach.
- Use assistive devices to save energy (bathing and grooming organizers, long-handled sponges, grabbers, combs, canes, walkers, and the like).
- Avail yourself of community resources like Meals on Wheels to get a well-balanced diet.

- Have a cart or wagon to help with moving things.
- Get clothes with pockets for carrying things.

I see supplements being advertised as energy boosters. Should I take them?

Many supplements are marketed as "anti-aging," suggesting they can reverse aging and restore your energy and vitality. Studies don't support these claims, however. Aging is associated with a decline in blood levels of many hormones and micronutrients, but there's little evidence that increasing these levels to what they were when we were younger is safe or improves our strength and energy. We learned this with estrogen replacement therapy, where those taking it developed an increased risk of cancer, blood clots, and other problems. Similar side effects can occur with human growth hormone (see below). Aging is much more complex than replacing a series of compounds that decline with age. Multiple systems are involved, so supplementing a single agent is unlikely to make a difference and may result in serious harm, both from the active ingredient as well as from whatever else may be in the supplement (see chapter 3).

Vitamin B$_{12}$ Shots

If you're not vitamin B$_{12}$ deficient, these shots are of no value. People with a true vitamin B$_{12}$ deficiency may have fatigue, weakness, depression, memory impairment, or numbness and tingling of their hands and feet. Vitamin B$_{12}$ deficiency can be diagnosed with blood tests, and can usually be treated with oral supplements that are easily absorbed.

Human Growth Hormone

Not worth it. Although injections of human growth hormone (HGH) decrease fat mass and increase lean body mass when given to otherwise healthy older people, the common side effects—which include swelling, joint pain, carpal tunnel syndrome, and prediabetes or actual diabetes—outweigh the potential benefits. In the United States, it is illegal to use HGH made from recombinant human DNA as an anti-aging intervention.

Testosterone

The story here is a little more complicated. Testosterone concentrations decrease with age. Low testosterone can affect libido, energy, mood, bone density, and anemia. Replacing it, for men or women, depends on the degree of deficiency and the symptoms you're trying to improve. There are many potential risks to testosterone supplementation, including prostate cancer, worsening of benign prostatic hypertrophy and sleep apnea, and making an overabundance of red blood cells, which is associated with an increase in heart attacks and strokes.

If you are considering testosterone replacement, see an endocrinologist to make sure the diagnostic tests, replacement dose, and monitoring are right for you. There is a lot of variation in testosterone blood levels, so don't consider replacement based on the results of one test. If you choose to try testosterone, work with your doctor to determine what symptoms you are hoping to address, and stop taking testosterone if these symptoms do not improve. For better energy, libido, and hemoglobin, taking testosterone for a few months is an adequate trial. If trying to improve bone density, it could take two years. See chapter 16 for more on testosterone and sexual function.

What Isn't Normal Aging?

Having less energy is part of normal aging, but it can also be a warning sign.

 Red Flags: Symptoms Needing Prompt Medical Attention

Seek prompt medical attention if you have any of the following symptoms at rest or when walking or exercising:

- new or worsening shortness of breath
- chest pressure or pain
- irregular or rapid heartbeat
- lightheadedness or feeling that you might pass out
- exhaustion
- thigh or calf pain that occurs routinely after you've walked a certain distance, say several city blocks; this could be a symptom of claudication, a type of angina in leg arteries (see chapter 9)
- severe abdominal, pelvic, or back pain
- unintentional weight loss

- extreme fatigue, lack of energy, or reduced stamina that interferes with your ability to do your daily activities

 Yellow Alerts: Common Conditions That Can Mimic or Worsen Energy Levels and Exercise Tolerance

Medications

Medications can affect energy and exercise ability in many different ways (see table 7.1). As discussed in chapter 3, the standard dose may cause older adults to experience a greater effect than expected, such as developing symptoms of low blood sugar from your diabetes medication or dehydration from your diuretic (water pill). Occasionally, medications that enter the brain can cause fatigue, depression, or fogginess. Review your medications with your health care provider, especially if you think they're contributing to your symptoms. Decreasing the dose or switching to a different medication may result in feeling more energetic and having greater exercise tolerance.

Depression

Depression should be considered early, when someone is concerned about low energy, not only after a physical cause cannot be found. Not infrequently, it coexists with other medical conditions, and treatment can improve one's energy level. As discussed in chapter 8, older adults are less likely than younger people with depression to feel sad or guilty. Instead they are more likely to be uninterested in things they previously enjoyed; preoccupied with physical symptoms; and irritated, short tempered, or anxious.

Deconditioning

Deconditioning is a loss of muscle and bone that occurs when you stay in bed or are much less mobile for any reason (see box 7.3). It causes weakness, fatigue, and an increased likelihood of falling. Deconditioning can occur quickly, and its negative effects are cumulative, whereas regaining strength and mobility take much longer.

CAUTION *Bed rest is only for dead people, and a few others.* Obviously, there are times when you feel really sick and need to be in bed, and naps are fine (see chapter 10). But just like the astronauts, without gravity you rapidly lose muscle and bone. So even if you're depressed, fatigued, or hospitalized, try to spend your time sitting up in a chair or, even better, moving. Many years ago, it was widely accepted that people who were ill needed bed rest. But in fact the opposite is true, and the consequences of bed rest can be devastating to older adults. Complications include blood clots, skin breakdown, joint contractures (tightening that causes a loss of joint movement), bone loss, cardiovascular problems, dehydration, malnutrition, loss of muscle mass, and weakness. Making an effort to sit up, even if it is just getting into a chair or eating at the dinner table, is important and can significantly reduce the risks associated with bed rest.

TABLE 7.1
Drugs That Can Cause Symptoms of Low Energy or Exercise Intolerance

Drugs and Examples	Symptoms
Cardiac and diuretic medications	
ACE inhibitors and ARBs: lisinopril (Zestril); ramipril (Altace); candesartan (Atacand); Losartan (Cozaar)	Low blood pressure; reduced kidney function, which can cause medications and toxins to build up.
Beta-blockers: metoprolol (Toprol); atenolol (Tenormin); carvedilol (Coreg)	Slow heart rate; depression.
Calcium channel blockers and renin inhibitors: amlodipine (Norvasc); diltiazem (Cardizem); verapamil (Calan); aliskiren (Tekturna)	Low blood pressure.
Central adrenergic agonists: methyldopa; clonidine (Catapres)	Low blood pressure; depression.
Diuretics: hydrochlorothiazide (Microzide); metolazone (Zaroxolyn); furosemide (Lasix)	Dehydration, electrolyte loss, and/or low magnesium with loss of appetite, fatigue, and muscle weakness.
Statins: pravastatin (Pravachol); simvastatin (Zocor); atorvastatin (Lipitor); rosuvastatin (Crestor)	Decreased exercise tolerance (reason unknown); muscle weakness and aches.
Pain relief	
GABA-ergic neurogenic pain medications: gabapentin (Neurontin); pregabalin (Lyrica)	Fatigue, oversedation, weakness, confusion.
NSAIDs: ibuprofen (Motrin, Advil); naproxen (Naprosyn, Aleve)	Heart failure; high blood pressure; reduced kidney function, which can cause medications and toxins to build up.
Opioid analgesics: morphine; oxycodone (in Percocet); hydrocodone (in Vicodin); tramadol (Ultram)	Fatigue, oversedation, weakness, confusion.
Muscle relaxants: cyclobenzaprine (Flexeril); methocarbamol (Robaxin); carisoprodol (Soma); metaxalone (Skelaxin)	Muscle weakness, fatigue, confusion.

TABLE 7.1 *(continued)*

Drugs and Examples	Symptoms
Neurological, psychological, and sleep	
Sleep and anxiety: diazepam (Valium); alprazolam (Xanax); zolpidem (Ambien); zaleplon (Sonata)	Fatigue, oversedation, weakness, confusion.
Tricyclic antidepressants: amitriptyline (Elavil); imipramine (Tofranil); doxepin (Sinequan) doses over 6 mg	Fatigue, oversedation, weakness, confusion.
SSRI and SNRI antidepressants: paroxetine (Paxil); citalopram (Celexa); fluoxetine (Prozac); duloxetine (Cymbalta); venlafaxine (Effexor)	Low sodium, causing weakness and confusion (more common with SSRIs).
Antipsychotics: chlorpromazine (Thorazine); olanzapine (Zyprexa); quetiapine (Seroquel)	Fatigue, oversedation, weakness, confusion.
Anti-dizziness: meclizine (Antivert, Bonine); dimenhydrinate (Dramamine); scopolamine (Trans-scop)	Fatigue, oversedation, weakness, confusion.
Gastrointestinal medications	
Gastrointestinal antispasmodics: atropine; dicyclomine (Bentyl); propantheline	Fatigue, oversedation, weakness, confusion.
Proton pump inhibitors for GERD: omeprazole (Prilosec); esomeprazole (Nexium); pantoprazole (Protonix)	Low magnesium and B_{12}, causing fatigue and weakness.
Other drugs	
Diabetic hypoglycemics: glipizide (Glucotrol); glyburide (Micronase); insulin	Low blood sugar symptoms including confusion and unresponsiveness.
Alcohol overuse	Heart problems; malnutrition.
Alpha-blockers for blood pressure and BPH: doxazosin (Cardura); terazosin (Hytrin); alfuzosin (Uroxatral); tamsulosin (Flomax)	Low blood pressure, particularly when standing up, causing light-headedness and potentially loss of consciousness.

Note: If you're not sure whether a drug you're taking is in one of the drug classes listed, ask your pharmacist or health care provider. Abbreviations are as follows: ACE, angiotensin-converting enzyme; ARB, angiotensin receptor blocker; BPH, benign prostatic hyperplasia; GABA, gamma amino butyric acid; GERD, gastroesophageal reflux disease; NSAID, nonsteroidal anti-inflammatory drug; SNRI, serotonin-norepinephrine reuptake inhibitor; SSRI, selective serotonin reuptake inhibitor.

What else could be causing my exercise intolerance and low energy?

There are many different conditions, physical and emotional, that can contribute to a feeling of low energy. Some common causes are:

- heart and circulatory conditions such as heart failure, rhythm disturbances, uncontrolled high blood pressure, coronary artery disease, or valve problems
- pulmonary (lung) conditions such as emphysema, asthma, or chronic bronchitis
- anemia
- liver or renal disease
- endocrine conditions such as diabetes or adrenal or thyroid disease
- infections and inflammatory conditions such as Lyme disease, rheumatoid arthritis, or human immunodeficiency virus (HIV)
- undiagnosed cancer
- sleep disorders (chapter 10)
- Parkinson's disease
- anxiety, grief, or stress (chapter 8)
- poor nutrition or obesity (chapter 15)
- uncontrolled pain (chapter 14)
- dehydration

Getting Evaluated for Low Energy

Exercise intolerance and low energy can affect your quality of life. You don't want to delay diagnosis; not only will you run the risk that the underlying conditions may worsen, but if not attended to, depression or the cycle of frailty can be triggered. While some degree of decreased energy may be normal with aging, medical problems in older adults oftentimes present with vague symptoms like decreased energy.

Make sure your health care provider understands what's normal with aging (or show them that part of this chapter!). My patients often tell me they don't have the energy or exercise tolerance they used to, and their health care provider told them that this is due to old age. Don't buy this explanation without questioning.

See chapter 4 for a discussion on how to make sure your providers know what your health care goals and priorities are, and take these into account when decisions are made on what diagnostic tests and treatments to pursue. At the same time, get their advice on how to maintain or improve the energy and exercise tolerance you have.

Should I See a Specialist?

Start with a generalist. The causes of your symptoms may not be immediately obvious, and it can take some time and investigation to determine them. Both you and your loved ones may feel frustrated or worried, which can eventually lead to doctor shopping, where you go from physician to physician looking for an answer, or to doctor avoidance, where fear of the unknown keeps you from finding out what's going on. Have patience—it can take time to sort out your symptoms. Depending on what is found, your primary care provider may refer you to a specialist. If you're concerned about a specific problem, ask your primary care provider about a referral.

Preparing for Your Visit

Complete this chapter's pre-visit checklist on page 371 in Appendix 3. Bring the completed checklist and all your medications and supplements with you to the appointment (use table 7.1 as a guide). Your health care provider should review these, do a thorough physical examination, and order blood tests and possibly other studies. Depending on the results, you may get some answers, additional tests may be ordered, or you may be referred to a specialist. You may also receive dietary or exercise recommendations.

Advice for Loved Ones

Nonspecific concerns like having less energy or stamina can be frustrating for both the older adult and their loved ones. Older adults may stop participating in activities they enjoy, become isolated, or believe this is the "beginning of the end." Sometimes you can see that they're not themselves, but other times it's hard to tell if something is different. Watching your loved one lose interest in the things they once enjoyed can lead to a lot of concern, and occasionally you may feel angry or impotent. This is where it helps to get a professional opinion. It's important to know whether there is an underlying medical or psychological problem causing your loved one's sense of low energy.

At the same time, there are real changes that occur with aging that affect how fast someone walks, their energy, and their exercise tolerance. Diet and physical activity can help. Spend the time you're together actively—having a good meal, taking walks around the block, going to museums or shopping. See if you can become partners in better fitness and diet. For example, you can compare your daily step counts. If you're like most worker bees, you're spending an inordinate amount of time sitting in front of your computer. Make it a friendly competition! Encourage your loved ones to build up their strength and endurance by increasing the number of steps or distance walked weekly. Help them identify what exercise classes are available at local senior and community centers. Perhaps you can even join one with them.

Loving someone who is frail can be more difficult. It is a visual reminder that life and strength are finite. Encourage eating regularly, and suggest protein-calorie supplements if your loved one is having trouble eating enough (chapter 15). Similarly, encourage socialization and participating in stimulating mental activities. Work with them to make their environment safer (chapters 9 and 18).

Most importantly, help your loved ones achieve what they decide is most important and what they want to expend their limited energy on (see chapter 4). Don't sweat the small stuff, as the book says—identify what's really important, and go for it. Help them conserve their energy by reminding them of SOC: select (prioritize) what really matters to them, optimize (plan one's time based on what works for them), and compensate. Do whatever's necessary to make things easier.

Bottom Line

Feeling some decrease in energy or increase in fatigue can be normal with aging. We can't do at 85 all that we could at 20. But at age 85, we usually can do most of what we could do at 84. If there's been a significant change, get checked out by your primary care provider. Meanwhile, don't let yourself get into the cycle of frailty. Make sure you eat well, including enough protein, get physical activity, and do regular exercise to preserve the energy and exercise tolerance that you do have.

RESOURCES

Guidelines

Centers for Disease Control and Prevention. *Physical Activity Guidelines for Americans*, 2nd ed. Washington, DC: Department of Health and Human Services, 2018. https://health.gov/PAGuidelines/.

National Academies of Sciences, Engineering and Medicine. "DRI [Dietary Reference intakes] Calculator for Healthcare Professionals." https://www.nal.usda.gov/human-nutrition-and-food-safety/dri-calculator.

For additional nutritional guidelines, see the Resources section in chapter 15.

Fitness Programs for Older Adults

National Association of Area Agencies on Aging
(www.N4a.org)
Website with information on local resources for seniors, including senior centers and fitness programs.

National Institute of Aging
(https://www.nia.nih.gov/health/exercise-physical-activity)
This program for exercise and physical activity is designed to help you fit exercise and physical activity into daily life. The website provides free exercise materials and videos to help you get ready, start moving, and keep going.

Physical Therapists or Personal Trainers
Discuss with your medical provider whether you meet requirements for physical therapy. Always ask therapists and trainers about their previous experience working with older adults who have your functional abilities and medical conditions.

Tai Chi and QiGong Instructors and Classes
Tai Chi for Consumer Health Information Center (www.americantaichi.net)
Tai Chi for Health Institute (www.taichifor healthinstitute.org)

Silver Sneakers
(silversneakers.com)
Offers online exercise programs for seniors. Silver Sneakers also offers classes in local venues such as a recreation center or at the YWCA and YMCA. Many Medicare Advantage programs offer Silver Sneakers membership as part of their benefit package.

YMCA and YWCA
(www.ymca.net)
The official website for the YMCA of the United States. Offers information on locating your nearest YMCA or YWCA. Note that most local branches of the YWCA and YMCA offer discounts for seniors.

For information on evidence-based fall reduction programs, see the Resources section in chapter 9.

BIBLIOGRAPHY

Cesari, M., B. Vellas, F. C. Hsu, et al. "A Physical Activity Intervention to Treat the Frailty Syndrome in Older Persons—Results from the LIFE-P Study." *Journals of Gerontology, Series A: Biological Sciences and Medical Sciences* 70, no. 2 (2015): 216–22.

Chodzko-Zajko, W., D. N. Proctor, F. Singh, et al. *Exercise and Physical Activity for Older Adults. Medicine and Science in Sports and Exercise* 41, no. 7 (2019): 1510–30.

CHAPTER 8

Ups and Downs

Our moods and emotions change often. Sometimes life feels like it's smooth sailing, other times it feels like we're on a merry-go-round, or worse, a roller coaster, careening up and plummeting down. Does the cycle of positive and negative emotions change with aging? Is there truth to the negative stereotypes of aging, that older people are more likely to be depressed, cranky, afraid, angry? In fact, no. Depression and many anxiety disorders are actually less common in older adults than in any other age group.

Yet aging undeniably brings significant changes and challenges to one's life. Some of these changes are welcome, others not. How you spend your time, your family and friendship circles, your living arrangements, your health, what you think about, what you really enjoy doing, and what is meaningful to you may change as you age and stop working, become an empty nester, or lose friends to illness or relocation. As discussed in chapter 1, there are ways to manage this "new normal," which include trying to be more flexible and learning to be a better advocate for yourself.

But these efforts don't always work. Sometimes you may find it difficult to cope. Feelings and emotions can become overwhelming and may impact your interest in future events and ability to connect with others or to finish what you started. These feelings can affect your mood, function, health, and well-being. You may never have felt this way before, or these feelings may be reminiscent of prior times in your life.

In this chapter, we discuss what might be contributing to your ups and downs, including your own perceptions of aging, expectations, sense of self, response to loss, feelings of grief and bereavement, worries and concerns, mood disorders like depression and anxiety, and self-medication for these feelings.

For an overview of the biology of emotion, see box 8.1.

BOX 8.1

The Biology of Emotions 101

Emotions, Moods, and Stress

Emotions are intense, short-term feelings that arise in response to a situation or a trigger. Emotions include happiness, fear, sadness, disgust, anger, and surprise. *Moods* are less intense, more sustained, and can occur without a clear precipitant. Unattended emotions can develop into moods, and moods can affect emotions and behaviors.

Stress also contributes to emotions, anxiety disorders, and depression. Your response to stress significantly affects your body as well as your mood. Your brain releases stress hormones, particularly adrenaline, resulting in a racing heart, increased breathing, sweating, tense muscles, and a change in pupil size. Chronic stress can cause or exacerbate chronic diseases, including high blood pressure, asthma, diabetes, and immune system disorders.

Responses to emotions are often instantaneous, and they can be verbal, physical, or a change in facial expression or body language. *Emotional regulation* is the ability to respond in a socially appropriate manner to all types of situations, some of which may require delaying our responses. Without this regulation, we may scream at our spouse, exhibit road rage, be consumed by worry or anxiety, or even become physically violent.

Emotions and the Brain

Many, if not all, of our feelings can be traced to changes in the brain. Everything from good moods to anxiety to feeling down in the dumps stems from activation of specific regions of the brain. These regions and their connections mediate our perceptions of and reactions to emotions and stress. These areas are within the cerebral cortex and below it, within the limbic system. The limbic system is involved in our emotional and behavioral responses, and the cerebral cortex helps control these responses. Several of these areas are depicted in the figure on page 112. Box table 8.1 provides examples of the functions of these areas.

People with mood disorders like depression and/or anxiety have lower activity in certain brain areas and increased activity in others. In major depression, there is altered communication between cortical, limbic, and other subcortical brain regions, elevated markers of inflammation, decreased production of new nerve cells, and overactivity of the axis involved in cortisol release. In people who have had recurrent depressions, the hippocampus is smaller. It's not yet known which comes first, the moods or the brain changes. It may be that the brains of people prone to anxiety or depression differ from others in their response to emotional situations.

(continued)

BOX 8.1 *(continued)*

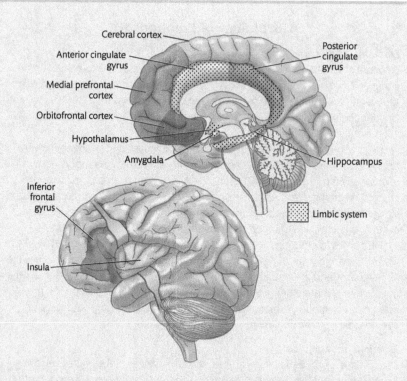

Stress reduction techniques change the brain as well as our responses to stress:

- *Mindfulness-based stress reduction (MBSR).* After eight weeks of training, certain brain areas show greater connection to others and their tissue density increases, suggesting the development and use of a different set of neural pathways. The amygdala becomes more efficient and better able to regulate emotions.

- *Meditation.* Brain changes similar to those discussed above in MBSR are also seen in people who are long-term meditators. Brain waves "calm down," and in mindfulness meditation, the brain areas associated with attention are activated.

Neurotransmitters and Brain Disorders

Neurotransmitters, the chemical messengers that nerve cells release and through which brain cells communicate, play a role in mood disorders and treatment. Changes in levels of neurotransmitters can affect brain functions including memory, sleep, appetite, mood, pain, anxiety, and motivation, as well as body functions like blood pressure and movement. Neurotransmitters attach to specific receptors on cell membranes. Medications developed to treat mental health and neurodegenerative diseases increase the levels of specific neurotransmitters by activating or inhibiting these receptors, thereby influencing which signals get passed along to other neurons and parts of the brain (see box table 8.2).

BOX 8.1 (*continued*)

Depression for many years was considered to be "simply" an imbalance of neurotransmitters in the brain. Antidepressants were thought to act as replacement therapy for the imbalance, much like thyroid medication does for hypothyroidism. There is some truth to this, but it's far from the whole story, as functional magnetic resonance imaging (MRI) and positron emission tomography (PET) scans have shown. It also takes much longer for antidepressants to alleviate depression than it takes for them to improve chemical balance.

BOX TABLE 8.1
Examples of Brain Areas Involved in Emotion and Behavior

	Examples of Functions
Limbic system	
Posterior cingulate gyrus	Recalling autobiographical memories, daydreaming, thinking about the future, involuntary awareness, and arousal.
Anterior cingulate gyrus	Coordinates emotion and thinking.
Amygdala	Central to emotional responses, including feelings like pleasure, fear, anxiety, and anger. Attaches emotional content to memories. Rapidly responds to significant threats (the fight-or-flight response) and activates sympathetic nervous system before you're even consciously aware of the threat.
Insula	Relays messages from the body to the emotional centers and recruits relevant brain regions for the processing of sensory information.
Cerebral cortex	
Medial prefrontal cortex	Involved in planning and anticipation, executive function, and empathic understanding.
Orbitofrontal cortex	Functions not verified; however, appears to modulate bodily changes that are associated with emotion (such as "butterflies" in the stomach and sweating linked to anxiety), and to be important in decision-making and impulse control.
Inferior frontal gyrus	Suppresses emotional reactions to stimuli.

(*continued*)

BOX 8.1 (continued)

BOX TABLE 8.2

Medications Used to Treat Neurodegenerative and Mental Health Disorders by Increasing Neurotransmitter Levels

Examples of Medications	Neurotransmitter(s)	Diseases Treated
Cholinesterase inhibitors: donepezil (Aricept); rivastigmine (Exelon)	Acetylcholine	Alzheimer disease
SSRIs: sertraline (Zoloft); escitalopram (Lexapro)	Serotonin	Depression
SNRIs: duloxetine (Cymbalta); venlafaxine (Effexor)	Norepinephrine and serotonin	Depression Note: may trigger anxiety
Most anti-Parkinsonian medications: levodopa/carbidopa (Sinemet); bromocriptine (Parlodel)	Dopamine	Parkinson's disease Note: may trigger psychosis, hallucinations
Benzodiazepines and benzodiazepine receptor agonists: lorazepam (Ativan); zolpidem (Ambien)	GABA	Anxiety and insomnia

Note: Abbreviations are as follows: GABA, gamma amino butyric acid; SNRI, serotonin-norepinephrine reuptake inhibitor; SSRI, selective serotonin reuptake inhibitor.

What's Normal with Aging?

It seems to me like old people have plenty of reasons to feel down. Their lives are filled with losses, physical illnesses, problems getting around, and memory glitches. I'm only 50, and I'm dreading getting older. How does anyone cope?

Actually, most older people are better adjusted emotionally than younger people. This is called the *paradox of positive aging*. Despite dealing with many significant losses, overall, older adults look at things through a more positive lens, and they're better able to control their emotions. It may be because older people have had lots of practice in developing better ways to handle emotional situations. But it also may be that in recognizing that you don't have all the time in the world left, you concentrate your time and energy on what matters and is important to you. This doesn't mean older people don't get upset, but in general it happens less often, is less intense, and doesn't last as long. For a deeper dive into age-related changes in behavior, personality, and emotions, see box 8.2.

My father died six months ago, and my mother is still overwhelmed with grief. Is this normal?

The deaths of important people in our lives become more common as we age. Grieving differs for each person; there is no set script. About 20 percent of people develop major depression or significant anxiety during the first year after a death, whereas mood improves for about 10 percent, likely those who were overburdened with caregiving or with their interpersonal relationship with the deceased. Most bereaved people experience distress after the death, but after the first year or so, they are able to find ways to reengage with life. For some, however, a condition called *complicated grief* develops, which continues to cause stress and difficulty establishing a new normal for their lives. See the Yellow Alerts section below for more on complicated grief.

My husband's personality has changed. When he was working, he was kind, considerate, and always even-tempered. Now he gets easily irritated and occasionally says inappropriate things in public. Is this his true personality coming through now that he no longer has to please his boss?

Personality refers to individual differences in patterns of thinking, feeling, and behaving that distinguish how people interact with others, deal with stressful situations, and approach daily tasks. In general, it remains stable throughout life. Behavioral changes such as irritation, withdrawal, and a condition called *disinhibition*—being impulsive and saying or doing things that are socially inappropriate—are *not* normal aging. People who start to exhibit these behaviors need an evaluation for medical, psychiatric, and substance use disorders.

What about self-esteem? I'm feeling less confident doing certain things, like public speaking or walking outdoors, than I used to be.

Self-esteem is your overall sense of self-worth or value, whereas *self-efficacy* is your belief that you can succeed in specific situations or in accomplishing a task. Self-esteem tends to be stable with age, although for some people, disabilities, loneliness, or feeling less in control can lead to a decrease in self-esteem. See the next section on what you might do to improve your self-esteem.

Self-efficacy plays a major role in how you approach goals, tasks, and challenges. There is often a physiological basis to a decreased sense of self-efficacy. For example, age-related changes in balance can result in your having a greater fear of falling (see chapter 9). As discussed in chapter 1, however, negative beliefs can contribute to a self-fulfilling prophecy where you perform worse than you could.

Deliberate practice can help improve your ability and confidence in public speaking or even walking. Deliberate practice is getting feedback on something you want to improve and then making efforts to improve it. You could do this yourself (videotape yourself talking to improve public speaking ability, for example). Or you could get input from a friend or professional, such as working with a physical therapist to improve your flexibility. These actions may improve your ability to do things that are important to you.

It seems to me that the older I get, the more people treat me either like I'm not there or like I'm a child, acting amazed that I can do anything at all. Can I do anything to counter this behavior?

What you're describing is called *ageism*, a prejudiced perception that older adults are senile, incompetent, rigid, or old-fashioned. Many older people say that at times they feel invisible, unseen by clerks, doormen, and even their doctors. Or they may feel infantilized, being told "You're so cute!" or called "Dearie" by perfect strangers. One of my friends who is in her seventies says this occurs because some people are shocked to see that you can still walk and talk after they know how old you are. Needless to say, this can be a downer. We see ourselves as we've been our whole lives, while others may be seeing us as stereotypes based on our age or appearance.

Don't let people get away with treating you this way, and work to combat ageism in your everyday life. Your response is most likely to hit home if you make it clear to doctors that they should be addressing their questions to you, not your daughter, and to the store clerk that you were in line before the person they chose to wait on. When told they're cute, some of my patients respond, "Don't call me cute—do I remind you of a baby or a child?" When they're called by their first name, some return the favor with the person with whom they're speaking, whether it's their doctor, a salesperson, or the bank manager. It often makes the other person take a step back and reconsider why they're being so familiar with a complete stranger.

Help other people know you as a full person, the way you see yourself. Should you have to do this? No. But if you do, you'll see a difference in how people treat you. I've found that doctors become more invested in my patients when they have a sense of the whole person and their life, not just their medical conditions.

BOX 8.2

What Happens with Aging: A Deeper Dive

Personality and self-esteem tend to be stable with age.
Although these characteristics are stable for most people as they age, disease and personal circumstances can cause them to change.

Most older people are better adjusted emotionally than younger people.
Studies find that, compared to younger people, older people remember positive images and statements more than negative ones, and what they got right more than what they got wrong. They're less likely to have negative emotions or react strongly to emotional events, and they're better able to control their emotions in general. This is despite the reality that some older adults are dealing with many significant losses. Dr. Laura Carstensen and her colleagues refer to this as the *paradox of positive aging*, which they attribute to the changes in motivations and goals that occur when one realizes that their time on earth is limited rather than limitless. To quote Carstensen, "people tend to take stock of life, live in the present and invest in things that are most important to them. Emotional meaning and satisfaction take precedence over achievement. [People] are less willing to accept negative experiences as a means to a long-term goal."

Some changes in areas of the brain that effect emotion and behavior appear to be part of normal aging.
For example, compared with younger adults, older adults typically show less activity in the amygdala in response to negative stimuli, decreasing the arousal response to those stimuli and reducing the likelihood that they will be remembered. This may be one explanation for the paradox of positive aging.

Many older adults experience "touch hunger."
Older people are often touched less often. In studies, older adults who received 3 minutes of a slow-stroke massage back rub or 5 to 10 minutes of a hand massage were less anxious, agitated, more relaxed, and had lower blood pressure, heart rate, and respiratory rate. Touch precipitates the release of oxytocin, a brain chemical that decreases stress hormone levels, lowering blood pressure, maintaining good moods, and increasing pain tolerance.

Older adults have lower rates of major depressive disorder (MDD) than middle-aged or younger adults.
One to five percent of older adults who live in the community have MDD, but about 10 to 15 percent suffer from *subsyndromal depression*; that is, they have symptoms of depression but not enough to meet the diagnostic criteria for MDD (see box table 8.3).

(continued)

BOX 8.2 (*continued*)

Older adults with MDD often have an anxiety disorder, and vice versa.
About 8 percent of older adults have an anxiety disorder, most often generalized anxiety disorder (GAD). Of older adults with MDD, more than 50 percent also have anxiety symptoms, while about 30 percent of older adults with anxiety symptoms also have MDD.

Many of the changes in behavior and emotional control that occur in older adults are due to disease, not normal aging.
Brain diseases, like strokes, ministrokes, Parkinson's disease, and dementia (including Alzheimer disease) can cause changes in one's behavior and ability to control emotions. Neurodegenerative disorders like Parkinson's disease or different types of dementia affect specific areas of the brain. Mood changes in these disorders appear to be associated with changes in specific brain networks. For example, in those with the apathy of dementia—in which people become uninterested in doing things, lose initiative, and have blunted emotions—studies have found decreased blood flow to the anterior cingulate cortex, inferior frontal gyrus, and orbitofrontal cortex.

BOX TABLE 8.3
Depression: Definitions from the *Diagnostic and Statistical Manual of Mental Disorders*, Fifth Edition *(DSM V)*

Major Depressive Disorder

Either of the following symptoms must be present for the same two-week period:
- Depressed mood
- Decreased interest or loss of pleasure in almost all activities (anhedonia)

Plus two or more of these symptoms:
- Significant weight change or appetite disturbance
- Sleep disturbance (too much or too little)
- Engaging in movements that serve no purpose, like pacing or rapid talking, or a slowing down of movement, thought, or speech
- Fatigue or loss of energy
- Feelings of worthlessness
- Decreased ability to think or concentrate; indecisiveness
- Recurrent thoughts of death or suicide with or without a specific plan for committing suicide

Subsyndromal Depression

Subsyndromal depression occurs when a person has some or many of the symptoms of major depressive disorder, but not enough to meet criteria for a diagnosis.

Adapting to Your New Normal

The brain is a muscle that requires both physical and mental conditioning.
—GARY J. KENNEDY, MD

I was always an active person with lots of friends and things to do. Now, times have changed. I'm retired, living alone, and many of my friends have moved away. I find myself spending my days (and nights) at home alone. I go out when my kids push me, and I have a good time, but I just don't feel like going out on my own.

Behaviors influence feelings. Increasing your engagement in pleasant and stimulating activities can improve your mood. As you say, when you do go out, you feel better. Make plans, identify specific goals—like taking a walk or going to a movie with someone—and notice how you feel while you're doing this compared to how you felt before you left the house. Add outings with friends or family into your regular schedule. Some suggestions? How about joining a book club, going out shopping, meeting friends for tea, or going to the gym? If you really can't get yourself going, discuss ways to get motivated with your health care provider.

You spoke above about things that may help with self-esteem. Are life review or reminiscence therapy ways to improve the way I feel about myself?

Life review is a term coined by my mentor, Dr. Robert Butler, who also coined the term *ageism*. It is a way of putting one's life in perspective, and it is similar to Erik Erickson's 8th stage of life, where we review what we've accomplished during our lives. The terms are sometimes used interchangeably, but some use the term *reminiscence therapy* to describe a memory, and life review to discuss the meaning the memory has for you.

Reviews and reminiscences may be done alone, in groups, or with a therapist or a lay leader. Various objects like photos, diaries, or mementos may be used as prompts. Reviews may be done chronologically or focus on topics that are important to you, such as family, love, achievements, regrets, and adjustments to life's changes. Studies have shown that those who complete a life review have an improvement in their mood, sense of well-being, and self-esteem.

I am feeling more stressed out than ever. It started with the COVID-19 pandemic and seems to be getting worse. I get easily upset and irritable when things don't go the way I want them to. Is this just cranky aging?

Not at all. Stress is inevitable, and we all need ways to cope. The pandemic stressed many of us out because it limited our ability to access some of the strategies we use to relieve stress. What you're experiencing may be the start of a depression, or it could be that your current coping mechanisms aren't working for you.

Coping mechanisms can be *active*, where we try to change the nature of the stressful circumstance or how we react to it, or *avoidant*, where we try to ignore or deny what's going on by distracting ourselves with other things or by increasing our use of alcohol or other mind-altering substances. *Active coping* involves identifying what's happening, acknowledging your feelings about it (anger, sadness, anxiety, and so on), and reappraising the situation, so that you feel less upset or even good about what happened.

I witnessed an example of a poor coping mechanism when I was meditating at a retreat center. Someone came in and took two pictures of the session. After the meditation, the person next to me confronted the leader, livid that the sound of the two camera clicks disrupted his meditation. The leader's response? The clicks had happened 45 minutes ago, but for this person, they were still happening. The lesson learned was that sometimes it's not the action itself that causes stress, it's how we react to it. Understanding what we're feeling and working on our reactions can help decrease our feelings of stress.

I have a friend who swears that exercise is her antidepressant. Could exercise cure my mood problems?

Regular exercise reduces depressive and anxiety symptoms in older adults. At the same time, it improves cardiovascular fitness, strength, and possibly prevents dementia. Even a single exercise session of 10 to 30 minutes can improve mood, although the more sessions over time, the longer the mood improvement lasts. Aerobic, mixed aerobic, and resistance exercise as well as progressive resistance training can

all be effective (see chapter 7). It can be easier to motivate yourself if you schedule a class ahead of time or have a partner to exercise with.

What else helps with stress reduction?

Relaxation techniques, yoga, and meditation can help reduce the psychological and physiological response to stress (see the Resources section at the end of this chapter). These techniques can also help you with the process of developing the active coping strategies discussed above. As with exercise, the more often these techniques are used, the greater the benefit you will achieve. These techniques do not substitute for treatment for anxiety disorders or major depression (see the Yellow Alerts below), but they can decrease day-to-day feelings of anxiety and depression. They can also be helpful in managing chronic insomnia and pain.

Relaxation techniques include progressive relaxation, guided imagery, biofeedback, self-hypnosis, and deep-breathing exercises. The goal is to help you feel calmer, breathe more slowly, lower your blood pressure, and increase your overall feeling of well-being.

Yoga is done in a number of different ways; however, all forms of yoga include controlled breathing, physical postures, and meditative techniques. Studies have shown that yoga can improve mood and decrease anxiety.

Meditation also has many different schools; however, *mindfulness meditation* has been studied most extensively, both for symptom alleviation and as a treatment for depression and anxiety. In mindfulness-based stress reduction, one learns to focus moment-to-moment attention on the experiences, sensations, and feelings one is having while trying to be accepting and non-judgmental about these experiences. In addition to the brain changes discussed in box 8.1, meditation practice decreases the tendency to overreact to certain stimuli and improves insight into behaviors.

I'm not much of a talker when it comes to what's bothering me. I also don't think I should pay someone just to hear me talk. Do you think talk therapy helps?

Talking about your concerns—particularly with those who are skilled at problem-solving and understanding your feelings—can be especially useful. Some find support groups to be helpful. Support groups may include others who are going through similar life situations as you are (such as bereavement, retirement, your own illness or that of a loved one). Group therapy guided by a professional can introduce you to new ways to think about and deal with your concerns, worries, mood, or feelings of stress. Certain individual and group psychotherapies are as effective as medication for many mood disorders. See the Resources section at the end of this chapter for evidence-based psychotherapies that have been shown to help older adults.

What Isn't Normal Aging?

 Red Flags: Symptoms Needing Prompt Medical Attention

Personality changes, including agitation, disinhibition, hallucinations, delusions, or paranoia, can be signs of depression, psychosis, dementia, other brain diseases, or of alcohol or drug abuse. Diseases that directly affect the brain (other than dementia or psychiatric disease), like strokes or brain tumors, can also cause these symptoms. People who exhibit sudden changes in behavior need medical evaluations, including imaging of the brain, usually with a computed tomography (CT) scan or magnetic resonance imaging (MRI).

Visual hallucinations are often a sign of brain disease and require evaluation. The one exception is when they occur in people with significant vision loss who have *Bonnet syndrome.* People who have Bonnet syndrome are aware that the hallucinations are not real and usually are not upset by them.

Manic behaviors in older adults are often manifested by confusion, disorientation, distractibility, and irritability more than a "high" mood. Those suffering from mania may be argumentative, certain that they are right, despite evidence to the contrary. They may be grandiose, have inflated self-esteem, not sleep much, be more talkative (often with pressured speech), over-engaged in work and other projects, or participate in pleasurable activities with high potential for painful consequences, like shopping sprees, sexual indiscretions, or foolish business investments. Mania that develops in later life is relatively uncommon and is often due to other medical disorders, most commonly stroke, dementia, hyperthyroidism, vitamin B_{12} deficiency, or medications, including antidepressants, steroids, or stimulants. Anyone displaying symptoms of mania needs a medical evaluation.

Suicidal thoughts or self-harm are never normal, and even less so in the mature adult. These behaviors need to be taken seriously and evaluated by a behavioral health professional. Of all Americans, older white men who attempt suicide are the most likely to die by their own hand. Persons 85 and older have a suicide rate three times that of the overall population. This is probably because they have a greater intention of dying and less physical resilience to survive an attempt. Firearms are the most common method of suicide for older adults. If guns are present in the home, they must be removed, or at the least unloaded and the ammunition hidden.

⚠️ **Yellow Alerts: Common Conditions That Can Mimic or Worsen Ups and Downs**

Medications

Feeling depressed or anxious—or experiencing any major change of mood—can sometimes be more than just the normal ups and downs that are part of aging. If you are taking medications, they could be causing your mood changes. See table 8.1 for a list of drugs and their possible side effects, including depression and anxiety. Abrupt withdrawal of some drugs can also precipitate depression or anxiety.

Complicated Grief

About 10 percent of people who have suffered the death of an important person in their lives develop *complicated grief*, where they experience intense feelings of loneliness and yearning, preoccupation with the person who died and the circumstances of their death, avoidance of reminders of the departed, a sense that their own life is meaningless, and difficulty with daily functioning that lasts more than a year (and often lasts for years) after the death. As one of my patients told me, "it is as if the loss happened just yesterday because the grief still feels so intense even a year later."

People who experience complicated grief oftentimes had a particularly close relationship to the deceased, such as being a hands-on caregiver, or live away from family members and their support. Several interventions can help, including medication and psychotherapy.

Depression

Both *major depressive disorder* (MDD) and *subsyndromal depression* can cause significant functional, cognitive, social, and health consequences for older adults (see box 8.2 for definitions). Those with subsyndromal depression are at a much greater risk of a future episode of MDD.

Depression can look different in older adults compared with younger people. There may be less sadness, tearfulness, and guilt, and more loss of interest and pleasure in activities (this is called *anhedonia*). Fatigue, poor appetite, difficulty sleeping, loss of interest in sex, and feelings of hopelessness are also common, resulting in difficulty with concentration, functional deficits, lack of motivation, and potentially accelerating the frailty cycle (see box 7.3). Other people may eat more and sleep more. Older adults with MDD often have coexisting anxiety. They are also more likely to have certain medical illnesses, such as stroke, cardiac disease, diabetes, Parkinson's, hypothyroidism, hearing loss, and dementia, and to be taking certain medications (see table 8.1). When depression is present, it may impede a person's recovery from medical illness. For example, heart attack survivors often develop MDD and, compared with their nondepressed peers, have slower recovery, more cardiovascular events, and an increased risk of death within six months.

In the past, depression was considered either "intrinsic"—that is, biological, or "extrinsic"—or situational. It's now recognized that most depressions have both biological (genetic and medical factors) and situational components. Certain situations can precipitate or worsen a depression. These include feeling a loss of control (when, for example, others are making decisions for you), disagreements with loved ones, grief or bereavement, and social isolation or loneliness.

Antidepressant medications can be used to treat all types of major depression. It is the severity of the depression that determines whether someone should be treated with antidepressant medications, not whether the depression is primarily intrinsic or extrinsic. In addition, short-term psychotherapy and physical exercise can improve mood and one's ability to cope with new or upsetting situations (see the Resources section at the end of this chapter). Some older adults with major depression may benefit more when treated with both medications and psychotherapy than from either alone. Subsyndromal depression may improve on its own or need treatment to avoid progression to major depression.

The cognitive impairment of depression, discussed in chapter 6, may be confused with dementia. The good news is that cognitive decline caused by depression often improves with treatment, and the improvement may persist for some time. For some people, however, late-onset depression, even if treatable, may be the first sign of a developing dementia.

Anxiety Disorders

About 8 percent of older adults have an anxiety disorder, most often generalized anxiety disorder (GAD). Almost half experience their first episode after age 50. People with GAD have excessive and uncontrollable anxiety and worry about everyday events or activities, causing them distress and functional impairment. They may also feel restless, on edge, irritable, tense, fatigued, or have sleep disturbances.

More than one-third of older adults with an anxiety disorder also have MDD. People with physical ailments are more likely to have an anxiety disorder, particularly those with cardiovascular disease, chronically painful conditions, lung disease, and gastrointestinal problems. Medications and medication withdrawal can also mimic these symptoms (see table 8.1).

Antidepressants help, as does physical activity. Benzodiazepines (like diazepam or lorazepam) should only be used in the short term, during crises, since they increase the incidence of falls, car accidents, and cognitive impairment in older adults. Cognitive behavioral therapy (see the Resources section at the end of this chapter) can be as effective as medication for GAD.

Alcohol Overuse and Abuse

Alcohol is often used for "self-medication" of a mood disorder, yet it increases the risk for depression, suicide, cognitive impairment, and social isolation. Warning signs of abuse include personality changes, mood swings, falls or bruises, headaches, sleep problems, memory difficulties, poor hygiene, poor nutrition, and social isolation. Remember, older adults become more sensitive to the effects of alcohol as they age (see chapter 3), so even if they just continue to drink as

they used to, they may begin to show signs of alcohol abuse. The National Institute on Alcohol Abuse and Alcoholism recommends no more than seven drinks a week and no more than three drinks at a time for older adults.

Substance Abuse

Some baby boomers continue to use recreational drugs into old age. Signs of misuse include personality changes, poor hygiene or grooming, withdrawal from others, taking medications at higher doses and for longer periods than prescribed, and using prescription medications for recreational or non-medical purposes. The opioid epidemic in our country does not spare the older adult population, particularly in rural areas. Older adults are prescribed more medications than younger people, and many of these are medications that can be abused, such as pain relievers (opioids) and benzodiazepines for sleep or anxiety.

TABLE 8.1

Medications That Can Cause Depression, Anxiety, and Mania

Drugs and Examples	Depression	Mania	Anxiety
Blood pressure, cardiac, and diuretic medications			
Beta-blockers, ACE inhibitors, central adrenergic agonists: metoprolol (Toprol); propranolol (Inderal); carvedilol (Coreg); enalapril (Vasotec); quinapril (Accupril); methyldopa; clonidine (Catapres)	X		
Pain relief			
GABA-ergic neurogenic pain medications: gabapentin (Neurontin); pregabalin (Lyrica)	?		

TABLE 8.1 *(continued)*

Drugs and Examples	Depression	Mania	Anxiety
Opioid analgesics: morphine, hydro-morphone (Dilaudid); hydrocodone (in Vicodin); tramadol (Ultram)	X		W
Muscle relaxants: carisoprodol (Soma); metaxalone (Skelaxin)	?		
Neurological, psychological, and sleep medications			
Sleep and antianxiety: diazepam (Valium); alprazolam (Xanax); lorazepam (Ativan); zaleplon (Sonata); eszopiclone (Lunesta); triazolam (Halcion)	X		W
Phenothiazine antipsychotics: thioridazine (Mellaril); perphenazine (Trilafon)	X		W
CNS stimulants: dexamphetamine (Dexedrine, Zenzedi); methylphenidate (Ritalin, Concerta); modafinil (Provigil); lisdexamfetamine (Vyvanse)	W		X
Anticonvulsant medications: topiramate (Topamax); lamotrigine (Lamictal); levetiracetam (Keppra)	?		
Antidepressants			
Tricyclic antidepressants: amitriptyline (Elavil); imipramine (Tofranil); nortripty-line (Pamelor); desipramine (Norpramin)		In people with bipolar disorder	W
Anti-Parkinsonian medications			
Decarboxylase inhibitor, dopamine agonists, anticholinergics: carbidopa/levodopa (Sinemet); pramipexole (Mirapex); amantadine (Symmetrel); bromocriptine (Parlodel); benztropine (Cogentin); trihexyphenidyl (Artane)			W
Diabetes medications			
Insulin and sulfonylureas: glimepiride (Amaryl); tolazamide; glyburide (Glynase); glipizide (Glucotrol); tolbutamide			Hypo-glycemia

(continued)

TABLE 8.1 (*continued*)

Drugs and Examples	Depression	Mania	Anxiety
Gastrointestinal medications			
Antispasmodics: dicyclomine (Bentyl); propantheline			W
H₂ blockers: cimetidine (Tagamet); famotidine (Pepcid); nizatidine (Axid)	?		
Proton pump inhibitors: pantoprazole (Protonix); lansoprazole (Prevacid); esomeprazole (Nexium)	?		
Prokinetic: metoclopramide (Reglan)			W
Cold, allergy, and itching medications			
First-generation antihistamines: diphen-hydramine (Benadryl); chlorpheniramine (Aller-Chlor, Chlor-Trimeton); hydroxyzine (Atarax); meclizine (Antivert, Bonine)			W
Decongestants: phenylephrine (SudafedPE); pseudoephedrine (Sudafed Sinus) (Sudafed); oxymetazoline (Afrin, Dristan)			X
Pulmonary medications			
Xanthine bronchodilator pills: aminophylline, theophylline			X
Inhaled beta agonists: albuterol (Proventil, Ventolin)			X
Leukotriene receptor antagonist: Montelukast (Singulair)	X		
Others			
Bladder relaxants: tolteradine (Detrol); oxybutynin (Ditropan); solifenacin (Vesicare)			W
Fluoroquinolone antibiotics: ciprofloxacin (Cipro); levofloxacin (Levaquin)	?		
Corticosteroids: prednisone, dexamethasone (Decadron); methylprednisolone (Solu-Medrol)	X	X	
Gonadotropin-releasing hormone agonists: leuprolide (Lupron); goserelin (Zoladex)	X		

TABLE 8.1 *(continued)*

Drugs and Examples	Depression	Mania	Anxiety
Vinca alkaloid chemotherapy: vincristine (Vincasar PFS); vinblastine; vinorelbine (Navelbine)	X		
Alcohol	X		W
Cocaine	W		X
Caffeine			X
Interferon	X		

Note: If you're not sure whether a drug you're taking is in one of the drug classes listed, ask your pharmacist or health care provider. X, may cause this condition; W, withdrawal symptoms occur when drug is abruptly stopped; ?, studies conflict as to whether these drugs cause this symptom. Abbreviations are as follows: ACE, angiotensin-converting enzyme; CNS, central nervous system; GABA, gamma amino butyric acid.

Getting Evaluated for Ups and Downs

Depression, anxiety, and other reasons for behavioral change are all underdiagnosed in older adults, even though there are often treatments that will alleviate the suffering of both those with these symptoms and those who care for them. This is partly because these disorders may present differently in older than in younger people, as discussed on page 122, and partly due to a fear or stigma that patients and families may have about mental health or neurodegenerative disorders like dementia. Yet most people with these behaviors and feelings would rather not have them; they'd rather feel better and be more active and engaged in life. This is a goal that might be achieved with treatment.

As discussed, feelings and emotions are often multifactorial and due to one's genetic makeup, brain connections and chemistry, life experiences, and reactions to the various stressors that accompany aging. I consider managing these disorders to be as important in my patients as managing their high blood pressure, diabetes, or asthma. If not attended to, they create suffering and can negatively affect well-being, health, and quality of life.

When your providers ask, "How are you feeling?" it's not just a question about your body but also your mind. If you are feeling "off" or not right in any way, tell them. Most primary care practitioners with an interest in mental health can provide an evaluation to determine whether an underlying medical condition is contributing to your feelings, and either provide initial treatment or refer you to a specialist.

Should I See a Specialist?

One should see a specialist—either a geriatrician, neurologist, or a psychiatrist—if there is a question about the diagnosis, whether the symptoms may be due to a neuropsychiatric disorder like Parkinson's or dementia, if the initial treatment doesn't work, or if the person has any of the following symptoms:

- suicidal thoughts
- mania
- personality changes, including agitation and disinhibition
- hallucinations or delusions
- paranoia

Let the specialist know if you are concerned that you or your loved one might harm themselves or others before the appointment. If so, the provider should be able to tell you how to access emergency psychiatric services.

Try to find a treatment provider with an interest or specialization in older adults, since the symptoms and treatments (especially medication dosages) are often different in older people than younger individuals. Each field has specialists with additional training in geriatrics, including psychiatry, social work, and clinical psychology.

Preparing for Your Visit

Complete this chapter's pre-visit checklist on page 374 in Appendix 3, bring it to your appointment, and review it with your provider. Someone familiar with your day-to-day moods and how you spend your time should come with you to the visit, if possible. It can be difficult to fully explain your feelings and the situations in which you find yourself. It's also possible that you and your loved one see things differently. It's important that the provider be aware of all points of view to be able to provide you with the best options. She will talk with you, ask many questions, and probably have you complete some questionnaires to get a sense of your mood, memory, and level of stress. She will also do a physical examination and order some blood tests to determine whether there is a disease or a medication contributing to the way you're feeling and behaving, and what medication, if any, would be best for treating you. The physical exam is a good time to make sure you have time alone with the provider to say things you may not be comfortable saying in front of those who came with you to the visit.

Advice for Loved Ones

It's tough to be with someone who seems to be constantly worrying, depressed, refusing suggestions that might improve things, behaving inappropriately, or who always sees the glass as half empty. Moods and behaviors like these can be contagious. Years ago, I realized that the anxiety and irritability I felt with certain patients came from my response to *their* anxiety or irritability. Just realizing that and grounding myself before I began the visit made it much easier for me not to succumb to the mood in the room. It also made me realize how painful it was to be that person.

Older people are often touched less often, a condition some call *touch hunger*. As described in box 8.2, back rubs or hand massages decrease anxiety, agitation, blood pressure, and respiratory rate. Think about this when you're with your loved one, and provide hugs, hold hands, or even give a massage.

When you're trying to convince an older adult to do something that will benefit them, remember that they will be more likely to respond if they're told the benefits than if they feel threatened with the negative consequences. To encourage walking, for example, tell them that walking will improve their mood and memory, and make it less likely that they'll have a heart attack or a stroke. Don't lead with how fat, weak, or frail they'll become if they continue being a couch potato.

For loved ones, spending time trying to get someone who feels down or anxious to accept that this isn't normal aging and that there are treatments that can help can be a struggle that you're unlikely to win alone. People with severe anxiety and depression may simply be unable to accept that anything might be able to help them, and this hopelessness is actually part of the disease process. Enlist help from others who care about the older adult—friends, family members, and their doctors—and from community resources like your state's Department of Aging.

And what about you? You need to take care of yourself during all of this, whether it's getting help dealing with difficult or potentially harmful situations, conflicts with the older adult or your other important relationships, or attending to the rest of your life, including your job. Being a caregiver for someone you love who has significant illness is a risk factor by itself for depression. Estimates put the chance of developing depressive symptoms at anywhere from 40 to 70 percent for primary caregivers, many of whom will neglect their own health and needs while caring for someone else's. Take advantage of support groups, therapy, and Internet-based interventions to reduce caregiver burden and depression while at the same time improving your caregiving skills and coping strategies (see the Resources section at the end of this chapter).

Bottom Line

Lots of things change as we age, and adapting to these changes can require conscious effort. In general, older people are emotionally well balanced, but at times depression, anxiety, and behavioral changes occur and greatly diminish the quality of life of both the older person and their loved ones. Both can benefit from evaluations and treatments, including support groups, psychotherapy, and medications. The most successful approaches combine keeping physically active, spending more time doing what you enjoy and less time in situations that bring you down, and teaching you to reappraise your emotional responses to decrease your reactivity or to create plans that may improve the situations you find yourself in. Medications can also be effective and give you the motivation to work on these behavioral and psychological skills. Remember—many ups and downs are part of life, but sometimes they aren't *normal* aging.

RESOURCES

Finding a Behavioral Health Professional Who Specializes in Older Adults

American Association for Geriatric Psychiatry
(www.aagponline.org)
National organization representing and serving members in the field of geriatric psychiatry.

Their website has portal that you can use to locate a geriatric psychiatrist in your area.

American Psychological Association (APA) Psychologist Locator
(https://locator.apa.org)
The APA is the main organization of psychologists in the United States. Its Psychologist Locator can help you find someone in your area with self-identified knowledge or interest in aging. Enter "senior" in the category of "age group specialization."

Area Agency on Aging (AAA)
Each part of the country has a local or state AAA that provides service information and referral to services for older adults, which may include mental health services.

National Register of Health Service Psychologists
(https://www.nationalregister.org)
The National Register of Health Service Psychologists is an organization of practicing and licensed psychologists. Click on the Find a Psychologist tab, then enter your zip code, and use the keyword "aging" to find a self-identified aging-knowledgeable psychologist near you.

Psychology Today's Find a Therapist Tool
(https://www.psychologytoday.com/us/therapists)
This search tool will help you locate clinical professionals, psychiatrists, treatment centers, and support groups that provide mental health services in the United States and internationally. Enter your address or zip code, and click on the age tab, 65+. These professionals provide therapy in your area, but they don't necessarily specialize in older adults.

Psychotherapies for Older Adults

The following therapies have been found to be effective in well-designed studies of older people. *Key:* **M**, effective in treating major depression; **S**, effective in treating subsyndromal depression; **A**, effective in treating anxiety; and **C**, effective in treating caregiver distress.

Problem-Solving Therapy (M, S)
Working with a therapist, the older person identifies the life problems that may be contributing to their depression and then develops and implements solutions to decrease their depression. A course of therapy usually involves six to eight meetings spaced one to two weeks apart. A virtual adaptation using Skype has also been shown to be effective.

Behavioral Therapy (M, S, C)
Behavioral therapy helps the older adult identify which life events are tied to depression. The therapist then helps the older person increase engagement in pleasant and stimulating events and decrease engagement in negative events to reduce depression. Participants may also learn relaxation techniques such as progressive muscle relaxation. Treatment is usually time limited, occurring over 12–16 weeks.

A self-directed workbook from the University of Michigan, titled *Behavioral Activation for Depression*, can be found at https://tinyurl.com/f58jrncj. This course helps you identify how your behavior can directly affect your mood, for better or worse, and teaches you skills to motivate you to put yourself into situations that are likely to improve your mood.

Cognitive Behavioral Therapy (M, S, A)
Cognitive behavioral therapy, or CBT, is based on the idea that certain thoughts and behaviors trigger depression and anxiety. The older person is then encouraged to change them. The cognitive part of CBT may involve reducing the frequency and intensity of maladaptive negative thoughts (such as taking things personally that may not be personal, guessing what someone else may be thinking when you don't really know, assuming that something will have a negative outcome). Treatment duration and length of sessions are similar to that of behavioral therapy. CBT can be done in individual and group formats. Internet-delivered CBT has been found to be effective in reducing anxiety and depression in older adults. Programs that provide some form of guidance (emails, phone calls, text communication) are much more effective than standalone, unguided ones.

Interpersonal Psychotherapy (S)
The focus of interpersonal psychotherapy is on interpersonally relevant life problems that appear to have triggered or maintained depression. The therapist works with the older adult to work on one or two life problems, with the goal of improving the person's ability to deal with that problem and reduce depression. The duration of treatment is 12 to 16 weeks.

Mindfulness-Based Stress Reduction (M, S, A, C)
This is an eight-week program aimed at reducing stress by learning mindfulness skills through regular meditation practices. The full program consists of weekly group-based meditation classes with a trained teacher, daily audio-guided home practice (approximately 45 minutes per day), and a daylong mindfulness retreat that takes place during the sixth week. One learns to mindfully attend to body sensations using various meditative practices. The group classes discuss how to apply this in daily life to help with stressors. Studies have found significant improvement in the emotional well-being of older adults, with large effects on anxiety, depression, stress, and pain acceptance. A free Internet-based class is available at: https://palousemindfulness.com/index.html.

Reminiscence Therapy (M, S)
Reminiscence therapy was developed specifically for older adults. This therapy can be provided individually or in groups, and there are several different versions. The therapist engages the older adult in discussion of both positive and negative life experiences in order to make better sense of them. The process may help to resolve long-standing internal conflicts about those experiences and help you develop a better sense of self and a deeper life meaning.

Therapy for Family Caregivers of Older Adults

Three additional approaches have been found effective in reducing distress in family caregivers of older adults with health or cognitive problems. Both support group and short-term programs can provide these therapies.

- *Psychoeducational skills-building* increases caregivers' knowledge of their relatives' health or cognitive problem; teaches behavioral, mood management, and problem-solving skills; and identifies ways to modify the home environment.
- *Psychotherapy counseling* tailored to caregivers is a primarily cognitive behavioral therapy delivered individually or in group.
- *Multicomponent approaches* involve combining two or more approaches. For example, a combination of support group, family counseling, and skills-building therapy.

Community Resources

Alcoholics Anonymous
(www.alcoholicsanonymous.com; 800-839-1686)
Provides information on AA meetings and educational sessions.

Alzheimer's Association
(www.alz.org; 800-272-3900)
Provides information about resources, support groups, and educational seminars for those with memory loss and their families.

Alzheimer's Foundation of American
(https://alzfdn.org/)
The AFA offers support, services, and education to individuals, families, and caregivers affected by Alzheimer disease and related dementias nationwide.

Substance Abuse and Mental Health National Helpline
(800-662-HELP [4357])
Referral and information service in English and Spanish for individuals and families facing mental health problems or substance abuse disorders.

Meditation Resources

Clark, G. Ross. "MBSR Formal Breathing Meditation 15 Min." YouTube video, 15:39. https://www.youtube.com/watch?v=Q7vn JEFOf7Y.

"Guided Meditation-Spanish." Dropbox audio, 14:28. https://www.dropbox.com/s /ggtgs8jbg9kv9tn/Guided%20Relaxation %20-%20Spanish.mp3?dl=0.

Kabat-Zinn, Jon. "Guided Mindfulness Meditation, Series 3, Breathscape Meditation." YouTube video, 20:21. https://youtu .be/524RMtfHKz8.

Matza, Deborah. "Breath Meditation." Dropbox audio, 10:13. https://www .dropbox.com/s/ozkopxsw8lg1fl8/01%20 MATZA%20Track%201_1.mp3?dl=0.

"Meditation on Compassion Guided Meditations for Love and Wisdom by Sharon Salzberg." YouTube video, 10:58. https:// www.youtube.com/watch?v=UZrVB943N2 Y&ab_channel=HighDesertHealingLLC .MindandBodyTherapy.

"Mindful Breathing Meditation (5 Minutes)." YouTube video, 5:22. https://youtu.be/nm FUDkj1Aq0.

"Mindful Breathing with Dr. Daniel J. Siegel." YouTube video, 45:53. https:// youtu.be/DEd1YP-TQt0.

UCLA Mindful Awareness Research Center. "Guided Meditations." Accessed December 3, 2021.http://marc.ucla.edu /mindful-meditations.

Meditation Apps

Breath Ball (Breathing practices)
Breathe2Relax
Calm
Headspace
Insight Timer
Meditation Time
Oak (meditation and breathing practices)
Simple Habit
10% Happier
UCLA Mindful (English and Spanish)
Wise at Work

Baumgart, P., and T. Garrick. "Assessment of Depressive Symptoms in Medically Ill Patients." *JAMA* 325, no. 24 (2021): 2497–98.

Bonanno, G. A. *The Other Side of Sadness: What the New Science of Bereavement Tells Us about Life after Loss.* New York: Basic Books, 2009.

Carstensen, L. L. "Integrating Cognitive and Emotion Paradigms to Address the Paradox of Aging." *Cognition and Emotion* 33, no. 1 (2019): 119–25.

Cole, P. M., M. K. Michel, and L. O. Teti. "The Development of Emotion Regulation and Dysregulation: A Clinical Perspective." *Monographs of the Society for Research in Child Development* 59, no. 2–3 (1994): 73–100.

Kroenke, K., R. L. Spitzer, and J. B. Williams. "The Patient Health Questionnaire, 2. Validity of a Two-Item Depression Screener." *Medical Care* 41, no. 11 (2003): 1284-92.

Spitzer, R. L., K. Kroenke, J. B. Williams, and B. Lowe. "A Brief Measure for Assessing Generalized Anxiety Disorder." *Archives of General Medicine* 166 (2006): 1092–97.

CHAPTER 9

Balancing Acts

Mobility, independence, and safety are important goals for most older adults and their loved ones, but these goals can be in conflict when walking is unsteady and falls result. Some falls are caused by acute medical conditions, such as when a person is seriously ill, loses consciousness, or has a seizure. These falls are not what we're discussing in this chapter. Here we're considering falls as a geriatric syndrome (see chapter 2). Syndromes are usually due to multiple, not single, causes. The more possible causes that you address, the less likely it is that you will fall and hurt yourself.

In the movie Swing Time, Fred Astaire and Ginger Rogers show us how to respond when we fall by dancing and singing "Pick Yourself Up" (lyrics by Jerome Kern and Dorothy Fields).

Nothing's impossible I have found,

For when my chin is on the ground,

I pick myself up,

Dust myself off,

Start all over again.

Wouldn't it be great if we could do this whenever we fell, either physically or emotionally? And most of the time we can—the majority of falls don't cause serious injuries, although they may cause pain, bruises, and lacerations. Only 10 percent of falls result in fractures or head trauma. Although infrequent, falls are the major cause of accidental death in older adults. One of my colleagues keeps a file of obituaries of celebrities who died from falls. It's an impressive list and includes the comedian George Burns, Dr. Robert Atkins of Atkins Diet fame, and Katharine Graham, the editor of the *Washington Post* who decided to publish the Pentagon Papers. This is not a list you want to join.

In this chapter, we'll discuss age-related changes in walking, balance, and bone structure. We will also cover common conditions that affect gait and balance as we get older, what increases the risk of falling or breaking a bone, and who to see and what you can do to improve your mobility, balance, and safety. A deep dive into assistive devices and how to use them can be found in Appendix 2.

For an overview of mobility, walking, and balance control, see box 9.1. A description of the anatomy and regulation of balance is provided in box 9.2.

BOX 9.1

Mobility 101

Mobility
Mobility is the ability to move purposefully in one's environment. Most adults are independently mobile, getting around without the need for help from another person or a device. Walking is our primary method of mobility, but when you were a baby, you didn't start with walking. You learned how to walk by first turning over in bed, moving from lying to sitting, to sitting up unassisted, standing, and finally, once able to stand, taking a few steps. The ability to walk is key to remaining independently mobile, but we also need to be able to stand up, maintain our balance, and have enough energy to move and propel ourselves where we want to go.

Walking
When we walk, we alternate the movement of each leg to provide support and momentum. One foot is on the ground at all times. Normal walking starts with both feet on the ground, then lifting one foot and swinging it forward until its heel touches the ground, at which point the other foot lifts up and swings forward. A normal gait has a regular pattern, with each foot on the ground about 60 percent of the time. *Gait speed* is a measure of how quickly you walk and is tied to success and survival in aging, including better health and functional status.

Balance Control
Maintaining balance is complex, whether you're walking, changing position, or turning. We're most steady when our bodies and heads are perpendicular to our feet, and when we have a solid base of support. We call our first steps "baby steps" because babies initially walk with their feet far apart, providing a more solid base of support for their bodies. Balance is harder when our base of support is narrower, that is, when our feet are closer together, or when we perform tasks that require us to move our bodies away from our feet. This is one of the reasons it can be harder for some older people to get up from a chair, climb stairs, or run.

Balance
Balance is controlled by the brain, which gets information on where you are in space at a given time from your eyes, inner ears, muscles, joints, and feet, and uses this input to adjust your posture, eye movements, and muscle activity to keep you upright. See box 9.2 for more on balance.

Energy
Discussed in detail in chapter 7, your heart, lungs, muscles, and nutrition are key to providing the energy that fuels your movement, increasing your ability and endurance.

Musculoskeletal System
Muscles, bones, and joints provide you with the strength and flexibility to move independently. Chapter 14 discusses these in detail.

BOX 9.2

Balance: More Than You May Want to Know

As illustrated in the figure below, *visual information from the eyes and sensors in the muscles, joints, and skin* (particularly pressure on the soles of the feet) supply data on where parts of the body are in relation to each other and the environment, including the direction and how fast they are moving. *Proprioception* is the term for the awareness these sensors provide us of the movement and position of our body without our needing to directly look at our body.

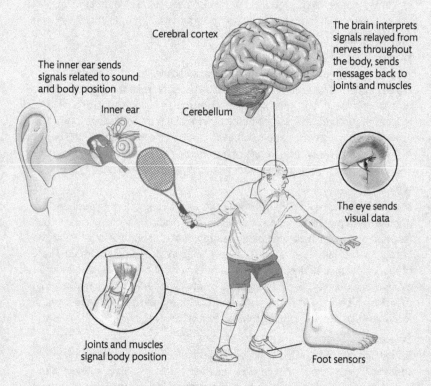

The inner ear sends signals related to sound and body position

Cerebral cortex

The brain interprets signals relayed from nerves throughout the body, sends messages back to joints and muscles

Inner ear

Cerebellum

The eye sends visual data

Joints and muscles signal body position

Foot sensors

Basics of balance. Adapted from American Institute of Balance

The *inner ear* transmits sound waves, which, like sonar, allow the brain to locate the origin of sounds. Sounds themselves and the relative distance of your body from these sounds are important pieces of information that help your brain adjust your body's position in space.

The *vestibular system* within the inner ear, as shown in the figure on page 137, relays information on head and body movements to the brain through detectors in its *semicircular canals* and the *saccule and utricle*, two organs contained within it.

BOX 9.2 (*continued*)

Each of the three semicircular canals is positioned to detect a different head movement: right to left, up and down, or side to side. Moving your head causes fluid to flow into the appropriate canal, stimulating hairlike cells that send messages to the brain through the vestibular nerve. The utricle detects when your body moves forward or backward, and the saccule when you get up or lie down. Small crystals are attached to the walls of these organs and stimulate their hairlike cells when you move in these directions.

The *cerebellum* is the part of the brain that controls balance. Information on movement collected by the eyes, inner ear, muscles, joints, and skin is sent to the cerebellum by way of the brain stem. The cerebellum works with the cerebral cortex, the "higher" brain where thinking and memory reside, to act on this information and instruct our eyes and muscles to adjust our body's position to maintain balance and coordination.

Your *center of gravity* is a hypothetical spot where your body would remain in balance if it were supported at just this point (think of balancing a ruler on the tip of your finger). Our center of gravity changes whenever we change position, at times resulting in loss of balance. The lower your center of gravity, the easier it is to keep your balance. Our center of gravity is slightly above our waists because the top of our body weighs more than the bottom.

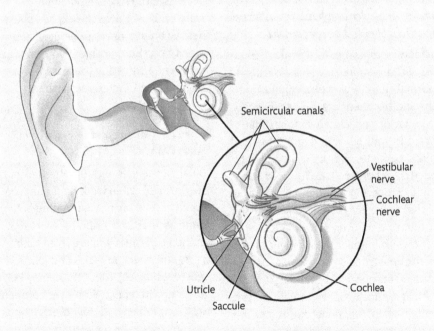

The vestibular system. Adapted from Thomas J. Balkany, MD, FACS, FAAP, and Kevin D. Brown, MD, PhD, *The Ear Book* (Baltimore: Johns Hopkins University Press, 2017)

What's Normal with Aging?

I looked in the mirror recently and noticed how much my posture has changed. Is this part of normal aging?

There are several changes in posture that occur with aging (see box 9.3). In general, much of your body moves forward. This includes your head and neck, thoracic spine, and your center of gravity. Over time, the muscles responsible for keeping the spine straight weaken. These biomechanical changes can increase your risk of falling, yet as discussed in the next section, there are things you can do to make that less likely and that will improve your posture.

For years, I've been walking daily with a younger neighbor. Lately, though, I'm finding it harder and harder to keep up with her. Should I be concerned?

To some extent, no. As discussed in box 9.3, walking more slowly is a part of normal aging, a way to compensate for the additional energy it takes to walk because of age-related changes that occur in your heart and lungs, muscle mass, strength, coordination and balance (see chapter 7). Arthritis or other joint or muscular conditions further increase the energy required for walking, resulting in an even slower gait.

Yet even though a slower *gait speed*, or the time it takes you to walk 10 meters (33 feet) at your usual pace, is "normal" with aging, faster speeds are linked to better health, functional status, and survival in aging. Slower walking speeds also can put you at risk for balance problems, falls, and an inability to get across the street before the light turns red.

So, what gait speed should you aim for? There are many factors that need to be considered, but in general, healthy older adults can usually safely walk around outside if their speed is 0.8 to 1.2 meters per second (m/s). The oldest among us and those using assistive devices walk at the lower end of this range. Most people can increase their speed if needed. For example, to safely cross most streets, you need a gait speed greater than 1.2 m/s. If your gait speed is low, you should try to increase it either on your own or with the help of a physical therapist. Increasing gait speed by 0.1 m/s has been shown to increase well-being; increasing to 1.0 m/s decreases the risk of a fall. If you're walking slower because of pain, shortness of breath, or other medical concerns, you should consult your medical provider. Addressing these issues may help you walk faster and farther.

I am finding it harder to keep my balance when I'm walking on the street or in the park. What's causing this?

Balance changes with age. It's harder to stay upright when walking on uneven paths or if you trip. Maintaining balance requires that your brain receive information on where you are from your eyes, inner ears, muscles and joints, and feet (see box 9.2). All of these may be affected with aging. Your eyes compensate for problems in the other systems, so your balance may be worse if your eyes are closed or your vision impaired (see chapter 12).

BOX 9.3

What Happens with Aging: A Deeper Dive

You walk more slowly.
With aging, it takes more energy to walk the same distance at the same pace than it did when you were younger. As discussed in chapter 7, this happens because of age-related changes in your heart and lungs, muscle mass, strength, coordination, and balance. Walking more slowly compensates for these changes. Each stride covers less distance, and your feet stay together on the ground for a longer time before you take your next step. Arthritis or other joint or muscular conditions further increase energy requirements for walking, resulting in an even slower gait.

Everyone shrinks.
Both men and women lose an average of one to three inches of height with aging. The spine shortens because, as we age, the discs that separate the vertebrae dry up and compress. The loss in height becomes more pronounced after age 70.

Your posture changes.
Your head and body start to lean forward and down. When your vertebral discs dry up, they also become less flexible, and the back curves forward. This is called *kyphosis*. The loss of muscle strength with age contributes by affecting the spinal erector muscles, whose job is to keep the spine straight. *Hyperkyphosis*, some-times called a *dowager's hump*, is an excessive curving of the upper back that can resemble a hunchback and affects 20 to 40 percent of older adults. Fractures of the spinal vertebrae due to osteoporosis can make a dowager's hump more pro-nounced (see chapter 13). Hyperkyphosis can make you more tired or short of breath because it restricts your lungs' ability to expand. It also causes your center of gravity to move forward, increasing your risk of falling unless you bend your knees as you walk.

It can be hard to get up out of a chair, especially if the chair is armless or low to the ground.
Getting up out of a low chair requires more oxygen, even for 30-year-olds. With age and decreased activity, leg, hip, and buttock muscles weaken—these are the muscles needed to stand up. Many of us need to retire couches and chairs we bought in our thirties and buy new ones with higher seats so that we can get up more easily. Physical therapy to strengthen the quadriceps (thigh), hip flexors, the glutes (buttocks), and hamstrings can greatly improve one's ability to sit and stand with less effort.

It's harder to keep your balance.
Most older adults will fail the "walk a straight line" test for impaired drivers even if they aren't intoxicated. The older you are, the worse your balance is. Half of older adults can't stand for 10 seconds heel to toe (one foot in front of the other with the heel of the front foot touching the toe of the back foot), let alone walk heel to toe, which is what is required when performing the "walk a straight line" test.

(continued)

BOX 9.3 (*continued*)

Balance is another multifactorial syndrome. With aging, the number of hair cells in the inner ear (which provide information on head and body motion) and the number of vestibular, cortical, and cerebellar neurons in the vestibular system and the brain decrease, making us less able to identify and compensate for shifts in our position and balance and to remain stable. Additionally, a quarter of older adults have lost some feeling in their feet, decreasing the brain's input from this area. As noted above, posture changes that move our center of gravity forward make it easier for us to topple over. Physical therapy can often help improve balance.

Balance worsens when your eyes are closed or you are in the dark.
Two-thirds of older adults can't stand for 30 seconds on a thick foam pad with their eyes shut without losing their balance. We count on our eyes to compensate for problems in the other systems that provide the brain with information on where we are in space.

You're more likely to fall.
Falls are yet another multifactorial syndrome associated with aging. This chapter discusses the good news that there are things you can do to ameliorate many of the individual factors associated with falling and to decrease your risk of injury.

Should I be using a cane, walker, or wheelchair? I'm embarrassed at the thought of being seen in public using one of these devices.

Many of us wouldn't be able to be seen in public or even get around our home safely if we *didn't* use an assistive device. Think of assistive devices like a pair of glasses, something that allows you to reenter and participate in the world. As you age, you may find that you're more unsteady when you're walking. To steady yourself and feel safer, you may touch walls, furniture, or another person as you walk. But walls and another person are not always available, and furniture (and you) can topple over. Assistive devices, especially canes and walkers, provide support and input to your brain, which then pro-

vides feedback to your muscles and feet so that you walk more steadily. By using an assistive device, you can also keep up your strength and endurance. With therapy and exercise, you can sometimes improve so that you no longer need a cane. Wheelchairs should only be used to transport you long distances, like in the airport, or if you really can't walk, as there is a risk of further deconditioning when you're not ambulating on your own at all.

See Appendix 2 for the basics of these devices. If you feel you need one, talk to your medical provider to make sure you get the device that is best for you. Resist the urge to borrow someone else's device or reuse your loved one's old walker or cane that you have been keeping in the closet. If the assistive device is not the right height or type for you, it may actually contribute to instability. If your cane or walker does not feel right, ask your health care provider or physical therapist to help modify it.

I often feel light-headed when I stand up. Sometimes it lasts just a moment, but sometimes I need to sit down or else I fear I may fall. Is this normal aging?

You have *postural hypotension*, a fancy way of saying that when you stand up, your blood pressure drops. This is also called orthostatic hypotension. You may feel light-headed as soon as you get up or a few minutes later. Your blood pressure measurements may not detect a change when you stand because postural blood pressure measurements vary greatly throughout the day. Regardless, people with postural lightheadedness are, like those with documented postural hypotension, at risk of losing their balance or falling.

Postural hypotension is *not* normal aging but is much more likely to occur in older people. It is a syndrome caused by diseases, medications, and blunting of the reflexes the body uses to increase low blood pressure. The most common cause is dehydration. I have a general principle that I teach medical professionals: older adults run dry (I'm not discussing bladders here). You and your health care provider need to keep in mind that older people are often on the brink of becoming dehydrated. One important reason is that even though they are becoming dehydrated, older adults don't feel thirsty, so they don't drink enough fluid to compensate. The resulting dehydration contributes to postural hypotension.

I'm 86 years old and often find that when I get up about 30 minutes after eating, I feel light-headed. Is this postural hypotension?

This is most likely a variation called *postprandial hypotension*, where light-headedness occurs when getting up 15–90 minutes after eating a large meal. Blood flow is shunted to the digestive tract after a meal, decreasing blood pressure. As we age, our body's reflex to then increase our blood pressure is blunted. As discussed below in the section on Selective Adaptation, preventive measures differ for postprandial and postural hypotension and light-headedness.

One of my greatest fears is that I won't be able to walk as I get older. How likely is this to happen?

Surveys of older Americans who live at home find that 11 percent of those 65–74, 15 percent of those 75–84, and 31 percent of those 85 plus say they have a lot of difficulty or are unable to walk or climb steps. The survey didn't ask about the use of assistive devices or whether they had done any of the things suggested below. Since being ambulatory is clearly important to most older people, I'd suggest starting now to "use it or lose it." There is good evidence that it is never too late to start an exercise routine. Also, identify and try to ameliorate risk factors as they come up. The survey only included those living at home, but remember, that's most older people, since only 5 percent of people 65 and over and 14 percent of those 85 and older live in nursing homes.

It seems like falls are common in older adults. Many of my friends have fallen, and some have seriously injured themselves. Senior centers and magazines have programs and articles to prevent falls. Are falls a part of normal aging?

Falls are *not* part of normal aging, but they are common. Each year, one-third of older people who live at home and more than half of those living in nursing homes fall. Those who have fallen have a 60 percent chance of falling the next year. As mentioned above, some falls can be caused by acute medical conditions. But most falls are a multifactorial geriatric syndrome, with several risk factors (see chapter 2). Multifactorial falls are due to the contributions of one or more risk factors that affect successful ambulation and balance. Many of these risk factors arise from age-associated changes, discussed in box 9.3.

What are the risk factors for falls?

Studies have identified hundreds of risk factors, but those most strongly associated with falling are having had a previous fall, being a woman, or being over 80 years old. People with cognitive impairment; depression; disorders of gait, strength, balance, the feet, or legs; who use psychotropic medications (antidepressants, sleeping pills, antianxiety medications, antipsychotics); and who have conditions such as Parkinson's disease, stroke, arthritis, postural hypotension, and impaired vision are also at higher risk.

I haven't fallen, but I'm worried that I will. I'm starting to stay home more as a result. Am I overreacting?

Believe it or not, there is a condition called *fear of falling* that affects not only people who have had a fall, but also those who haven't but are afraid they will fall and injure themselves like someone they knew or heard about. They restrict their activities and become isolated and deconditioned, increasing their risk of a fall. Their fears of falling become a self-fulfilling prophecy. The best thing you can do if you're afraid of falling is to face these fears and identify what you can do to improve your walking and decrease your risk of falls and injuries.

Are the risk factors for injury the same as those for falls?

Risk factors for injurious falls include those for falls, in particular a history of previous falls, but also include factors that make injury more likely, like taking anticoagulant medications (blood thinners), which can increase bleeding, and having osteoporosis, which can increase fractures. The greater the distance fallen, the harder the surface, and falling onto your head or hip also increase the chance of injury.

I've fallen once. What should I do to prevent another fall?

The number one risk factor for falling is having fallen before. *Falls beget falls.* There are two major reasons for this. The first is that whatever caused you to fall may cause you to fall again. So, it is very important to review what you were doing when you fell. Were you up on a ladder (something that might be called a *risky behavior*)? Or were you just walking within your home? Did you have a warning that you might fall—did you trip, lose your balance, or feel light-headed or dizzy? See the chapter 9 checklist on page 376 in Appendix 3 for ways to help sort this out. The second reason that a fall may presage another fall is that many people who fall more than once develop fear of falling (see page 142), limit their activities, and become deconditioned and even more likely to fall again. Breaking this cycle often requires physical therapy and family support.

How about preventing an injury from a fall?

Interventions shown to prevent injurious falls include combinations of exercise, vision evaluation and treatment, as well as home evaluation and modification. Additionally, fractures, including hip fractures, have been shown to be prevented by a combination of osteoporosis medications (discussed on page 147) as well as calcium and vitamin D supplementation.

What is osteoporosis? Is it part of normal aging?

Osteoporosis, which means porous bone, is a *disease* where bone density and quality decreases, making the bone more brittle and increasing the risk

of a fracture. During your life, bone is always turning over, with new bone being made and old removed. Bone density increases until one's late twenties and then starts to decrease because old bone is removed faster than new bone is laid down. This is especially true for women during the three to five years after menopause, and for both men and women after age 70.

How do I know if I'm at risk for osteoporosis?

You're at greater risk if you didn't do weight-bearing or strength-building exercises during your bone-building years or, if you are a woman, if you are small boned, white or Asian, or have a family history of fractures that occur after minimal trauma. Although less common, Hispanic and African American women also develop osteoporosis. It is also more common in smokers, drinkers, those who have taken certain medications (see table 9.1), and people who are inactive. Women should get a baseline bone mineral density test, called dual-energy x-ray absorptiometry, or DEXA, at least once after age 65, or at age 60 if high risk. Screening for men is controversial. See chapter 5, on prevention, for more detail on osteoporosis screening recommendations.

Adapting to Your New Normal

Some of the risk factors for mobility impairment, falls, and injury can't easily be changed, like age or sex. Some mobility changes are part of normal aging but still increase your risk for falls, while others are age-related disorders like Parkinson's, stroke, and dementia, all of which increase the risk of being injured in a fall.

This section covers *universal adaptations*—things everyone should do to decrease their risk of mobility impairment, falls, and injuries—and *selected adaptations*, which apply only to people with certain conditions. You and your medical provider should identify which of the selected adaptations apply to you.

Universal Adaptations

Revisit Your Choice of Footwear

Only you can decide which shoes you're willing to wear, but this is another vanity issue where the downside can literally be falling down and hurting more than your pride. You're most likely to fall when walking barefoot or in socks alone, or when wearing slippers, high heels, or shoes with open or loose heels (such as flip-flops and Crocs). The higher the heel, and the less surface area between the sole and the floor, the more your posture and balance will need to change, and the more likely you are to fall. Ideally you should get a well-fitting shoe that covers your whole foot and has a thin, firm sole that is mostly in contact with the floor, with a low heel and a back that can support your heel and ankle. Athletic shoes fit the bill for more casual occasions. Nonslip soles (those with rubber traction) help most people except those with shuffling gaits, like people with Parkinsonism, in whom nonslip soles can catch or stick and actually increase the risk of a fall. In this case, consider a shoe with a smooth but not slick sole.

Avoid Risky Behavior

This one can be hard, because we all think we should be able to do what we were previously able to do. But our balance and endurance aren't what they were when we were younger. Think twice before you climb up on a ladder, go skiing, try to beat the light when crossing the street, or drink too much. A grabber tool can allow you to access items that are on high shelves or low floors.

Have an Emergency Fall Plan

Anyone can have a bad fall, even those who are the most fit. About 50 percent of older people who fall can't get back up, even if they're not injured, and many remain on the ground for hours before they are found. These *long-lie falls* have consequences above and beyond the fall itself. If you get dehydrated, your muscles can start to break down and also cause kidney failure. You can develop pressure sores or pneumonia. How can you prevent spending hours on the floor if you fall? Make a plan for what to do should you fall and need help. Carry a cell phone or a cellular watch with you around the house, subscribe to a personal emergency response system (PERS) (Appendix 1), or work out a plan with someone that you know who will check in on you a few times a day. The latter approach may not be as useful if you fall at night, however.

Practice How to Fall and Get Up Safely

There is a right way to fall, although sometimes it happens so fast, it may be hard to remember what to do and not to do. When you fall, try to let your body go limp—don't stiffen up. Keep your knees, wrists, and elbows loose and bent. Don't try to break the fall with your hands and knees (this is a good way to fracture your wrist!). Tuck in your chin, and throw your arms around your ears to protect your head.

Don't get up quickly after a fall. Look around for a sturdy piece of furniture or the bottom of a staircase. Roll over onto your side by turning your head in the direction you are trying to roll, then move your shoulders, arm, hips, and finally your leg to that side. Push up your upper body. Lift your head and pause for a few moments to steady yourself. Slowly get up on your hands and knees and crawl toward a sturdy chair. Place your hands on the seat of the chair and slide one foot forward so it is flat on the floor. Keep the other leg bent with the knee on the floor. From this kneeling position, slowly rise and turn your body to sit in the chair. Sit for a few minutes before you try to do anything else. If you are not able to sit up safely after a fall, you need to call for help.

Fall-Proof Your Home

It can be easy to fall in your home if there's clutter, but there are many other hazards you might not think of, like the thresholds of doors and stairs, throw rugs that aren't tacked down, and cables and cords that can get in the way and cause slips and trips. Make sure you have good lighting, and consider getting a night light. Bathrooms are where many falls occur, so if you are worried about tripping on the way to the bathroom at night, consider using a bedside commode or urinal. Install grab bars and non-slip bathmats. Complete a home safety evaluation (see the Resources section at the end of this chapter) to maximize your safety.

Limit Yourself to One Alcoholic Drink a Day

As discussed in chapter 3, you get a bigger bang for your buck with alcohol as you age. Alcohol has a major effect on balance and can result in falls and accidents.

Review Your Medications

Many medications increase the risk of falls, often by making you feel light-headed or affecting your balance. The more medications you take, the more likely you will fall. With your doctor, try to decrease the numbers and doses of medications, particularly those listed in table 9.1.

Consider Vitamin D Supplementation

Falls decrease when vitamin D is replaced in those who are vitamin D deficient. It's less clear if supplemental vitamin D (800–1,000 international units) decreases falls in people who are not vitamin D deficient.

Get in Shape

Exercise has repeatedly been shown to reduce the risk of falling. The most effective types of exercise are strengthening, stretching, balancing, and functional exercises (see pages 98–99 for more details). Functional exercises mimic your everyday movement to improve your performance. Stretching is important because if your muscles are tight, it can be difficult to realign posture. If your ankles are too tight, your ability to balance can be affected.

Balance exercises strengthen your core muscles, lower back, and legs, and can also help retrain your ability to sense where you are in space (proprioception). You may need someone to assist you with these at first. Once you get comfortable with the exercises, try doing them with one or both eyes closed. Tai chi, a Chinese art form, also decreases falls. Tai chi teaches movements that flow into each other, shifting your weight and extending your limbs to challenge your balance. It's also meditative, as the movements are accompanied by slow, deep breathing. Participating in a yoga class may also help to improve balance and strength.

It's often a good idea to see a physical therapist to develop an exercise program tailored for you. Your physical therapist can introduce you to exercise videos or community exercise programs that are safe. Exercising by yourself can be hard, but there are many group exercise programs that have been shown to reduce falls while increasing socialization. These programs incorporate more than one type of exercise (gait training, balance, strengthening) as well as discussions of home safety and other tips. See the Resources section at the end of this chapter, and contact your local Department of Aging to find out where and when these programs are offered. If you're self-motivated, you can join an exercise program for older adults on the Internet or use DVDs to do classes in your own home.

Physical Therapy for Mobility and Balance

Medicare will cover physical therapy if you have moderate to severe mobility limitations, or minimal mobility restriction accompanied by leg weakness, abnormal gait, vestibular (balance/dizziness) symptoms, excessive fear of falling, need for device or brace modification, or symptoms of Parkinsonism.

Pay Attention to Your Posture

Physical therapy and some alternative therapies, like the Alexander technique, can help you become more aware of your posture and the alignment of your head, neck, body, and feet. Lumbar extensor and core muscle exercises help limit forward movement of your head and neck and increase your stability. This is particularly important when using a computer or phone, where you may unconsciously bend forward for long periods of time.

Selective Adaptations

Osteoporosis Prevention

If you have osteoporosis, you are at much higher risk of injury from a fall because your bones are weaker and more prone to fracture. The following activities can help keep your osteoporosis from worsening, while also reducing the risk of a fracture after a fall.

Stop smoking. Studies show that smoking can reduce bone density. It is not only a risk factor for osteoporosis, but it can also impede your body's ability to repair fractured bone. Stopping smoking isn't easy, but it can be done (I know what I'm talking about). Only 10 percent of older Americans still smoke. Speak with your doctor about the options now available to help you quit smoking.

Build bone through exercise. Weight-bearing exercises like walking, hiking, jogging, climbing stairs, playing tennis, and dancing, as well as strength-building exercises like lifting weights and using resistance bands, help to build bone. Note that swimming and bicycling, although great aerobic activities, are not weight-bearing exercises and do not build bone.

Ensure adequate calcium intake. Men aged 51–70 should ingest 1,000 mg of calcium per day. Men over 70 and women over 51 should ingest 1,200 mg of calcium a day. There is controversy over whether calcium supplements are associated with increased cardiac events, so the best way to get calcium is through food sources (see the Resources section in chapter 15).

Ensure adequate vitamin D intake. Vitamin D is needed to absorb calcium into the bones and to decrease fractures. Vitamin D levels may decrease if you don't get enough sunlight, especially during the winter. Intake should be 600 IU (international units) daily up to age 60 and 800 IU over age 70. Food sources of vitamin D include egg yolks, saltwater fish, and liver, as well as many dairy products that are supplemented with vitamin D.

Osteoporosis Treatment

In addition to quitting smoking, weight-bearing exercise, calcium and vitamin D supplementation, there are several medications available for treating osteoporosis. Most have been shown to decrease vertebral fractures, but only the bisphosphonates and zoledronic acid have been shown to reduce nonvertebral fractures (hip and wrist fractures). It takes 1.5–2 years before these medications are effective in decreasing the rate of fractures.

Many people worry about taking bisphosphonate medications because of the increased incidence of *atypical femoral fractures* and *osteonecrosis of the jaw*. Atypical fractures are stress fractures in the long bone of the femur. Studies show that of 1,000 people treated with bisphosphonates for three years, 100 will be prevented from having a "typical" fracture, while less than 1 person will have an atypical fracture, making it far more likely that an individual will benefit rather than be harmed from these medications. Osteonecrosis, bone death that occurs when blood flow to the bone is reduced, occurs in 1 in 10,000 bisphosphonate users. This risk is much greater in cancer patients taking higher doses, people who are also taking glucocorticoids (like prednisone) or immunosuppressive agents, and those with a history of complicated recent dental work.

Oral estrogen and estrogen-progestin are not first-line therapies to prevent osteoporosis, although they may be safe to take in the three to five years postmenopause and for those under 60 without heart disease. They are effective at decreasing fractures, but estrogen alone carries an increased risk for stroke and blood clots, while estrogen-progestin combinations increase the risk for cardiovascular disease and invasive breast cancer.

Pain Relief

Pain can interfere with walking or balance. Additional pain can come when we compensate for back or lower extremity joint pain by changing the way that we walk, putting excess strain on other joints. Discuss your pain with your medical provider, and see the discussion of nonpharmacologic and pharmacologic pain relief on pages 239–47. You may find that taking a pain medication before going out or starting a physical therapy session allows you to be able to do more.

Severe Knee and Hip Osteoarthritis

If pain medications, joint injections, and physical therapy don't improve your pain level or mobility, it may be time to consider joint replacement.

Joint replacement surgeries are performed commonly, and 95 percent of patients are satisfied with the outcome. That doesn't mean you should rush into them, but if your mobility is severely limited by knee or hip osteoarthritis, you should consider whether joint replacement makes sense for you. The surgeries last two to three hours, and the current prostheses last, in general, 20 or more years. Minimally invasive (or keyhole) surgery causes less trauma to the muscles and tendons and is associated with faster healing, but it isn't right for everyone and at times can make it harder for the surgeon to operate. Most hip replacement patients are able to resume light everyday activities within four to six weeks. Knee replacement patients take about three months to return to normal activities.

Discuss the pros and cons with your orthopedist and primary care provider. One concern with delaying surgery is that the muscles that support the joints may atrophy if you don't use them. *Prehabilitation*, which is rehabilitation done before surgery to strengthen the muscles in your legs, may help you

recover sooner. Prehabilitation also helps you learn how to do the exercises that you will do after surgery, making it easier for you to do them in recovery. If you're overweight, weight loss prior to surgery can also improve your outcome. If you decide to have surgery, make sure your surgeon does at least 50 of these procedures yearly, and ask about their complication rate.

Vision Impairment

Don't wear your reading, progressive, or multifocal glasses when you're walking outdoors or on the stairs. Reading glasses and the lower portion of progressive and multifocal lenses improve near-vision. Wearing them outdoors cause objects outside the near-vision range to blur, like the edges of curbs, stairs, or cracks in the sidewalk, increasing the likelihood of falling.

Consider having your first cataract removed. Cataract surgery has been shown to reduce your risk of falling by 33 percent (see chapter 12).

If your vision can't be corrected with glasses, get a referral to a low-vision center (see the Resources section in chapter 12).

Postural Hypotension

If you get dizzy or light-headed when you stand, work with your medical provider to see if there is a specific condition or medication responsible. In the meantime, your goal is to restore normal blood pressure when you stand and to avoid falling. The following are things you can do that may improve the situation.

On getting up in the morning

- Exercise gently before getting up (move your ankles up and down and clench and unclench your hands) and again after standing (march in place).
- Get out of bed slowly. First sit up, then sit on the side of the bed, then stand up and stay near the bed for a little while before starting to walk away.

When changing position

- Take your time when changing position, such as when getting up from a chair.
- Make sure you have something to hold on to when you stand up. Installing grab bars by the toilet and bathtub will help you stay balanced when you're moving about inside the bathroom.
- Try to sit down when washing, showering, dressing, or working in the kitchen.

Lifestyle changes

- If you're on a low-salt diet, ask your doctor if you can stop. Getting more salt in your diet will help you stay hydrated.
- Drink six to eight glasses of water or low-calorie drinks each day, unless you have been told to limit your fluid intake.
- Avoid taking very hot baths or showers, as these can further lower your blood pressure.
- Consider using compression stockings to decrease the pooling of blood in your veins when you stand up. These can be found in pharmacies and surgical/medical equipment supply stores and online. Nowadays they even come in colors and decorative patterns.

Postprandial Hypotension

If you get light-headed or dizzy when you stand 15–90 minutes after eating, have a cup of coffee or 100 mg caffeine with meals. Remember to get up slowly from your chair with nearby support if needed.

Peripheral Neuropathy

If you have decreased sensations or numbness and tingling in your feet and hands, you may have peripheral neuropathy, a disorder that affects the nerves that carry messages to and from the brain and spinal cord to the legs and the arms. This can result in pain, numbness and tingling, burning, or a loss of sensation. There are multiple causes, including diabetes, alcoholism, poor nutrition, some vitamin deficiencies, thyroid disease, Lyme disease, and medications (see table 13.3).

What can you do?

- Work with your medical provider to determine whether there may a treatable cause (see the Yellow Alerts in chapter 13, which discusses peripheral neuropathy).
- Wear shoes that are supportive and have thinner soles. These can increase your ability to feel with your feet.
- Use a cane to compensate (see Appendix 2).
- If you have diabetes, keep your blood sugar as close to your target

level as possible (see chapter 5). Poorly controlled diabetes can affect the nerves in your feet, making you less aware of foot infections or injuries. It can also impair your ability to feel where your feet are and put you at risk for falls.

Foot Abnormalities or Pain

Physical abnormalities such as a difference in the length of your legs, the presence of bunions or hammertoes, or the need for ankle braces, shoe inserts, shoe body, or sole modification can put you at risk for a fall. Podiatrists or physiatrists (rehabilitation medicine specialists) can often help with these problems, as well as help you identify where to buy shoes that can prevent falls.

What Isn't Normal Aging?

 Red Flags: Symptoms Needing Prompt Medical Attention

- Loss of consciousness
- Seizures (convulsions)
- Dizziness accompanied by any of the following: slurred speech, visual changes, one-sided weakness or loss of coordination (this could be a stroke or a transient ischemic attack)
- Sudden inability to stand or walk
- Falling and hitting your head
- Thigh or calf pain that occurs routinely after you've walked a certain distance, say, two or three blocks
- Shortness of breath or severe fatigue when walking usual distances

⚠️ **Yellow Alerts: Common Conditions That Can Worsen Balance and Mobility**

Medications. For a list of medications that can put you at risk of a fall, see table 9.1.

Pain in the back, buttocks, or legs when you stand or walk. Pain in these regions could be due to muscle strains or deconditioning, but it may also be due to one of the conditions in table 9.2.

Neurological diseases. Parkinson's disease, dementia, strokes, and ministrokes may have an effect on balance and can lead to falls.

Dizziness. Dizziness is one of those words that means different things to different people. For some it means feeling light-headed, for others it means feeling giddy, woozy, spinning, floating, or off-balance. Any of these sensations can impair your mobility or balance. To identify the reason for feeling dizzy, it's most helpful if you can describe it as (1) *vertigo*, where you or the room is spinning; (2) *disequilibrium*, where you feel off-balance or unsteady (like feeling drunk); (3) *lightheaded or feeling faint*; or (4) a combination of these.

TABLE 9.1
Drugs That May Cause Falls, Muscle Weakness, Dizziness, and Bone Loss

Drugs and Examples	Falls and Imbalance	Muscle Weakness	Dizziness	Bone Loss
Blood pressure, cardiac, and diuretic medications				
ACE inhibitors and ARBs: lisinopril (Zestril); ramipril (Altace); candesartan (Atacand); losartan (Cozaar)			X	
Beta-blockers: metoprolol (Toprol); atenolol (Tenormin); carvedilol (Coreg)			X	
Calcium channel blockers: amlodipine (Norvasc); nifedipine (Procardia); diltiazem (Cardizem)		X	X	
Diuretics: hydrochlorothiazide; triamterene-hydrochlorothiazide (Dyazide); furosemide (Lasix)	X	X	X	
Pain relief				
GABA-ergic neurogenic pain medications: gabapentin (Neurontin); pregabalin (Lyrica)	X		X	
NSAIDs: ibuprofen (Motrin, Advil); naproxen (Naprosyn, Aleve)			X	
Opioid analgesics: morphine; oxycodone (in Percocet); hydrocodone (in Vicodin); tramadol (Ultram)	X	X	X	
Muscle relaxants: cyclobenzaprine (Flexeril); methocarbamol (Robaxin)	X		X	
Neurological, psychological, and sleep medications				
Sleep and anxiety: diazepam (Valium); alprazolam (Xanax); clonazepam (Klonopin); zolpidem (Ambien); zaleplon (Sonata)	X	X	X	
Antipsychotics that are sedating: chlorpromazine (Thorazine); olanzapine (Zyprexa); quetiapine (Seroquel)	X	X	X	
*Antipsychotics that cause Parkinsonism**: fluphenazine (Prolixin); haloperidol (Haldol); risperidone (Risperdal).	X			
CNS stimulants: methylphenidate (Ritalin, Concerta); modafinil (Provigil)			X	

(continued)

TABLE 9.1 (*continued*)

Drugs and Examples	Falls and Imbalance	Muscle Weakness	Dizziness	Bone Loss
Anti-dizziness: meclizine (Antivert, Bonine); dimenhydrinate (Dramamine); scopolamine (Trans-scop)	X		X	
Anticonvulsants: phenytoin (Dilantin); valproic acid (Depakote); carbamazepine (Tegretol, Carbatrol); levetiracetam (Keppra)	X	X	X	X†
Dementia cholinesterase inhibitors: donepezil (Aricept); rivastigmine (Exelon); galantamine (Razadyne)	X		X	
Antidepressants				
Tricyclic, SSRI, and SNRI antidepressants: amitriptyline (Elavil); imipramine (Tofranil); escitalopram (Lexapro); sertraline (Zoloft); venlafaxine (Effexor); duloxetine (Cymbalta)	X	X	X	F
Other antidepressants: mirtazapine (Remeron); bupropion (Wellbutrin); trazodone (Desyrel)	X		X	F
Anti-Parkinsonian medications				
Decarboxylase inhibitor: carbidopa/levodopa (Sinemet)	X	X	X	
Dopamine agonists and COMT inhibitor: pramipexole (Mirapex); amantadine (Symmetrel); bromocriptine (Parlodel); tolcapone (Tasmar); entacapone (Comtan)	X		X	
Diabetes medications				
Insulin and sulfonylureas: glyburide (Glynase); glipizide (Glucotrol)	X		X	
Biguanides: metformin (Glucophage, Glumetza)		X	X	
Thiazolidinediones: pioglitazone (Actos); rosiglitazone (Avandia)				F
Others: dulaglutide (Trulicity); exenatide (Bydureon, Byetta); repaglinide (Prandin)			X	
Gastrointestinal medications				
Antispasmodics: atropine; dicyclomine (Bentyl); propantheline	X	X	X	
Antidiarrheal: hyoscyamine (Levsin, Levbid), atropine/diphenoxylate (Lomotil)	X	X	X	

TABLE 9.1 (continued)

Drugs and Examples	Falls and Imbalance	Muscle Weakness	Dizziness	Bone Loss
H₂ blockers: cimetidine (Tagamet); famotidine (Pepcid)			X	
Proton pump inhibitors: pantoprazole (Protonix); omeprazole (Prilosec); esomeprazole (Nexium)			X	X/F
Others: ondansetron (Zofran); metoclopramide (Reglan)	X		X	
Cold, allergy, and itching medications				
First-generation antihistamines: diphenhydramine (Benadryl); chlorpheniramine (Aller-Chlor, Chlor-Trimeton)	X			
Decongestants: phenylephrine (SudafedPE), pseudoephedrine (Sudafed Sinus), oxymetazoline (Afrin, Dristan)		X	X	
Urinary medications				
Bladder Relaxants: tolteradine (Detrol); oxybutinin (Ditropan); solifenacin (Vesicare)	X		X	
Beta-3 agonist: mirabegron (Myrbetriq)			X	
Others				
Fluoroquinolones: ciprofloxacin (Cipro); levofloxacin (Levaquin)			X	
HIV therapy: tenofovir disoproxil fumarate, also known as tenofovirDF (Viread)				X
Corticosteroids: prednisone; dexamethasone (Decadron); methylprednisolone (Solu-Medrol)				X
Aromatase inhibitors: anastrazole (Arimidex); exemestane (Aromasin); letrozole (Femara)				X
Alcohol	X		X	X

Note: If you're not sure whether a drug you're taking is in one of the drug classes listed, ask your pharmacist or health care provider. X, may cause this condition; F, bone fracture warning. Abbreviations are as follows: ACE, angiotensin-converting enzyme; ARB, Angiotensin Receptor Blockers; CNS, central nervous system; COMT, catechol-O-methyltransferase; GABA, gamma amino butyric acid; HIV, human immunodeficiency virus; NSAID, nonsteroidal anti-inflammatory drug; SNRI, serotonin-norepinephrine reuptake inhibitor; SSRI, selective serotonin reuptake inhibitor.

*Symptoms of Parkinsonism are rigidity, hesitant gait, tremor, and poor balance.

†All drugs listed may not have this adverse effect.

TABLE 9.2
Causes of Back or Leg Pain When Standing or Walking

	Pain Location(s)	Pain Worsens With	Pain Improves With	What Causes the Pain?
Hip osteoarthritis	Groin, thigh, buttocks, knee on the same side as the arthritic hip	Walking, bending over to tie a shoe, rising from a chair	Rest	The shock-absorbing cartilage in the joint gradually wears away, decreasing the protective space between the bones. The friction of bone rubbing on bone can produce pain, swelling, stiffness, and the formation of bone spurs.
Knee osteoarthritis	Knee	Getting in or out of cars, using the stairs, walking	Rest	
Lumbar stenosis	Back and buttocks Can also be similar to sciatica (see below)	Standing, walking	Bending forward, sitting, or lying down	The spinal canal narrows, usually due to osteoarthritis, and puts pressure on the spinal cord and the spinal nerve roots. Symptoms may occur because of inflammation, compression of the nerve(s), or both. Bending forward increases the space available for the nerves between the vertebrae and relieves the pain.
Sciatica	From lower spine to hip, buttock, and down the back of the leg, usually on only one side of the body Leg may feel numb, weak, or tingly	Coughing or sneez-ing; prolonged sitting	Lying down	The sciatic nerve is a large nerve that runs from the lower back down the back of each leg. Osteoarthritic bone spurs and herniated discs are two common reasons for pressure on this nerve.
Intermittent claudication	Calves or thighs	Walking a certain distance, say, several blocks	Stopping walking	Leg arteries narrow and cause pain similarly to how heart arteries narrow and cause angina. This often improves with physical therapy or other treatment. Claudication can also be a sign that you are at risk for cardiac disease. Tell your medical provider.

Getting Evaluated for Mobility, Balance, and Falls

As discussed above, for most people, losing mobility is one of the greatest fears of aging. There can be many possible causes, and most can be managed to allow you improved mobility, with or without an assistive device. Your primary care provider can usually help you identify the issues that are interfering the most with your mobility and provide referrals if needed to specialists, including physical therapy, to help improve these limitations and implement the adaptations discussed above.

When to See a Specialist

Discuss any possible visit to a specialist with your primary care provider. Geriatricians do comprehensive fall assessments in their offices as part of primary or consultative care. This may be a good first place to start and can help guide the next steps as well as what type of further work-up you may need. For a list of other specialists who may need to be consulted, see table 9.3.

TABLE 9.3

Specialists to Consider Consulting for Specific Causes of Mobility or Balance Concerns or Falls

Symptom	Specialist
Vertigo	Ear, nose, and throat (ENT) doctor; vestibular rehabilitation
Poor vision, cataracts	Ophthalmologist or optometrist, low-vision center
Painful knee or hip arthritis	Rheumatologist, orthopedist, or physiatrist
Lumbar stenosis or sciatica	Physiatrist, Physical therapy
Painful or disfigured feet that interfere with your ability to walk or balance	Podiatrist or physiatrist
Abnormal gait and balance; rigidity or shuffling gait	Neurologist
Intermittent claudication (reproducible pain in calves or thighs after walking a certain distance)	Vascular medicine or surgery doctor
Decreased exercise tolerance, shortness of breath with exertion	Cardiologist or pulmonologist

Preparing for the Visit

Your doctor will ask you several questions and evaluate your gait, balance, strength, take your blood pressure while lying and standing; inspect your feet; and review your medications. Fill out the chapter 9 pre-visit checklist on page 376 in Appendix 3 to help identify the risk factors most likely to be affecting your mobility and risk of falling. Bring it with you to your appointment, and review it with your provider.

Advice for Loved Ones

Not every fall or injury can be prevented, even if you have someone with you around the clock. Achieving a balance between safety, happiness, independence, and peace of mind for both of you can be difficult. Many older adults don't want someone else in their home, and they don't necessarily want to live with their children (see chapter 18). They also may not want to leave a home they've lived in for decades. I worked out a deal between my Aunt Julie and her son to allow her to live alone, as long as she got *and used* a personal emergency response system. In cases like these, a lot depends on your relationship with each other and whether you can reach a compromise you both can live with.

What can you do? Start with a complete home safety assessment, and implement what you find lacking (see the Resources section at the end of this chapter). Have the older adult's mobility assessed, and make sure the referrals and suggestions are followed up on. Go for walks with them when you're visiting. Things may not change overnight. I find it can take six months to get someone to regularly use an assistive device they need, and longer than that to accept help in the house. Most importantly, don't let differences on this issue ruin your relationship and the time you have together.

Bottom Line

Maintaining mobility is important to older adults, as loss of mobility can lead to isolation, depression, and deconditioning. Each person has different risk factors for losing mobility, falling, and injuring themselves. Identifying and addressing these factors, both individually and in combination, can improve one's mobility and independence. Use assistive devices—they can give you your life back and allow you to do the things that are important to you. Don't worry about how they make you look. It's how you feel and what you can do that will really make the difference in your life.

RESOURCES

Improving Safety

Home Fall Prevention Checklist
(https://www.cdc.gov/steadi/pdf/check_for
_safety_brochure-a.pdf)
This guide from the Centers for Disease
Control and Prevention (CDC) helps seniors
identify and fix hazards within the home.

Home Modifications
(www.homemods.org)
The University of Southern California's
School of Gerontology offers the Stop
Falls program, which contains education,
resources, and low-cost brochures and
DVDs on fall-proofing your home.

For more information on personal emergency response systems, see Appendix 1.

Evidence-Based Fall Prevention Programs

National Council on Aging
(https://www.ncoa.org/healthy-aging/falls
-prevention/falls-prevention-programs
-for-older-adults-2/)
The National Council on Aging can help
you find information on fall prevention
programs that are proven to reduce the
risk of falling. These programs include:
- A Matter of Balance
- Bingocize

- CAPABLE
- Enhance Fitness
- FallsTalk
- FallScape
- Fit & Strong!
- Healthy Steps for Older Adults
- Healthy Steps in Motion
- The Otago Exercise Program
- Stay Active and Independent for Life
  (SAIL)
- Stepping On
- tai chi for arthritis
- Tai Ji Quan: Moving for Better Balance
- YMCA Moving for Better Balance

Older Adult Fall Prevention
(https://www.cdc.gov/falls/index.html
?CDC_AA_refVal=https%3A%2F%2Fwww
.cdc.gov%2Fhomeandrecreationalsafety
%2Ffalls%2Findex.html)
Facts, resources, and interventions from
the CDC to help older adults prevent falls.
STEADI Older Adult Fall Prevention Program
(https://www.cdc.gov/steadi/patient.html)

The CDC's STEADI program (STEADI
stands for Stopping Elderly Accidents,
Deaths, and Injuries) provides patient
education material to help reduce the risk
of falls.

BIBLIOGRAPHY

Black, D. M., and C. J. Rosen. "Postmenopausal Osteoporosis." *New England Journal
of Medicine* 374 (2016): 254–62.

Fritz, S., and M. Lusardi. "Walking Speed:
The Sixth Vital Sign." *Journal of Geriatric
Physical Therapy* 32, no. 2 (2009): 46–49.

Rabenda, V., D. Nicolet, C. Beaudart,
O. Bruyère, and J.-Y. Reginster. "Relationship
between Use of Antidepressants and Risk
of Fractures: A Meta-Analysis." *Osteoporosis
International* 24, no. 1 (2013): 121–37.

Reuben, D. B., C. Roth, C. Kamberg, and
N. S. Wenger. "Restructuring Primary Care
Practices to Manage Geriatric Syndromes:
The ACOVE-2 Intervention." *Journal of
the American Geriatrics Society* 51, no. 12
(2003): 1787–1793.

Rizzoli, R., C. Cooper, J.-Y. Reginster, et al.
"Antidepressant Medications and Osteoporosis." *Bone* 51, no. 3 (2012): 606–13.

CHAPTER 10

Sleep Cycles

We spend a third of our life asleep, or at least trying to sleep. When we succeed, we wake up refreshed and ready to start the day. When we don't, we feel tired, unable to think clearly, and we are more likely to fall or have a car accident. When we're sleep deprived, we may eat more, and our chronic medical and inflammatory conditions can get worse. You may not even be aware that you're sleeping poorly—many people with sleep apnea think they've slept soundly through the night.

How we sleep changes with age. The good news is that there's a lot you can do to improve the amount and soundness of your sleep that doesn't require taking sleep medications or using alcohol to help you fall asleep.

This chapter discusses age-related changes in sleep, what's myth and what's reality, causes of sleep problems, primary sleep disorders, and methods to improve the quality and duration of your sleep.

For an overview of circadian rhythm and the stages of sleep, see box 10.1.

What's Normal with Aging?

For a deeper dive into age-related changes in sleep and sleep behaviors, see box 10.2.

I've heard that older people don't need as much sleep as younger people. Is this true?

No. You need same amount of sleep as you did when you were younger, but you may end up getting less for the reasons discussed below. To function optimally, most older adults need seven to eight hours of sleep a night, although some may need less and others more.

I don't wake up as alert and ready to start the day as I did when I was younger. Does sleep itself change with aging?

It definitely does. As you age, it takes longer to fall asleep. More importantly, as described in box 10.2, as we age, we become lighter sleepers, wake up more during the night, and often have difficulty falling back to sleep. We're more likely to be awakened by faint amounts of light, noise, or touch. *Circadian rhythm* often shifts, so preferred bedtimes become one to two hours earlier than when younger, and older adults are more likely to become "morning" people, waking earlier and favoring the early hours for getting things done.

Medical and psychological conditions can also cause us to awaken during the night (table 10.1).

BOX 10.1

Sleep 101

Why do we feel sleepy? Many of us have found that the longer we're awake, the sleepier we get. Yet there are also times of the day, like after lunch, where we feel sleepy before getting a second wind, and then we find we're awake and ready to go again. If time awake were the only factor that controlled sleepiness, this wouldn't happen.

Circadian rhythm accounts for getting that second wind. Circadian rhythm is a natural, internal system that regulates feelings of sleepiness and wakefulness over a 24-hour period. It controls a variety of functions, including two that promote sleep: the lowering of core body temperature and the release of melatonin as bedtime approaches. The circadian rhythms of all these functions are synchronized by light, which travels through the optic nerve to the hypothalamus that then controls the rhythms generated in other parts of the brain. The important role of light explains why we are most awake while the sun is shining and feel ready for sleep when it's dark outside. Circadian rhythms are strongest when we keep regular hours, so we sleep best when we try to go to bed and wake up at about the same time every day.

SLEEP STAGES

The quality of your sleep varies throughout the night, cycling every 1.5–2 hours through rapid eye movements (REM) and the three stages of non-REM sleep (stages N1–N3).

Stage N1 is when you feel drowsy and initially fall into a light sleep.

Stage N2 is a slightly deeper sleep where your heart rate slows and your body temperature drops; you spend about half of each cycle in Stage N2 sleep.

Stage N3 is a deep sleep also known as slow-wave sleep; when awakened during slow-wave sleep, you may be groggy or disoriented for a few minutes.

REM sleep is when you dream, and it accounts for about 20 percent of each cycle. Brain activity is similar to being awake, and skeletal muscle tone is markedly decreased.

As the night progresses, the amount of time spent in each stage changes. Slow-wave sleep (Stage N3) occurs mainly during the first half of the night, while the amount of REM sleep increases throughout the night, so that the last third of sleep is spent primarily in Stage N2 and REM, the stages where it appears that memory consolidation occurs.

BOX 10.2

What Happens with Aging: A Deeper Dive

Older people sleep about an hour less each night than younger adults.
The amount of sleep we get decreases each decade as we age. A study that measured sleep in healthy people in sleep labs found that those aged 18–34 slept an
average of 7 hours, while those aged 65–79 slept an average of 5.8 hours. These
are likely underestimates of total sleep time, since most people sleep longer when
they're in their own bed than when they're in a sleep laboratory.

It takes older adults only a few minutes longer to fall asleep than younger adults,
but they spend more time awake during the night.
After age 20, the average time to fall asleep increases about 1 minute per decade,
while the increase in time awake is about 10 minutes per decade. This probably
accounts for the hour difference in total sleep time. Older adults spend more of
the night in the lightest stage of sleep, Stage N1, and they awaken more from
minor disturbances, like a partner getting out of bed. For details on other conditions that can cause older adults to awaken at night, see table 10.1.

When in bed trying to fall asleep, older adults spend more time awake than
younger adults.
This is called *sleep efficiency*, and as discussed later in this chapter, remaining
in bed when you can't fall asleep actually makes it less likely you'll fall asleep.
Younger adults have around a 90 percent sleep efficiency; that is, 90 percent of
the time they spend in bed they're asleep, while for older adults, it's about 78
percent.

With aging, older adults are more likely to go to bed and wake up earlier.
Changes in circadian rhythm are common in older adults, often resulting in their
going to bed and waking up one to two hours earlier than middle-aged adults.
A decrease in core body temperature induces sleep, and with aging this happens
earlier in the night and correlates with the earlier bedtimes.

Older adults are more likely to become morning people.
Even some people who were "night owls" when they were younger prefer to do
things in the morning as they get older. Changes in circadian rhythms prompt this
shift, and the result is they perform certain tasks better in the morning, like tests
of recognition memory (see box 6.2 in chapter 6).

The numbers of awakenings, limb movements, and respiratory events like
gasping or apnea (stopping breathing) increase with age.
Even when these issues don't meet criteria for the primary sleep disorders
(see the Yellow Alerts section below), they interrupt sleep and cause oxygen
levels to decrease further at night.

My husband and I disagree on whether taking a nap during the day is a good thing. Will napping interfere with getting a good night's sleep, or can it help us catch up on the sleep we need?

Naps are not intrinsically bad. We all have a "nap zone," usually after lunch, when we could easily fall asleep. This is due to circadian rhythms that cause us to feel the sleepiest between 1:00 and 3:00 p.m. (and between 2:00 and 4:00 a.m.) each day. Surprisingly, we may feel this way even if we don't eat a big lunch; our core body temperature drops, and we get sleepy at this time during the day. Countries that allow for a siesta recognize this natural rhythm, closing businesses in the afternoon and allowing people to nap and then go back to work later in the day.

Naps can help us regain our alertness or allay fatigue. They're fine so long as you're not turning to sleep because you're bored, taking sedating medications, or depressed. You also don't want to nap within two to three hours of your regular bedtime, as doing so can interfere with your sleep. Be sure to determine whether you need a nap because you're sleep deprived—if so, you need to be evaluated for conditions that interfere with sleep (see the Getting Evaluated for Sleep Concerns section below).

TABLE 10.1
Disorders That Interfere with Sleep

Symptoms or Conditions	Why Worse at Night?	What Can You Do?
Any pain: toothache, arthritis, muscle aches, etc.	Body position Lack of distraction	See chapter 13.
Skin disorders: itching, bug bites, allergies, medication reactions, or medical conditions such as kidney disease	Itching gets worse with dry skin. The hormone cortisol, which decreases itching, is at its lowest level at night. Skin gets drier because we urinate more and drink less at night, and circadian rhythm causes skin temperatures to be higher at night.	• Keep skin hydrated with moisturizer. • Drink more fluids. • Keep bedroom cool. • Use ice to help with itching. • Try nonprescription corticosteroid cream or spray if the area is inflamed. • Mentholated lotions may help. • See your health care provider if the reason for your itching is unclear and symptoms do not respond to the treatments above.

(continued)

TABLE 10.1 (*continued*)

Symptoms or Conditions	Why Worse at Night?	What Can You Do?
Shortness of breath or cough		
Heart failure	Lying down causes an increase in circulating fluid that can result in fluid entering the lungs, interfering with oxygen exchange and causing shortness of breath.	• Sitting up can help as a temporary measure, but doing so will cause you to have a less restorative sleep. Don't get used to sleeping in a chair. • Speak with your doctor about adjusting your medications to make it easier for you to breathe while lying down.
COPD or asthma	Oxygenation decreases when we lie down. With these conditions, lying down can further decrease oxygenation and cause airway secretions to collect, resulting in more shortness of breath and wheezing.	• Same as for heart failure. • If you use stimulant inhalers at night, they may keep you from sleeping. Speak with your doctor.
Allergies, postnasal drip	Bedroom allergies, such as to dust mites. Room may be very dry, especially when the heat is on in winter.	• Discuss allergy testing with your doctor. • Use a humidifier in the bedroom.
Medications	Depends on the medication.	• See table 10.3 for a list of medications that can cause cough.
Heartburn/GERD	Gravity helps food and drink move through the GI tract. When lying down, these can reflux into the esophagus and pharynx.	• See chapter 14. • Don't lie down within one or two hours of eating.
Other conditions		
Nighttime urination: urge incontinence, prostate enlargement, diuretics, leg swelling	See chapter 11.	See chapter 11.

TABLE 10.1 (*continued*)

Symptoms or Conditions	Why Worse at Night?	What Can You Do?
Numbness and tingling (pins and needles): nerve compression, CTS, neuropathy	Sleeping position puts pressure on nerves (feet fall asleep) and can compress nerves that are already compromised, as in CTS.	• Relieve the pressure by changing positions or using pillows. • Wrist splints can help with CTS. • Get an evaluation if you can't get comfortable or the numbness and tingling are present during the day.
Leg cramps: sudden painful muscle contractions in the leg or foot where you can feel the muscle hardening.	Unknown	• Pain is relieved by forcefully stretching the affected muscles to release the contraction and relieve pain. • Routine daily stretching exercises can decrease the occurrence and strength of the contractions.
Psychological concerns: anxiety, depression, worrying	Lack of distraction	• Write down your concerns before bed, or keep a notebook at bedside and jot them down if you wake up thinking about them, so you'll be able to remember them in the morning. • See chapter 8.

Note: Abbreviations are as follows: CTS, carpal tunnel syndrome; COPD, chronic obstructive pulmonary disease; GERD, gastroesophageal reflux disease; GI, gastrointestinal.

Adapting to Your New Normal

Many of my friends have developed difficulty sleeping as they age. What can I do to avoid having the same problem?

The first step to a good night's sleep is to establish a *healthy sleep routine*.

- Plan to sleep seven to eight hours nightly.
- Go to bed and wake up at about the same time every day to maintain your circadian rhythm.

- Exercise and get bright light or sunlight exposure daily. But don't exercise two to three hours before bed. Doing so will increase your core body temperature, which interferes with falling asleep.

- Stop caffeine intake, in any form, by early afternoon. Remember that there's lots of stealth caffeine in sodas, tea, chocolate, nonprescription medications, and energy drinks.

- Within two to three hours of bedtime, avoid heavy meals, alcohol, drinking lots of liquids, and taking a nap. Alcohol may initially make you sleepy, but as your body processes the alcohol, you may feel restless, interfering with your sleep. If hungry before bedtime, skip protein and have a light snack of carbohydrates or dairy products.

- Wear comfortable bedclothes.

- Keep your bedroom
  - *Cool* (if your feet are cold, wear socks).
  - *Quiet* (soothing sounds such as a white noise machine or a fan may be of benefit)
  - *Dark* (cover the light-emitting devices, use black-out shades, wear a mask to keep the light out of your eyes, buy the dimmest night-light possible).

I get into bed at a reasonable time, but I have a hard time falling asleep. I toss, turn, read, worry . . . everything but sleep. Then I'm exhausted the next day. What can I do to get a better night's sleep?

Maintaining a regular sleep schedule is important, but it's even more important that you don't go to bed if you're not sleepy. It may help to wind down with a hot bath, relaxation tape, glass of warm milk, or cup of chamomile tea. Take advantage of the fact that sleep comes when your core body temperature starts to decrease. Taking a long, warm bath or exercising moderately about three to four hours before bedtime will help. Avoid naps, or limit them to 30–60 minutes early in the afternoon. If thoughts or worries are keeping you awake, take some time early in the evening to write down your concerns, or keep a notebook at bedside and jot them down if you wake up thinking about them. Putting your worries on paper can reassure you that you'll remember them and take care of them when you are awake. The best time to think through life concerns is during the day, when your brain is fully functioning. If these suggestions don't work, discuss your sleep problems with your health care provider. There are multiple medical and psychological conditions that cause insomnia (table 10.1).

Life itself can get in the way of sleep, especially when there are major changes or decisions looming. These can consume your thoughts and energy, which may result in difficulty sleeping. Anxiety is the most common psychological condition associated with difficulty falling asleep and early awakening. It is particularly common in those who are caregivers. Sometimes insomnia is the first sign of depression, which can cause a delay in falling asleep, nighttime wakefulness, and early morning awakening where you can't get back to sleep. But this isn't true for all depression. Sometimes people who are depressed sleep much more than usual (see chapter 8).

I find I can't get back to sleep if I wake up to go to the bathroom, or for most any reason. I just lie in bed waiting for sleep to come. It's driving me crazy.

Don't stay in bed it you don't fall asleep within 15–20 minutes. Get out of bed and do something calming that won't get you excited or agitated, like listening to peaceful music, reading, doing relaxation exercises, or meditating. *Don't use the computer or tablet*—the blue light from the screen will only help keep you awake. *Don't try to fall asleep in a chair*—lying down is the best cue to your body that it's time to sleep. Only get back in bed when you're tired enough to sleep.

Some people with chronic insomnia begin to associate the bedroom with feeling anxious and alert rather than relaxed and calm. **Stimulus control therapy (SCT)** attempts to reassociate the bedroom with relaxation so that it becomes easier to fall asleep and stay asleep. The key here is to *use the bed only for sleep and sex, not arousing activities* like worrying, checking your phone, reading, or watching television. *Remember:* if you're not asleep in 20 minutes, get out of bed and do a soothing activity as described above.

Are sleeping medications as bad as everyone says they are? I've been taking them for years.

Sleeping medications can be a major bone of contention between patients and their doctors. Prescription sleeping pills like zolpidem (Ambien) and temazepam (Restoril) can help improve sleep quality, increase total sleep time, and decrease nighttime awakenings. But these benefits are fairly small and short-lived compared with the increased risks of these medications in older adults, including daytime sleepiness, cognitive impairment, agitation, confusion, problems with balance, and

an increased risk of falls and fractures. Other prescription drugs like mirtazapine (Remeron), trazodone (Desyrel), and amitriptyline (Elavil) are sometimes prescribed off-label for sleep, but their effectiveness is not proven, and they may have significant side effects, particularly amitriptyline.

The risks of all sleeping pills, whether prescription or over-the-counter, increase with aging, even if you've been taking them for years without problems (see chapter 3). Antihistamines like diphenhydramine, found in Benadryl, Tylenol PM, other "PM" medications, and doxylamine (Unisom, Nytol Maximum Strength) are nonprescription medications that are associated with the same risks as the prescription sleeping medications in older adults.

What about nonpharmacologic treatments for insomnia?

Cognitive behavioral therapy for insomnia (CBT-I) is the most effective treatment for chronic insomnia. CBT-I has no side effects and is more effective than medications. In CBT-I, misconceptions and maladaptive behaviors around sleep are identified and attempts made to change them through education and behavioral change. A critical part of CBT-I is *sleep restriction*, which involves initially limiting the amount of time in bed to the hours that you currently sleep. CBT-I improves sleep quality, and restriction makes it easier to fall asleep, stay asleep, and not wake up earlier than desired. Most people who take part in CBT-I won't need to take sleeping pills. There are trained therapists who can do CBT-I in person or by telephone; there are also effective Web-based courses (see the Resources section at the end of this chapter). SCT, discussed on page 165, is part of CBT-I, but it can also be done independently.

I used to go to sleep at 11:00 p.m. and get up at 7:00 a.m. Now I'm falling asleep at 7:00 p.m. and getting up for the day at 3:00 a.m. Even if I force myself to stay up until 9:00, I still wake up at 3:00. What's going on?

You may have a *circadian rhythm disorder*, a condition that can occur if you don't spend enough time exposed to bright light during the day. As mentioned above, it's not uncommon for older people to go to sleep earlier than when younger. But if you have a circadian rhythm disorder, your sleep changes are extreme, more than expected from normal aging alone. People who have a circadian rhythm disorder may be ready to go to sleep between 7:00 and 9:00 p.m. (or they may fall asleep while watching television or reading in the early evening), and then awaken for the day between 3:00 and 5:00 a.m. And staying up later doesn't help—they just become more sleep deprived. Some people have a different circadian rhythm disorder where they're not ready to go to sleep until very late at night and awaken later in the morning.

Exposure to bright light is the main treatment for circadian rhythm disorders. This can come from a morning walk outdoors, sitting by the windows or on a porch, or by using a light box. The optimal dose of light and exposure time when using a light box is not clear. Experts suggest the following.

- If you fall asleep very early (6:00–9:00 p.m.), try to get two hours of exposure to either sunlight (without sunglasses) or 30–60 minutes from a light box of 1,000–10,000 lux (the units for light intensity) during the late afternoon or early evening. The lower the light intensity, the longer you need to be in front of the light box. The light box should be at eye level and 1.5 to 2 feet away from you. Direct your gaze toward the box, but don't stare directly into it. Avoid bright light in the morning by wearing sunglasses; exposure to bright light in the morning will make you want to go to sleep even earlier in the evening.

- If you don't get sleepy until late at night and want to go to bed and wake up earlier, two hours of morning sunlight or 1,000–10,000 lux for 30–60 minutes upon awakening may help. Also, reduce evening light, especially the blue light that is emitted by computer screens.

There are behavioral approaches that can help gradually shift the biological clock by changing long-standing sleep patterns. *Melatonin* may be used as an adjunct to these. However, supplements are not regulated, so be sure you get one with a seal of approval (see the Resources section at the end of chapter 3) to be sure you're buying the real thing, or ask your health care provider for a prescription brand.

What Isn't Normal Aging?

 Red Flags: Symptoms Needing Prompt Medical Attention

- Excessive daytime sleepiness, including falling asleep when you're watching TV, sitting in a car stopped in traffic, or after eating lunch.
- A bed partner or family member shares concerns about your snoring or notes that you kick your legs or stop breathing during the night.
- Sleeping many more hours than usual.
- Having some daytime sleepiness along with any of these concerns:
  - Depression or irritability
  - Attention or concentration problems
  - Fatigue, malaise, lack of energy
  - Reduced motivation
  - Increased errors or accidents
  - Hyperactivity, impulsivity, or aggression

Note: These symptoms may happen occasionally and be totally normal. If they are happening often, though, you should be evaluated. See the Getting Evaluated for Sleep Concerns section below.

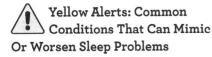 **Yellow Alerts: Common Conditions That Can Mimic Or Worsen Sleep Problems**

Medications

Some medications and supplements are stimulants that can make it difficult for you to fall asleep. Others interfere with sleep by increasing anxiety, nighttime urination, nightmares, coughing; interfering with normal stages of sleep; or exacerbating a primary sleep disorder (table 10.3). Review your medications with your health care provider, and discuss alternatives if you believe your medications may be affecting your ability to sleep.

 Don't stop sleeping medications cold turkey. **Sudden withdrawal can produce a rebound effect where your sleep and anxiety get much worse than they were before you were on the drugs. You can, however, with your health care provider's help, taper them slowly and successfully over time.**

Primary Sleep Disorders

Primary sleep disorders increase with age, but they're not "normal." As shown in table 10.2, there are four major types.

Obstructive Sleep Apnea

People with obstructive sleep apnea, or OSA, temporarily stop breathing (apnea) 5 to 30 times an hour, waking up each time they resume breathing. Usually they are not aware of these episodes. Blood oxygen decreases, and carbon dioxide accumulates over the course of the night. All of this results in sleep deprivation, daytime exhaustion and napping, morning headaches, poor memory, confusion, distractedness, and irritability. People with OSA are at increased risk for stroke, heart attack, irregular heart rhythms (arrhythmias), traffic accidents, repeated falls, cognitive impairment, and difficult-to-control high blood pressure.

In OSA, apnea results from the upper airway collapsing partially or completely during sleep. Although usually associated with obesity, which affects the airway's soft tissues, OSA in older adults is more often due to decreased muscle tone (another example of how everything sags as we age). Sleep apnea can also occur when your breathing muscles don't get the right signals from your brain. This is called central sleep apnea, and it is much less common than OSA and treated differently.

The mainstay of treatment for OSA is the use of a continuous positive airway pressure (CPAP) machine connected to a mask that is worn throughout the night. Many people are unwilling to try CPAP, concerned that they will look strange or ridiculous, or that it will interfere with their relationships with their bed partner or their comfort in bed. I've been using CPAP for more than 20 years and can testify that the masks keep getting more comfortable and less intrusive.

My CPAP Story

I was exhausted. I had to pull over to sleep after driving for about an hour, and I was spending three hours each weekend afternoon sleeping. Everything was an effort. I knew that I snored, and maybe even had periods where I stopped breathing. It wasn't until I took a trip with my cousin and she refused to share a room with me that I finally saw a sleep specialist. I did an overnight sleep study, was diagnosed with sleep apnea, and started using CPAP. Initially, I was embarrassed to be seen wearing it, but that quickly went away when I got my weekends back, could drive for hours without stopping to nap, and realized that I had added 20 additional hours of awake time each week by using the CPAP. Since then, my machine goes with me wherever I go.

If you find you really can't tolerate CPAP, work with your sleep doctor to identify some alternative ways to deal with OSA. Some less effective options include the following.

- Sleep on your side, not on your back. You may find it helpful to sew a pocket on the back of your pajama top and put a soft foam ball inside to help keep you from sleeping on your back.

- Avoid alcohol or sedatives.

- Exercise regularly.

- Discuss with your sleep doctor if you should try nighttime oxygen supplementation. This can sometimes reduce the apnea and increase oxygen saturation.

- If you are obese, consider weight loss or bariatric surgery.

- Discuss with your sleep doctor or dentist whether a mouth appliance may decrease your apnea.

Restless Legs Syndrome

The unpleasant and uncomfortable leg sensations that people with restless legs syndrome (RLS) feel occur mainly at night, or when at rest or inactive. These sensations and the urge to move improve with walking around.

RLS can be a sign of iron deficiency, kidney or neurological disease, arthri-

TABLE 10.2
Symptoms of Primary Sleep Disorders

Sleep Disorder	Symptoms
Obstructive sleep apnea (OSA)	Loud snoring, intermittent periods where breathing stops or there are gasping or choking sounds preceding an abrupt awakening from sleep.
Restless legs syndrome (RLS)	Uncontrollable urge to move legs, particularly at night. Abnormal feelings like pins and needles, itching, something crawling on the legs.
Periodic limb movement during sleep (PLMS)	Repetitive jerking leg movements where the foot or leg forcefully moves upward for a few seconds every 20–40 seconds.
REM sleep behavioral disorder (RBD)	Repeated episodes of acting out dreams through vocalization, hand gestures, thrashing, or kicking, lasting less than one minute.

tis, or vitamin or mineral deficiency, but most often no cause is identified. The condition can be aggravated by some medications used for nausea and vomiting, psychiatric medications (antidepressants, antipsychotics, and lithium), diphenhydramine (Benadryl), caffeine, alcohol, and beta-blockers.

There are medications that may help, but the first line of treatment for RLS is nonpharmacological.

- Improve your sleep habits, as described earlier in this chapter.

- Avoid caffeine, alcohol, and nicotine, and see if your symptoms improve.

- Exercise regularly.

- Apply counter-stimuli, such as rubbing your legs, taking a hot or cold bath, or using a whirlpool before sleep. The Relaxis vibrating pad has been shown to improve sleep quality in those with RLS. It requires a prescription and usually costs more than $500.

Periodic Limb Movements during Sleep

The jerking movements of periodic limb movements during sleep, or PLMS, occur hundreds of times during the night, and each causes a brief awakening. PLMS occurs in about 85 percent of people who have RLS. Treatment is similar. The common sudden jerking contractures of limbs that occur during the transition to, or shortly after, falling asleep are not PLMS. These are called *hypnic, or myoclonic, jerks*, are benign, and may decrease when caffeine is removed from the diet.

REM Sleep Behavioral Disorder

Because muscles lose their tone during rapid eye movement (REM) sleep, you don't act out your dreams. In REM sleep behavioral disorder, or RBD, muscles retain tone during REM sleep, and dreams are acted out with vocalizations and limb movements. These involuntary movements can be harmless, or

TABLE 10.3

Drugs That Can Cause Sleep Disturbances

Drugs and Examples	Effect	How to Minimize Effect
Blood pressure, cardiac, and diuretic medications		
Beta-blockers: metoprolol (Toprol); propranolol (Inderal); nadolol (Corgard); sotalol (Betapace, Sotylize, Sorine)	Daytime somnolence, difficulty falling asleep, increased awakenings, vivid dreams, or nightmares; exacerbation of RLS	Discuss changing medications with your prescriber.
	RBD	Don't take at bedtime.
Diuretics: hydrochlorothiazide; furosemide (Lasix); chlorthalidone (Hygroton)	Increased nighttime urination	Take last dose before 4:00 p.m.
	Leg cramps	Ask prescriber to check your magnesium and potassium levels.
ACE inhibitors: lisinopril (Zestril); enalapril (Vasotec); ramipril (Altace)	Cough	Discuss changing medications with your prescriber.
Statins: rosuvastatin (Crestor); atorvastatin (Lipitor); pravastatin (Pravachol); simvastatin (Zocor)	Leg cramps	May respond to lower doses; discuss with your doctor.
Nifedipine (Procardia)	Leg cramps	Discuss changing medications with your doctor.
Endocrine medications		
Thyroid hormones: levothyroxine (Synthroid); liothyronine (Cytomel)	Sleeplessness	Ask prescriber to check thyroid levels.
Corticosteroids: prednisone; dexamethasone (Decadron); methylprednisolone (Solu-Medrol)	Increased nighttime wakefulness (common with prednisone)	Discuss dose with your doctor. Do not stop abruptly; taper the dose slowly.
	Withdrawal: insomnia, vivid dreams, anxiety, irritability, tiredness	
Hypoglycemics: glipizide (Glucotrol); glyburide (Micronase); pioglitizone (Actos); insulin	Low blood sugar, causing anxiety and awakening	Discuss medications with your doctor.

TABLE 10.3 *(continued)*

Drugs and Examples	Effect	How to Minimize Effect
Pulmonary medications		
Aminophylline, theophylline	Sleeplessness	Discuss time of last dose with your doctor.
Bronchodilators: albuterol (Ventolin, ProAir, Proventil); terbutaline	Sleeplessness when used at bedtime	Speak with your doctor about other rescue inhalers that can be used in the evening.
	Leg cramps	Ask your provider to check your magnesium and potassium levels.
Neurological, psychological, and sleep medications		
Chronic antianxiety or sleeping medications: diazepam (Valium); lorazepam (Ativan); clonazepam (Klonopin); zolpidem (Ambien); eszopiclone (Lunesta)	Can cause fragmented sleep **Withdrawal**: insomnia, vivid dreams, anxiety, irritability, tiredness, RBD	Speak with your provider about slow taper of medication. Do not stop abruptly; taper the dose slowly.
SSRI and SNRI antidepressants: paroxetine (Paxil); escitalopram (Lexapro); citalopram (Celexa); duloxetine (Cymbalta); venlafaxine (Effexor)	**Withdrawal**: insomnia, vivid dreams, anxiety, irritability, tiredness RBD	Do not stop abruptly; taper the dose slowly. May occur when starting medication.
Other antidepressants: particularly protriptyline (Vivactil); fluoxetine (Prozac); bupropion (Wellbutrin); and venlafaxine (Effexor)	Sleeplessness Exacerbation of RLS	Discuss changing medications with your doctor.
Antipsychotics: haloperidol (Haldol); risperidone (Risperdal); lithium (Eskalith, Lithobid)	Exacerbation of RLS	Discuss changing medications with your doctor.
Anti-Parkinsonian medications: Sinemet; bromocriptine (Parlodel); ropinirole (Requip); pramipexole (Mirapex)	Can induce nightmares and impair sleep	Discuss changing medications with your doctor.

(continued)

TABLE 10.3 *(continued)*

Drugs and Examples	Effect	How to Minimize Effect
COMT inhibitors: tolcapone (Tasmar); entacapone (Comtan)	Leg cramps	Discuss changing medications with your doctor.
CNS stimulants: caffeine, methylphenidate (Ritalin); dexamphetamine (Dexedrine, Zenzedi); modafinil (Provigil)	Sleeplessness Exacerbation of RLS	Don't use in the afternoon or evening. Taper and stop medication.
Dementia medications: donepezil (Aricept)	Can induce nightmares and impair sleep Leg cramps RBD	May improve with lower dose (may also affect drug's effectiveness). Discuss switching to galantamine (Razadyne) or rivastigmine (Exelon). Don't take at bedtime.

Others

Alcohol	May initially cause drowsiness but can impair sleep later in the night Exacerbation of RLS **Withdrawal**: RBD	
Decongestants: pseudoephedrine (Sudafed Sinus) and phenylephrine (SudafedPE); oxymetazoline (Afrin, Dristan)	Sleeplessness	Don't use in the afternoon or evening.
Diphenhydramine (Benadryl)	Exacerbation of RLS	
Antinausea and vomiting: droperidol	Exacerbation of RLS	

Note: If you're not sure whether a drug you're taking is in one of the drug classes listed, ask your pharmacist or health care provider. Abbreviations are as follows: ACE, angiotensin-converting enzyme; CNS, central nervous system; COMT, catechol-O-methyltransferase; RBD, REM sleep behavioral disorder; RLS, restless legs syndrome; SSRI, selective serotonin reuptake inhibitor.

they can injure a bed partner or the person with RBD, including falling out of bed. Movements look meaningful; vocalizations may be loud or profane.

RBD is common in people with Parkinson's disease and some other neurodegenerative diseases. RBD may predate symptoms of Parkinson's by months to many years. Antidepressants, beta-blockers, and cholinesterase inhibitors taken in the evening or before sleep may precipitate RBD (table 10.3). Treatment starts with slowly decreasing the dose of precipitating medications. Many people with RBD respond to higher doses of melatonin.

Symptoms and Disorders That Worsen at Night

At night there's not much to distract us from our pains, concerns, or itches, all of which can feel more intense when we're trying to get to sleep. Certain pains get worse with lying down, and some are caused by our sleeping positions (see table 10.1). Lying down also decreases blood oxygen levels and causes fluid that has entered our tissues during the day (for example, swollen legs or, in those with heart failure, the lungs) to reenter circulation, increasing urination. Recognizing and treating these conditions can improve your sleep.

Sleep Disorders in People Living with Dementia

About 25–33 percent of people with dementia have difficulty sleeping. Their sleep tends to be lighter, with more arousals, fragmentation, circadian rhythm disorders, nighttime wandering, and agitation. It's particularly important to make sure that a person with dementia is not being kept awake by symptoms that she can't communicate, particularly pain. Increasing daytime social interactions and physical activity, and decreasing nighttime noise and light may help. In those living with dementia, melatonin has been shown to improve circadian rhythm problems. People living with dementia may also have primary sleep disorders.

- Consider RLS if you see the person rubbing or massaging their legs, pacing more, or wandering, especially if these behaviors occur mainly in the evening or when inactive and improve with leg movement.

- OSA patients with mild to moderate dementia can tolerate CPAP, possibly benefiting their cognition.

- Sleep and behavior problems may be signs of circadian rhythm disorders and may respond to sunlight or bright light containing 1,000–10,000 lux (see the discussion of circadian rhythm disorders on page 166).

Getting Evaluated for Sleep Concerns

Do you have problems falling or staying asleep, or do you awaken feeling unrefreshed? Do you have overwhelming bouts of sleepiness during the day that interfere with activities you'd like to do? Have people complained about your snoring, or that during sleep your breathing is irregular or that you kick? Do you have symptoms that force you to awaken during the night? If so, you should discuss your concerns with your health care provider.

Remember, you're not the only one your sleep problems affect—your bed partner, family, and friends may end up suffering along with you. You may be cranky, have difficulty concentrating, and be unable to spend quality time with them because you are tired. People who live with you may become sleep deprived. An evaluation might help both of you, resulting in ways to improve both your sleep and your relationship.

Should I See a Specialist?

Most primary care doctors and geriatricians are skilled at identifying the medical and psychological factors that can interfere with a good night's sleep, including medications, unrelieved pain, and other symptoms. If your sleep doesn't improve with the measures discussed in this chapter, or if there is concern that you might have a primary sleep disorder, they can refer you to a sleep specialist. These doctors can be board certified in pulmonary medicine, neurology, internal medicine, or psychiatry. If your primary care provider or specialist is concerned that you might have OSA, RLS, or PLMS, she may have you spend a night in a sleep laboratory to undergo a sleep study (polysomnography), where your breathing, brain waves, and muscle tone will be monitored as you sleep. Sometimes it is possible to be evaluated for OSA with a home machine, or to wear a wrist activity monitor to estimate when you go to sleep and wake up to identify circadian rhythm disorders. A sleep specialist may also be able to refer you for CBT-I training.

Preparing for the Visit

Keep a sleep log (table 10.4) for a week or two before the appointment. A sleep log provides valuable information about your sleep patterns, particularly whether you have difficulty falling asleep, wake up too early, or have habits or symptoms that could be modified to improve your sleep. Fill out the chapter 10 pre-visit checklist on page 378 in Appendix 3, bring it to your appointment, and review it with your provider. Ask your family or nighttime companions whether you snore, breathe irregularly or stop breathing, or kick during the night. Bring all medications you take to the appointment; include over-the-counter medications and the supplements and vitamins you get from the health food or drug store.

At your appointment, your health care provider will review your sleep log, medications, and your answers to the questions in the checklist. She will also conduct a physical exam, screen for depression or cognitive impairment, and may order blood work. If possible, bring someone to the appointment who can describe your sleep—we are often not aware of our own breathing or other behaviors during the night. Recognize that it may take some time to make the changes needed to improve your sleep.

Advice for Loved Ones

Depending on whether you live together, share a bed or bedroom, or live apart, the sleep problems of the older person in your life will affect you differently. Your own sleep quality may be impaired, and you or your loved one may be sleep deprived, irritable, or easily triggered. You need to take care of yourself. This may require sleeping in separate beds or separate bedrooms—a difficult change at this point in life, but one that is necessary if you're not getting good sleep yourself. Encourage the older adult to adopt behaviors that might improve sleep (see "Adapting to Your New Normal" above) and to get help for symptoms that interfere with sleep. Try to stay away from the easy fixes, like asking for sleeping medications.

For people living with dementia, especially those unable to verbalize their distress, it is important to search for cues and clues that they may be having symptoms like pain that interfere with their sleep. It is important to work with health care providers and aides to identify the underlying reasons for sleep problems, as nighttime restlessness and wandering are often what drives families to place their loved one in a nursing home or other institution. Sometimes caregivers may put someone to bed at 6:00 or 7:00 p.m. because it's convenient or the person seems tired. Remember, it's unlikely that they will sleep for 12 or 14 hours, and they may get up and wander. Try some of the suggestions in this chapter to help improve sleep.

Bottom Line

A good night's sleep for an adult is usually seven to eight hours, but as we age, it can be hard to achieve because of difficulty falling asleep, staying asleep, or recurrent brief awakenings during the night. Poor sleep and sleep deprivation can result in daytime exhaustion, irritability, and even falls, injuries, or worsening cognition. Healthy sleep routines, understanding what can make sleep better and worse, and determining whether you have a primary sleep disorder can help you get a better night's sleep. Work with your health care providers to address possible factors interfering with your sleep. Also, check out some of the resources on behavioral interventions at the end of the chapter, including CBT-I.

TABLE 10.4
Daily Sleep Log

	Date						
	Fill out before you go to sleep						
Did you nap? If yes, for how long?							
What time of day?							
Did you exercise? If yes, for how long?							
What time of day?							
Did you get exposure to bright light or sunlight? If yes, for how long?							
What time of day?							
How many caffeinated beverages did you drink?							
What time of day was the last one?							
What time did you get into bed to go to sleep?							
Within two to three hours of bedtime, did you:							
Eat a heavy meal?							

TABLE 10.4 (*continued*)

Date							
Drink alcohol?							
Take a nap?							
Exercise?							
Fill out upon awakening							
What time did you wake up?							
What time did you get out of bed for the day?							
Did you wake up feeling tired?							
How many times did you wake up during the night?							
Were you able to easily get back to sleep?							
Did you stay in bed for more than 20 minutes if you couldn't fall asleep?							
Did you take something for sleep?							
Note medication, dose, and time.							

CBT-I

CBT-I Provider Directory
(https://www.med.upenn.edu/cbti
/provder_directory.html)
The Perelman School of Medicine at the
University of Pennsylvania has a directory
of self-identified providers of CBT-I that
can be searched by state.

CBT for Insomnia
(https://www.cbtforinsomnia.com
/about-us/)
Dr. Gregg D. Jacobs, a behavioral sleep
specialist, offers (for a fee) a five-week
online CBT-I program.

Stress and Relaxation Resources

*National Center for Complementary and
Integrative Health*
(https://www.nccih.nih.gov/health
/sleep-disorders-in-depth)
This website offers information on stress
and relaxation techniques, as well as on the

usefulness of complementary approaches
for improving sleep.

Elder, J. D. "Meditation on Body with Music."
Dropbox audio, 34:37. https://www.dropbox
.com/s/t12vig8wm8sj60z/01%20ELDER
%20Track%201_1.mp3?dl=0.

Elder, J. D. "Meditation on Body without
Music." Dropbox audio, 26:40. https://www
.dropbox.com/s/x7qwx3gl5cmw431/02
%20ELDER%20Track%202_1.mp3?dl=0.

"Jon Kabat Zinn Body Scan Meditation."
YouTube video, 45:27. July 18, 2016.
https://youtu.be/u4gZgnCy5ew.

Matza, Deborah. "Body Scan." Dropbox
audio, 10:13. https://www.dropbox.com/s
/ozkopxsw8lg1fl8/01%20MATZA%20
Track%201_1.mp3?dl=0.

See the Resources section at the end of
chapter 8 for meditation resources and
how to find mental health professionals
for older adults.

BIBLIOGRAPHY

Boulos, M. I., T. Trevor, and T. Kendzerska.
"Normal Polysomnography Parameters in
Healthy Adults: A Systematic Review and
Meta-Analysis," *Lancet Respiration Medicine* 7, no. 6 (2019): 533–43.

Hood, S., and S. Amir. "The Aging Clock:
Circadian Rhythms and Later Life." *Journal
of Clinical Investigation* 127, no. 2 (2017):
437–46.

CHAPTER 11

Urine Trouble

Sorry for the play on words, but one of life's ironies is that as you age, you often do feel like you're "in trouble" when it comes to your ability to control when and where you urinate. Most of us haven't concerned ourselves with this since we were toddlers, but worrying about having an accident can interfere with your daily life, causing you to think twice about leaving the house or doing activities you love. Having to go multiple times during the night can cause sleep deprivation.

For reasons discussed below and in box 11.2, all older adults are more vulnerable to developing *incontinence* (urine loss) and *nocturia* (getting up at night to urinate). These are *geriatric*

syndromes (see chapter 2) that occur when a vulnerable person is exposed to one or more precipitating factors. For this reason, the line between normal and not normal is blurred when it comes to aging and urination.

This chapter explains the age-related changes that increase vulnerability to developing urinary frequency, incontinence, and nocturia. It also provides information and strategies on how to prevent or reduce these problems, and discusses medical evaluations for these concerns.

For an overview of the anatomy of the urinary system, urine flow, and bladder control, see box 11.1.

What's Normal with Aging?

For a deeper dive into age-related changes in urine production, bladder function and control, and the prostate, see box 11.2.

I was asked to give a urine sample at my Medicare annual wellness visit. After the visit, my medical provider called to tell me I had a urinary tract infection and prescribed antibiotics. I felt fine and didn't have any urinary symptoms. Is this typical for older people?

Asymptomatic bacteriuria occurs when bacteria are present in a urine sample, but the person doesn't have symptoms of a urinary tract infection (see box 11.2). This is normal in many in older adults and should not be treated with antibiotics unless there are urinary symptoms. Urine studies should not be done unless an older adult has symptoms or there is a need to check the urine for other substances, such as protein, blood, or glucose.

BOX 11.1

Urination 101

Urine is made in the kidney and then flows through the ureters and into the bladder, where it is stored (see the figure below). Urine leaves the body through the urethra, which is opened and closed by the sphincters, voluntary muscles within the urethra and the pelvic floor. In men, the prostate sits between the bladder and the penis, and the urethra runs through the center of the prostate and the penis. In women, the urethra is much shorter and ends in the vulva (female external genitalia).

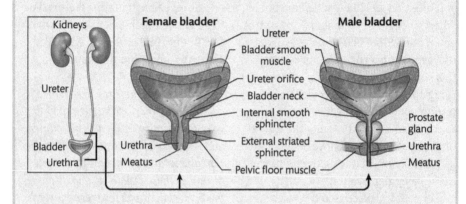

Bladder control depends on coordination between the muscles and nerves of the urinary system and the brain. The key structures involved in urination and its control are the bladder, urethra, internal and external urethral sphincters, pelvic floor muscles (see the figure above), and of course the brain and spinal cord. Think of the bladder as a muscular balloon that stores urine, and the urethra as the flexible pipe that drains it. The bladder muscle remains relaxed as the bladder fills with urine. The muscles of the bladder neck—also known as the internal *sphincter*—remain closed, and the separate muscles of the external sphincter contract to prevent urine from leaking through the urethra. When the bladder is full, nerve signals pass this information to the brain, which then signals the bladder to contract and the internal and external sphincters to relax, allowing urine to exit the body. For both men and women, the external sphincter is within the pelvic floor muscles and is under voluntary control, meaning you can learn to contract and relax it to help control urination.

A full bladder triggers a reflex for the bladder to contract. Toilet training teaches us to inhibit this reflex—the brain overrides it, and urination is delayed. As the bladder continues to fill, it sends messages to the brain that it's going to need to empty soon. To stay dry, these messages need to be recognized, and you need to get to a toilet. You can disregard these messages to a point, but if bladder volume or pressure is too high, the reflex will fire, and you'll urinate, whether you want to or not.

BOX 11.2

What Happens with Aging: A Deeper Dive

Your urine tests may suggest you have a urinary tract infection (UTI) when you don't.
The urine of 10 percent of community-dwelling older men, 20 percent of community-dwelling women, and 50 percent of people who live in nursing homes contains bacteria, even in people who have no symptoms of a UTI. This is called *asymptomatic bacteriuria.* Antibiotics have no benefit here, and in fact they can cause bacteria to become antibiotic-resistant, making the infection harder to eradicate if the person does develop a symptomatic UTI. Antibiotics are indicated for people with bacteria in the urine if they also have symptoms like new or worsening urgency, incontinence, frequency, pain with urination, or blood in the urine.

For the reasons below, incontinence and nocturia are more common.

You need to urinate more often.
As we age, the urge to void may be triggered by lower urine volumes than when we were younger. Additionally, the bladder may not fully empty when you urinate because its flow is impeded by weakened bladder muscles and age-related conditions, including (1) an enlarged prostate (see below), (2) impaired vaginal supports that cause the uterus or bladder to fall (prolapse) into the vagina, and (3) severe constipation. This means it will take less time after you've urinated for your bladder to fill up and you again feel the need to urinate.

You feel sudden intense urges to urinate.
These sudden urges come from *uninhibited bladder contractions (UBCs)*, bladder spasms that come without warning and cause you to feel an urgent need to void. Exactly why older adults have more UBCs is not clear. One reason is that the older brain is more sensitive to bladder sensations and produces UBCs in response to bladder irritants like an infection or a stone. UBCs can also be triggered by changing position, hearing running water, going out in the cold, or getting close to a bathroom.

Laughing can lead to accidents.
For many older adults, "I laughed till I peed" isn't hyperbole. Pelvic floor muscles and sphincters weaken with age, losing their ability to stop urine that has leaked out of the bladder from leaving the body. Age-related conditions such as chronic constipation, general deconditioning, menopause, childbearing, and prostate removal can also weaken these muscles.

You urinate more during the night.
Both UBCs and incomplete emptying contribute to an increase in nocturia, the need to urinate at night. In addition, however, there is a decrease in the nighttime secretion of antidiuretic hormone (ADH). ADH decreases urine volume by

(continued)

BOX 11.2 *(continued)*

increasing the amount of fluid reabsorbed by the kidney. In younger people, ADH is released mainly at night, and thus urination occurs primarily during the day. This doesn't occur in older people, resulting in a greater proportion of their urine output occurring during the night.

Getting to the toilet takes more time.
Gait speed slows, and hand and finger dexterity may decrease, so it takes longer to manipulate buttons and zippers, and to pull down undergarments.

Prostates enlarge.
In men, the prostate enlarges with aging, a process called benign prostatic hyperplasia (BPH). The enlarged prostate can impinge on and narrow the urethra. As a result, the bladder has to generate a higher pressure to start urination, and the bladder thickens and at times weakens. This is one of the reasons the bladder may not empty completely. Urgency occurs because these bladder changes precipitate UBCs, triggering frequency and increased nighttime urination. These changes also can cause hesitancy at the start of urination, a weak stream that stops and starts, and dribbling at the end of urination.

I feel like the ads on TV. I've "gotta go, gotta go," and I'm worried that I'm going to have an embarrassing accident. My life is beginning to revolve around figuring out where the closest bathroom is, watching how much I drink, and crossing my legs so that I can get to the bathroom on time. Don't tell me this is part of normal aging!

Aging increases the likelihood of urinary leakage, accidents, and having to get up at night to urinate. Some of these symptoms are due to age-related changes, and some are due to lifestyle, medical conditions, or medications. As discussed in the next section, this doesn't mean there's nothing you can do about it.

With aging, the bladder contractions you learned to inhibit with toilet training come back, sometimes with a vengeance, pelvic floor muscles and sphincters weaken, bladder capacity decreases, you urinate more at night than during the day, prostates enlarge, and you move more slowly, so you may not be able to get to the toilet on time. Each of these alone may not affect your ability to control your urine, but in combination they can cause urinary symptoms and incontinence.

Lifestyle changes can prevent or reduce urinary urgency, frequency, leakage, and nocturia, regardless of the underlying bladder condition. Continence products like pads and underwear can help, but they shouldn't replace making lifestyle changes or seeing a medical provider to figure out why you are having urinary problems and what else might be done about them.

I'm a 70-year-old woman who used to sleep soundly through the night. Now I get up several times each night to urinate. Is there something wrong with me?

As we age, we eliminate more fluid at night than during the day (see box 11.2 for more details). Some of this is due to age-related changes in physiology, and some is due to conditions that are more common with aging. The result is that most older people get up once or twice a night to urinate, but some are up far more often. If the need to urinate is interfering with your sleep, see the discussion on nocturia on page 194.

If I drink less, will I have less of a problem with leakage, frequency, and getting up at night?

Unfortunately, if you drink less, you'll be trading one problem for another. It's understandable that the first thing many people do when incontinence or frequency become a problem is to drink less in order to make less urine. The problem is that reducing your liquid intake can lead to unintended consequences like dehydration, falling, constipation, dry skin and mouth, getting confused, and feeling weak. Staying hydrated yet continent requires some skills and determination that will be discussed in this chapter's next section.

Do all older men develop urinary problems from prostate enlargement? Could my urinary symptoms be due to prostate cancer?

No, and really unlikely. The prostate does enlarge in all men as they age, a condition called benign prostatic hyperplasia (BPH), but only about 50 percent develop clinical symptoms. See the Yellow Alerts below for more on BPH. An enlarged prostate causes the part of the urethra that passes through the prostate to narrow and causes symptoms of obstruction, including urge. Prostate cancer, however, usually occurs in portions of the prostate away from the urethra and so *rarely causes urinary symptoms.*

Adapting to Your New Normal

⟨CAUTION⟩ If you have *new-onset incontinence* (the involuntary leakage of urine) or *bothersome nighttime urination*, get an initial medical evaluation, as discussed later in this chapter.

Are there things I can do to help me avoid urine troubles?

There are several steps you can take to make it less likely that you'll have an accident.

Don't Wait to Urinate

Some people delay going until their bladders are so full that any movement sets off a bladder contraction or overcomes their ability to keep their urethra closed, resulting in leakage. Repeatedly delaying urination can also cause the bladder to become overstretched and weaker over time. If you are incontinent, even occasionally, it may help to void every two to four hours whether you feel the need or not. This will also decrease the amount of urine spilled if you do have an accident.

Avoid Constipation

Hard stool can push against the urethra and cause it to narrow or close, decreasing or even stopping urine flow. For more information, see chapter 14.

Simplify Toileting

Slow walking speeds and poor balance can make it more difficult to get to the toilet in time. Improve your mobility through physical therapy and walking aids (see chapter 9 and Appendix 2), alter your environment to make it easier and safer to get to the bathroom, and use equipment to help with toileting (bedside commodes, urinals, high toilet seat, or grab rails around the toilet) and undressing (Velcro attachments).

Review Your Medications and the Time of Day You Take Them

Ask your medical provider if any of your medications could be contributing to your urine troubles (see table 11.1). You may need to change medications or adjust the dosage or schedule.

Could something I eat or drink cause me to need to urinate more frequently?

Absolutely! Some fluids are diuretics, causing you to urinate more, and some foods and fluids irritate the lining of the bladder, causing increased frequency, urgency, and incontinence.

Fluids

- Alcohol.
- Caffeinated beverages, including coffee, tea, energy drinks, colas.

- Acidic fluids like juice, alcohol, and caffeinated beverages. Try decaffeinated drinks, low-acid coffees, and non-citrus herbal teas instead.
- Carbonated liquids, such as fizzy soft drinks, club soda, seltzer, and sparkling waters may irritate sensitive bladders.

Foods

- Caffeine
- Chocolate
- Citrus fruits and juice
- Spicy foods
- Artificial sweeteners
- Uncooked onions
- Condiments that contain acid, such as soy sauce, vinegar, ketchup, mayonnaise
- Processed foods with artificial flavors, preservatives, monosodium glutamate (MSG), and benzyl alcohol

If you think a certain food might be setting off your symptoms, remove it from your diet for a while and see if your symptoms improve. Then slowly add small amounts back to see if the symptom recurs.

It feels like I'm not totally emptying my bladder. I often leak or need to go again soon after urinating. Is there anything I can do about this?

There is. It's called *double voiding*. Incomplete emptying results in urine remaining in the bladder despite having just urinated. If you are unable to empty your bladder completely, tell your medical provider so that he can make sure there's not another reason for the problem.

TABLE 11.1

Medications That Can Cause Urinary Incontinence

Drugs and Examples	Stress	Urge	Overflow	Nocturia	Functional
Blood pressure, cardiac, and diuretic medications					
ACE inhibitors that cause cough: enalapril (Vasotec); lisinopril (Prinivil, Zestril); ramipril (Altace)	X				
Alpha-blockers: doxazosin (Cardura); Terazosin (Hytrin)	X*				
Calcium channel blockers: amlodipine (Norvasc); nifedipine (Procardia); diltiazem (Cardizem); verapamil (Calan)			X	X†	
Diuretics: hydrochlorothiazide (Microzide); furosemide (Lasix)		X		X	
Pain relief					
GABA-ergic neurogenic pain medications: gabapentin (Neurontin); pregabalin (Lyrica)				X†	
NSAIDs: indomethacin (Indocin); ibuprofen (Motrin, Advil); naproxen (Naprosyn, Aleve)				X†	
Opioid analgesics: morphine; oxycodone (in Percocet); hydrocodone (in Vicodin); tramadol (Ultram)			X		
Muscle relaxants: cyclobenzaprine (Flexeril); methocarbamol (Robaxin)			X		
Neurological, psychological, and sleep medications					
Antianxiety and sleep medications: alprazolam (Xanax); clonazepam (Klonopin); triazolam (Halcion); zolpidem (Ambien); zaleplon (Sonata)	X				X
Tertiary tricyclic antidepressants: amitriptyline (Elavil); imipramine (Tofranil); doxepin (Silenor)			X		
SNRIs: venlafaxine (Effexor); duloxetine (Cymbalta)			X		
Antipsychotics: haloperidol (Haldol); thioridazine (Mellaril); olanzapine (Zyprexa); quetiapine (Seroquel)			X		X

(continued)

TABLE 11.1 (*continued*)

Drugs and Examples	Stress	Urge	Overflow	Nocturia	Functional
Cholinesterase inhibitors for dementia: donepezil (Aricept); rivastigmine (Exelon); galantamine (Razadyne)		X			
Cold, allergy, and itch medications					
First-generation antihistamines: diphenhydramine (Benadryl); chlorpheniramine (Aller-Chlor, Chlor-Trimeton); hydroxyzine (Atarax)			X		
Decongestants: pseudoephedrine (Sudafed Sinus); phenylephrine (Sudafed PE); oxymetazoline (Afrin, Dristan)			X		
Hormones					
Estrogen (oral, transdermal)	X				
Corticosteroids: prednisone, dexamethasone (Decadron); methylprednisolone (Solu-Medrol)				X†	
Thyroid medication: thyroxine (Synthroid)				X	
Urinary medications					
BPH alpha-blockers: terazosin (Hytrin); alfuzosin (Uroxatral); tamsulosin (Flomax)	X				
Bladder relaxants: tolteradine (Detrol); oxybutinin (Ditropan); solifenacin (Vesicare)			X‡		
Other medications					
Alcohol	X			X	X
Anticholinergics (see table 3.2 for list)			X		
Thiazolidinediones for diabetes: pioglitazone (Actos); rosiglitazone (Avandia)				X†	

Note: If you're not sure whether a drug you're taking is in one of the drug classes listed, ask your pharmacist or health care provider. Abbreviations are as follows: ACE, angiotensin-converting enzyme; BPH, benign prostatic hyperplasia; CNS, central nervous system; GABA, gamma amino butyric acid; NSAID, nonsteroidal anti-inflammatory drug; SNRI, serotonin-norepinephrine reuptake inhibitor.

*Causes stress incontinence in women (used to treat overflow in men).

†Increases fluid retention, causing increased urination.

‡Causes overflow incontinence in men (used to treat urge incontinence).

Instructions for Double Voiding

Both men and women should sit for a few minutes after urinating, then try to void again. Lean forward and backward. You may find that the sound of running water or softly stroking the area of your lower back above the buttock crease will get the urine to start flowing again.

My mouth feels dry at night, so I'm drinking a lot of water. I then need to get up several times a night to urinate. I'm getting really sleep deprived. Any thoughts on what might help?

Dry mouth itself may benefit from artificial saliva sprays or discs. See if one of the treatments below helps to decrease your nightly fluid intake.

- Avoid tobacco and alcohol, including mouthwash that contains alcohol.
- Discuss your medications and dosages with your medical provider to see if there are substitutes for those that can cause dry mouth, like anticholinergics (see table 3.2) and some blood pressure and anticonvulsant medications.
- Consider using a humidifier, especially during the winter, when your heating system may make your home more dry.
- Mouth breathing causes dry mouth. Find out if you have nasal congestion or obstructive sleep apnea (see chapter 10).
- You may lose fluid if you sweat heavily at night. Sweating is usually caused by the use of bed clothes or covers that are too heavy or sleeping in an overheated bedroom. Keep

your bedroom temperature cool. If the sweating persists, discuss with your medical provider.

I'm a 55-year-old man who doesn't have any prostate problems, but my father and uncle both needed procedures for benign prostatic hyperplasia. Is there anything I can do to reduce my chances of following in their footsteps?

The rate of prostate growth is dependent on many things other than age, including hormone levels and genetics. The risk of BPH is much greater in those who are obese, and the prostates of obese men are less responsive to 5-alpha reductase inhibitors, medications like finasteride that decrease the size of the prostate. Some studies have suggested that smoking can also increase the risk BPH. Physical activity decreases the risk of BPH. So, what can you do? Stop smoking, be physically active, and, if you are overweight, try to lose weight.

Incontinence

All incontinence is not the same. Knowing the *type(s) of incontinence* you have will inform you about the options that exist to improve your control. Use the figure on page 188 to identify which type best fits your symptoms: stress, urge, mixed, overflow, or functional.

Each type of incontinence is a different geriatric syndrome, with its own predisposing and precipitating factors. Some of these factors are not part of normal aging and may need additional medical evaluation.

Two important provisos to remember as you begin to better understand and treat your incontinence:

- *Medications* cause all sorts of urinary symptoms, so be sure these aren't contributing to your problems before adding still another to your list. See table 11.1.

- *Behavioral treatments—including pelvic floor exercises, or Kegels, and urge suppression techniques—are worth learning to do properly.* They are effective in about 75 percent of patients with urge, stress, and mixed incontinence. Even a year after prostatectomy, men who do pelvic floor

and urge suppression exercises are able to decrease their incontinence episodes by half.

Stress Incontinence

Every time I am out with my friends and we get to laughing, I feel myself lose a little urine. Why does this happen?

Coughing, sneezing, straining, laughing, changing position, or exerting yourself are all actions that increase pressure on your bladder. If your urethral sphincters and pelvic floor

Of the following, when are you most likely to leak urine? (check only one)

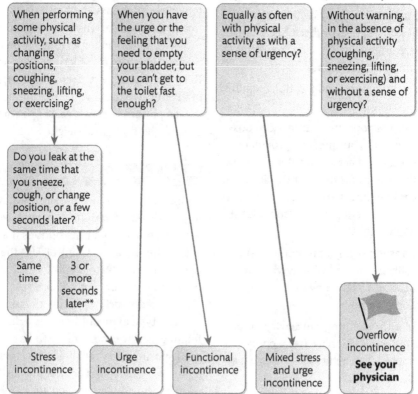

When performing some physical activity, such as changing positions, coughing, sneezing, lifting, or exercising?

When you have the urge or the feeling that you need to empty your bladder, but you can't get to the toilet fast enough?

Equally as often with physical activity as with a sense of urgency?

Without warning, in the absence of physical activity (coughing, sneezing, lifting, or exercising) and without a sense of urgency?

Do you leak at the same time that you sneeze, cough, or change position, or a few seconds later?

Same time

3 or more seconds later**

Overflow incontinence
See your physician

Stress incontinence

Urge incontinence

Functional incontinence

Mixed stress and urge incontinence

**These maneuvers trigger a UBC that causes you to void a few seconds later

Types of urinary incontinence. Adapted from J. S. Brown, C. S. Bradley, L. L. Subak, et al., "The Sensitivity and Specificity of a Simple Test to Distinguish between Urge and Stress Urinary Incontinence," Annals of Internal Medicine 144, no. 10 (2006): 716

muscles aren't strong enough to stop it, you'll leak small amounts of urine. With stress incontinence (SI), urine leaks within a second or two of these actions. If it takes longer, you're probably triggering an uninhibited bladder contraction (UBC), and you have urge incontinence (see below). With urge incontinence, the amount of urine leaked is much greater than with stress incontinence.

Precipitating Factors for Stress Incontinence

Medications like antianxiety drugs, sleeping medications, and oral estrogen decrease urinary sphincter and urethral tone, leading to increased leakage when you cough, sneeze, and the like.

Chronic cough—which can be caused by smoking, chronic obstructive pulmonary disease (COPD), asthma, gastroesophageal reflux disease (GERD), postnasal drip, and medications—can contribute to incontinence. In particular, angiotensin-converting enzyme (ACE) inhibitors, commonly used to treat high blood pressure and other cardiac concerns, can cause chronic cough. Ask your doctor for help if coughing is making your SI worse.

Being overweight can also be a factor in incontinence. Studies have shown weight loss to be effective at decreasing SI, especially for women under 75.

Treatments for Incontinence

Behavioral treatments include strengthening the pelvic floor muscles, such as with Kegel exercises. These exercises take 5–10 minutes a day and can be done anywhere. I do them in the car

whenever I'm stopped at a traffic light, and I tell my New York City patients they can do them on the subway and no one's the wiser. For a step-by-step guide to Kegel exercises for both men and women, see box 11.3. *Hint:* Doing a pelvic floor muscle contraction before an activity like standing up, which can cause SI, will decrease leakage.

Medications are currently not approved in the United States to treat SI.

Surgical treatments may be indicated if behavioral treatments aren't effective or your quality of life is severely compromised. See a urologist or gynecologist to discuss the pros and cons of surgery.

Urge Incontinence

I see ads all the time for overactive bladder. Is this the same as urge incontinence?

Overactive bladder (OAB) is the term used to describe the overwhelming sense of urgency that comes from an uninhibited bladder contraction. *Urge incontinence* happens when you can't stop urine from flowing after a UBC. The contraction empties the bladder, so the volume of urine lost can be substantial.

Precipitating Factors for Urge Incontinence

Medical conditions that irritate the bladder or genitals can increase UBCs, resulting in urge incontinence. Examples include a urinary tract infection (UTI), a bladder tumor or stone, atrophic vaginitis, or a prostate infection. Men should see a urologist to determine whether their symptoms are due to prostate disease. Neurologic conditions

BOX 11.3

Exercises That Strengthen Pelvic Floor Muscles, or Kegels for All

Pelvic floor muscles surround the vagina, rectum, and urethra, and for women and men, they stop leakage from both stress and urge by strengthening urethral support. After doing these exercises for two to four weeks, you'll notice some improvement, and by three to four months, you should be able to rely on them to decrease leakage.

Step one: identify the correct muscles

a. Isolate the muscles you use to:
   - Stop urination in midstream
   - Keep you from passing gas

b. Tighten these muscles without tightening your stomach, legs, or buttocks or holding your breath.

How do you know you're doing this right?

You will feel a pulling upward and inward in your abdomen. Men can see movement of their penis and testicles as the muscles are tightened and relaxed. Women will feel a slight pulling in the rectum and vagina, the skin around the anus tightening and the anus itself being pulled up. Women can also insert a finger or two into the vagina and squeeze. If the correct muscles are being used, there will be a tightening around the fingers. Anyone who can't identify the right muscles or is having difficulty doing the exercises should ask to be referred for special training using biofeedback, electrical stimulation, or both.

Step two: lift and squeeze

a. Start the exercises while lying down, so you don't have to deal with gravity. Once you've mastered them while reclining, do the exercises when sitting, standing, or walking.

b. Slowly pull up your pelvic muscles, lifting toward your belly button, and squeeze for a count of 3, then relax the muscles the same amount of time. Make sure you're breathing and not tightening your stomach, leg, or buttock muscles. Don't lift and squeeze while urinating, as doing so can cause other bladder problems. Use your imagination to picture stopping a urine stream.

c. Work up to a set of 10 contractions, each lasting six to eight seconds, and do them three times a day, three to four times a week. *Remember: take as much time relaxing the muscles as you spend contracting them.*

d. Finally, do the exercises in the positions and conditions that mimic when you leak, such as standing up or when you cough, laugh, or sneeze.

such as stroke, dementia, Parkinson's disease, multiple sclerosis, and diabetic neuropathy also increase the frequency of UBCs.

Medications can also lead to urge incontinence. Diuretics, by increasing urine volume, can cause increased frequency and urgency. Cholinesterase inhibitors used for the treatment of dementia occasionally can cause increased urge incontinence.

Treatments for Urge Incontinence

Behavioral treatments can help keep you dry. In addition to doing daily exercises that strengthen pelvic floor muscles, *urge suppression* can help prevent the urges related to UBCs. An urge is a wave that increases in intensity, peaks, and subsides, as shown in the figure below. If you can work through it, you'll have time to get to the bathroom. As my colleague Dr. Catherine DuBeau says, "It's mind over bladder."

Voiding frequently during the day will keep your bladder volume low, so if

Instructions for Urge Suppression
When you feel the urge:
1. *Freeze and squeeze.* Stay still, and do five rapid pelvic floor muscle (Kegel) contractions to reduce the urge. Lift the pelvic floor muscles and squeeze for just a second or two, then release. Doing several of these quick flicks in a row can help stop UBCs.
2. *Suppress the urge.* After the rapid pelvic muscle contractions, distract yourself with something else, like slow, deep breathing, until the urge subsides and you can walk to the bathroom.

you can't overcome the urge, you'll at least have less leakage. You can start by scheduling bathroom breaks every two hours. As you become more proficient at stopping the urge, you'll be able to go longer without leaking. Increase the time by 15–30 minutes until you can stay dry for three to four hours. It may take several weeks, but eventually you'll begin to notice a difference.

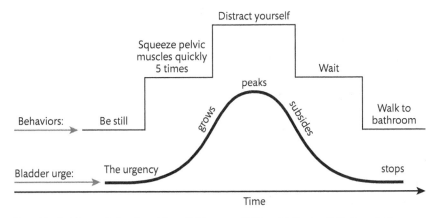

Note: Used with permission from Diane K. Newman, DNP, and Catherine E. DuBeau, MD

Urge suppression. Modified from D. K. Newman and A. J. Wein, *Managing and Treating Urinary Incontinence*, 2nd ed. (Baltimore: Health Professions Press, 2009)

Why should I bother with exercises when I can just take a medication?

Medications can be as effective as behavioral treatments for urge incontinence; however, they are not a cure. The incontinence will recur once the medication is stopped. Some people use them as a bridge while they work on their pelvic floor muscle strength and urge suppression techniques.

Medications decrease the urge sensation, help inhibit bladder contractions, and increase bladder capacity. The two most common types of oral medications are anticholinergics and beta-3 agonists. As noted in chapter 3, anticholinergic drugs can cause many side effects in older adults. But some bladder anticholinergics like tolterodine and solifenacin have fewer side effects and are better tolerated than others, like oxybutynin. Mirabegron and vibegron are beta-3 agonists and newer drugs, so less is known about their side effects, although high blood pressure, fast heart rate, and headache have been reported in some people.

◇CAUTION◇ If your incontinence worsens when using these medications, it may be because you have some urinary retention. Immediately stop the medication, and speak with your doctor.

Mixed Stress and Urge Incontinence

My incontinence is triggered by laughing and by standing up. Sometimes when I stand, I feel an urgency that I can't control, and I lose a lot of urine. Do I have stress incontinence or urge incontinence, and what can I do to avoid these embarrassing accidents?

A check of the figure on page 188 indicates that you most likely have mixed stress and urge incontinence. Urge incontinence is what's causing the large urine loss, so that's what you should concentrate on by using the pelvic muscle exercises and urge suppression techniques above.

Overflow Incontinence

I'm freaked out. I recently leaked a large volume of urine and had no idea that I needed to go. What's going on?

Overflow incontinence occurs when the urethra or bladder outlet is narrowed or partially obstructed, resulting in dribbling, a weak urinary stream, hesitancy, frequency, or nocturia. There's usually no sensation of an urge to void, and leakage can be continuous because the bladder doesn't fully empty. Depending on its cause, this may progress to complete urinary retention, an inability to urinate. *Complete urinary retention is an emergency that requires immediate medical attention.*

Precipitating Factors for Overflow Incontinence

Medical conditions can be risk factors for overflow incontinence. Obstruction can be caused by medications, an enlarged prostate, a narrowing of the urethra (called a stricture), bladder or uterine prolapse, or neurologic conditions such as diabetes, multiple sclerosis, and vitamin B_{12} deficiency.

Severe constipation can cause urinary retention by mechanically obstructing the urethra.

I'm a healthy 75-year-old guy who took Sudafed for a cold and then couldn't pee. I ended up in the ER, where they had to put a tube into my bladder to get the urine out. What happened?

Medications can exacerbate urinary obstruction, particularly in men. Treatments for colds and sinus conditions may contain decongestants and/or antihistamines, which can close down a partially obstructed urethra, requiring a tube (catheter) to be inserted through the penis to drain the bladder. The narrowing is usually from BPH. Speak with your medical provider if you have BPH symptoms like a weak or hesitant stream, dribbling, frequency, or nocturia. Review table 11.1 for drugs to avoid.

Treatments for Overflow Incontinence

Behavioral treatments like the double void technique (see pages 184 and 187) to empty the bladder as much as possible may help to decrease the urine volume available for leakage.

Medications may help treat overflow incontinence. For men with urge incontinence due to an enlarged prostate, a class of medications called alpha-blockers relax prostate smooth muscle, improving flow through the urethra (see table 11.1 for a list of these medications). In addition, 5-alpha reductase inhibitors like finasteride can shrink the prostate, but it takes several months before you'll see any results.

Surgery or self-catheterization may help people who have mechanical reasons for overflow incontinence (including neurologic issues or urinary outlet obstructions, for example). You should discuss these and other options with a urologist.

Functional Incontinence

My mom has had some accidents at home and when we're out. It seems that she can still control her urine, but she can't get to the toilet on time. She moves so slowly. Any suggestions?

Physical and environmental barriers combine with age-related changes to interfere with the ability to get to the toilet on time. This combination of circumstances is called functional incontinence, in contrast to the physiologically based problems discussed above.

Precipitating Factors for Functional Incontinence

Medications can contribute to functional incontinence by causing confusion, rigidity, immobility, and balance disorders. For more information, see tables 6.2 and 9.1.

Environmental barriers like cluttered hallways and living spaces can make it difficult to get to the bathroom quickly.

Cognitive status can sometimes play a role in functional incontinence. People living with dementia may be physically able to get to the bathroom but lack the understanding that it's time to go. Regular toileting schedules can be helpful for them. Prompting them to go to the bathroom before leaving the house or before leaving one activity and heading to the next one may also help.

Physical disabilities can make it harder to get to the bathroom. Create a clear straight path to your bathroom or commode. At times, a caregiver may need to assist.

Treatments for Functional Incontinence

Physical and occupational therapists can help improve mobility, dexterity, and evaluate the environment. Equipment can be obtained to make it easier and safer to get to and use the toilet, such as bedside commodes, urinals, high toilet seats, or rails around the toilet, and to make it easier to undress (such as Velcro fasteners on clothing). Review medications from time to time with your medical provider to see if any may be contributing to functional incontinence.

Nocturia

Mike is concerned that he's up multiple times each night going to the bathroom. He says it makes him sleep deprived and irritable. "Can't you just give me a pill so I can sleep through the night?"

Most older people get up once or twice a night, but some are up far more often. I find that people usually get concerned when they're getting up three or more times a night, or when they feel that they're not getting enough sleep either because they're up so often or because they can't fall back asleep.

The problem here is figuring out which comes first—waking up or the need to urinate. Sleeping pills may make your problem worse. As with incontinence, there are often factors that can be modified to decrease nocturia.

Precipitating Factors for Nocturia

Urge incontinence, overactive bladder, and incomplete emptying can each exacerbate nocturia (see the discussions of these conditions and management strategies above).

Excessive urine output can be caused by the following.

- *Leg swelling*, especially that which worsens throughout the day but improves overnight. When you lie down, this fluid reenters the circulation and goes through the kidneys, increasing the amount of urine you make at night. Varicose veins, heart failure, and certain medications can cause your legs to swell.

- *Medications* that increase fluid retention, like nonsteroidal anti-inflammatory drugs (NSAIDs), GABA-ergic pain medications, calcium channel blockers, thiazolidinediones for diabetes, and corticosteroids (see table 11.1), or drugs that increase urine production, like diuretics.

- *Out-of-control diabetes*, which increases urine production to help eliminate excess blood sugar from the body.

- *High levels of calcium* in the blood can interfere with the kidneys' ability to concentrate urine, resulting in excessive urine output.

Sleep disorders such as obstructive sleep apnea or restless legs syndrome can wake us up several times a night (see chapter 10), as can pain. Some medications interfere with sleep, while other medications cause insomnia when abruptly stopped (see table 10.3).

Treatments for Nocturia

- Drink less fluid in the late afternoon and evening, especially alcohol, caffeine, and carbonated beverages (see the Adapting to Your New Normal section above).
- Take your last dose of diuretic medication no later than 4:00 p.m.
- If you have leg swelling, elevate your legs for 30 minutes around dinnertime so that some of this fluid is eliminated before going to bed.
- Speak with your medical provider to determine whether there are alternatives to the medications you're taking that cause fluid retention, or if there are other ways for you to reduce leg swelling.

Mike's doctor changed some of his blood pressure medications and had him lie down with his feet elevated for 30 minutes each night after dinner. Things got better, but he still woke up and urinated several times a night. Often the volume of urine was small, leading his doctor to wonder if Mike had a sleep disorder. He was tested and found to have obstructive sleep apnea (see chapter 10). It turned out that he was waking up more from the sleep disorder than from his need to urinate. Mike's doctor prescribed a CPAP machine, and since using it, Mike urinates two to three times a night, sleeps much better, and is much more fun to be around.

Mike's care points to the fact that nocturia is a geriatric syndrome. Mike was vulnerable to developing incontinence because he's older, so he eliminates more of his urine at night, sleeps more lightly, and has BPH. The precipitating factors that tipped him over into nocturia were his swollen legs, blood pressure medication, and sleep apnea. Addressing these issues decreased how often he needed to get up to urinate at night and improved his sleep.

What Isn't Normal Aging?

 Red Flags: Symptoms Needing Prompt Medical Attention

- Inability to urinate.
- Urine loss without warning, not preceded by a sense of urge, movement, coughing, sneezing, or laughing.
- Blood in the urine.
- Sudden incontinence in a man.
- Pelvic pain.
- Pain with urination.

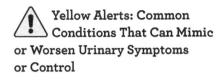 **Yellow Alerts: Common Conditions That Can Mimic or Worsen Urinary Symptoms or Control**

Medications

The medications associated with each type of incontinence are listed in table 11.1. If you're taking one of these drugs, discuss whether you should taper or change medications with your medical provider.

Symptoms of Benign Prostatic Hyperplasia

The symptoms of BPH are not specific to prostate problems. They could also be due to infection, bladder problems, or neurologic disease, among others. These symptoms may be related to *voiding*, like hesitancy, delay starting a stream, having a weak stream, or being unable to void; *storage*, like frequency, nocturia, urge, or incontinence; and/or occur *after voiding*, like dribbling or feeling that the bladder doesn't fully empty. If these problems are bothering you, speak with your medical provider.

Prostatitis

In men, prostatitis, an infection of the prostate gland, and a UTI may be diffi-cult to differentiate, but doing so can be important because the course of treatment is generally six weeks for prostatitis. Men with acute prostatitis have fever, chills, pain when urinating, and a tender prostate. Those with chronic prostatitis have varying urinary symptoms and pain.

Vaginal Atrophy

Postmenopausal vaginal atrophy is a common condition that can cause UBCs and urge incontinence. Vaginal estrogen applied as a cream or as an intravaginal ring may help with overactive bladder as well as urge incontinence. It may also reduce the recurrence of urinary tract infections.

Getting Evaluated for Urinary Concerns

Fewer than one in four people who experience incontinence discuss it with their medical providers. And it's the rare provider who spontaneously asks whether you're having "accidents" or difficulty getting to the bathroom on time. But as you've learned in this chapter, there's a lot that can be done to improve the situation. And there are real downsides to not getting help. People with incontinence and nocturia often decrease their fluid intake, get dehydrated, and then fall or become confused. They also stop going out, afraid that they'll be caught unawares, resulting in isolation and depression. Some use pads or other products, but sometimes these aren't enough. They also worry about odors and discomfort. As Mike showed us, an evaluation with your medical provider can help identify the precipitating factors and develop a plan to address them, decreasing episodes of incontinence or nocturia.

Take the initiative and make an appointment with your primary care provider to find out if you might have a urine infection, another medical condition, or are taking medications that can cause incontinence or nocturia.

Should I See a Specialist?

You should see a specialist—a urologist, a gynecologist, or a urogynecologist— if you have any of the following.

- Recurrent urinary tract infections.
- Incontinence with new onset of neurologic symptoms such as rigidity, loss of sensation, and/or muscle weakness.
- Marked prostate enlargement that doesn't respond to medications.
- Pelvic organs that protrude out the entrance to the vagina.
- Pelvic pain with incontinence.
- Persistent blood in the urine.
- A large amount of urine remaining in the bladder after you void.

Preparing for the Visit

Fill out this chapter's pre-visit checklist on page 379 in Appendix 3, bring it along with a list of all your medications and supplements to the appointment, and review it with your provider. Based on this information, your health care provider may ask additional questions and examine your mobility, fluid status (heart, lungs, leg swelling), cognition, abdomen, or do a rectal and/or pelvic examination. They may also order blood work to measure your sugar, calcium, and vitamin B_{12} levels; ask for a urine sample to examine under the microscope; and send a culture to see if there is an infection. If trying to detect whether you completely empty your bladder, they may get a post-void residual—a measure of how much urine is left in the bladder after you double void. This can be done by ultrasound or by inserting a bladder catheter.

Advice for Loved Ones

Incontinence can affect a person's sense of dignity and self. After all, adults aren't supposed to be incontinent—that's for babies and toddlers. Interrupted sleep from nocturia can result in sleep deprivation, crankiness, and fatigue. Follow the older adult's lead on the subject so that you don't infantilize them. Encourage them to adopt some of the prevention and symptom reduction strategies described in this chapter. Suggest that they discuss their symptoms with their medical provider. Normalize the topic by talking about your own concerns; many middle-aged women have over-active bladders, stress incontinence, and urge incontinence, and many middle-aged men experience symptoms of an enlarged prostate.

If the older person is living with dementia, remind them to go, or take them to the bathroom every few hours to decrease the likelihood and volume of incontinence. For the families of these older adults, incontinence can be the straw that breaks the camel's back, resulting in nursing home placement. Try to get ahead of this by availing yourself of resources like those at the end of the chapter.

Bottom Line

Urinary symptoms are common in older adults. Behavioral treatments are often helpful, and there are also medications and surgical treatments, but you first need to discuss the problem with your medical provider. The initial evaluation focuses on identifying conditions that can be treated or need further evaluation, starting you on the road to having more control of your urine trouble.

RESOURCES

Associations

National Association for Continence (https://www.nafc.org)
The NAFC is a nonprofit organization providing information and resources related to incontinence.

Simon Foundation for Incontinence (https://simonfoundation.org/)
This advocacy organization is committed to reducing the stigma associated with urinary and fecal incontinence.

Incontinence in People with Dementia

Alzheimer's Association (https://www.alz.org/help-support /caregiving/daily-care/incontinence)

Visit this website for tips on managing incontinence in people with dementia.

Andrews, J. "Maintaining Continence in People with Dementia." *Nursing Times* 109, no. 27 (2013): 20–21.

Books

Genadry, Rene, and J. L. Mostwin. *A Woman's Guide to Urinary Incontinence*. Baltimore: Johns Hopkins University Press, 2007.

Haag, Sarah. *Understanding and Treating Incontinence: What Causes Urinary Incontinence and How to Regain Bladder Control*. Minneapolis: Orthopedic Physical Therapy Products, 2019.

BIBLIOGRAPHY

Brown, J. S., C. S. Bradley, L. L. Subak, et al. "The Sensitivity and Specificity of a Simple Test to Distinguish between Urge and Stress Urinary Incontinence." *Annals of Internal Medicine* 144, no. 10 (2006): 716.

D'Silva, K. A., P. Dahm, and C. L. Wong. "Does This Man with Lower Urinary Tract Symptoms Have Bladder Outlet Obstruction? The Rational Clinical Examination: A Systematic Review." *JAMA* 312, no. 5 (2014): 535–42.

Newman, D. K., and A. J. Wein. *Managing and Treating Urinary Incontinence*, 2nd ed. Baltimore: Health Professions Press, 2009.

CHAPTER 12

All Eyes and Ears

I expected that all five of my senses would start on a permanent downhill course as I aged. Yet, surprisingly, some improved! In my thirties, my sense of smell returned. In my forties, I stopped having to stretch my arms out and squint to focus when reading the paper. In my fifties, I was shocked to realize how many of my old friends suddenly had blue eyes. And in my sixties, people stopped mumbling and I heard birds chirp once more. What happened? I stopped smoking, got progressive lenses, had cataract surgery, and began using hearing aids.

These actions taught me a lot about aging. There's often a tendency to put off medical "interventions" until they are absolutely needed, if ever. This may be a good sentiment at times and for some people. But I am finding, and studies support, that certain early interventions may provide greater or equal benefit with less risk.

Our senses provide input into many functions that are increasingly important to us as we age. For example, as discussed in chapters 6 and 9, seeing and hearing play major roles in cognition, especially memory and spatial perception, and in balance.

In this chapter we'll review what to expect and how to adapt to the normal age-related changes and common diseases that occur with your vision and hearing. The other senses are discussed elsewhere—smell and taste in chapter 15, touch (peripheral neuropathy) in chapters 9 and 13, and pain in chapter 13.

VISION

For an overview of the anatomy of the visual system, see box 12.1.

For a deeper dive into how vision changes with age, see box 12.2.

What's Normal with Aging?

I've been told that I should see an eye doctor every year. My vision isn't changing that quickly, so why do I need to go so often?

Many eye diseases like glaucoma or macular degeneration are asymptomatic until vision has already been lost. Small cataracts can increase your risk of a fall. Although these diseases aren't part of normal aging, they occur frequently in older adults (see the Yellow Alerts section below). Seeing an ophthalmologist or optometrist every one to two years allows earlier detection and treatment of these diseases, decreasing vision loss and falls.

I've been having lots of problems with my vision. I can't read newspaper print, let alone the patient instructions that come with my medications, and my grandchildren laughed at me the other day because one of my socks was brown and the other blue. I could swear they were the same color when I put them on. Is this normal?

Everyone's vision changes with age (box 12.2). Print becomes blurry and too small to read. Glasses help but may not fully correct the problem. You may need more light. Healthy 60-year-olds need about twice as much light to read as 20-year-olds; 80-year-olds need three times more. Color and contrast perception decreases, making it harder to differentiate between colors or distinguish the outlines of objects. Your eyes are more sensitive to glare, and it takes longer to adapt to sunlight as well as darkness. Your eyes may feel dry or sandy.

These changes can affect your ability to read, use the computer, paint, or walk or drive safely. Dimly lit areas can be hazardous, increasing the risks of stumbling and falling. Decreased color perception explains the sock problem (yellows, oranges, and reds are easier to identify). You'll have little trouble reading print that is black on a white background, or vice versa, but it can be hard when there's less contrast, like when trying to read red letters on an orange page, noticing stains on clothing, and being confident you know where the edge of a step is.

Some of this is normal aging, and some is due to conditions that can be treated. As discussed below, a new prescription for glasses, cataract surgery, artificial tears for dry eyes, and additional lighting with brighter bulbs can greatly help. Be glad you live in a time where low- and high-tech devices can be harnessed to help you.

BOX 12.1

Vision 101

When we see an object, our brain is actually interpreting an image made from the light reflected by the object. This light passes through the *cornea* and enters the eye via the *pupil*, traverses the *lens*, and then travels through the *vitreous*, a clear gel that fills the eyeball, to the *retina*, a thin tissue that layers the inside of the eye. The retina contains special cells that convert light into electrical signals that the brain can understand. These signals travel through the *optic nerve* to the brain.

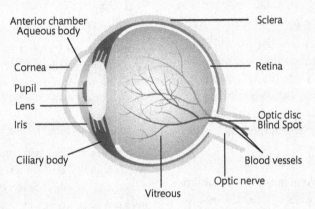

Anatomy of the eye. Courtesy of Dreamstime.com

The eye has special functions to adapt to different conditions when we're trying to see. The pupil, under the control of the iris (the colored portion of the eye), changes size to control the amount of light that enters the eye, dilating (enlarging) when it's dark and constricting when it's sunny or there's glare. The lens is a clear part of the eye that changes shape to further focus light, or an image, onto the retina. The *macula* is the central area of the retina that allows you to see what is directly in front of you, like when you're reading a book. The *peripheral retina* is responsible for side and night vision.

How about driving? Will these changes to my vision affect my ability to drive?

Age-related vision impairment makes night driving challenging because of the difficulty adapting to darkness, changes in lighting, and the glare of oncoming headlights. Many states require corrected vision of at least 20/50 for an unrestricted license; vision worse than this can result in a restricted license that only allows you to drive during the day, having to make modifications to your car, or losing your driver's license.

A vision score of 20/50 means that one needs to be 20 feet away to clearly see an object that a person with normal vision could see from 50 feet away. In other words, the person with 20/50 vision needs to be 30 feet closer to see as well as a person with 20/20. Most older adults can meet this standard, but 10 percent of people age 70–79 and 25 percent of those over 80 years old cannot (see chapter 19 for more on driving).

Adapting to Your New Normal

Is there any truth to the belief that sunglasses can help prevent vision loss?

Absolutely. Several eye disorders, including both cataracts and macular degeneration (see the Yellow Alerts section below), have been linked to sun exposure. When in the sun, wear sunglasses or a brimmed hat to block ultraviolet rays.

What can I do to maximize my ability to see in the wake of these age-related vision changes?

Increase lighting levels. This is especially important where you do close-up work or where safety could be an issue, like near the bathroom or stairways. Nightlights, lights that are activated by motion, and flex-armed lamps can be particularly helpful.

Use watches, telephones, and clocks with large numbers. A larger display will help you see more clearly.

Control glare by using matte finishes and avoiding shiny surfaces. Don't aim for a shine when you wax your floors—it will increase glare and falls. In fact, you may notice that hospital units specifically designed for older adults use non-glare, low-shine floors to reduce the risk of falls.

Match colors near a sunny window or in a well-lit area.

Increase the color contrast to differentiate edges. For example, use a dark placemat with white dishes. Put colored tape on the edge of steps to improve their visibility.

Sometimes my eyes sting and burn, feel sandy or gritty, and my vision gets blurry. I thought this might be dry eye, but my eyes are actually watery. Any thoughts on what I can do?

These symptoms *may* be due to dry eyes. Dry eyes occur when your tears can't adequately lubricate your eye, either because you don't produce enough tears or the tears you produce are of poor quality. Watery eyes can be a response to the irritation that you describe.

Tears are important. They bathe the surface of the eye, keeping it moist, and wash away dust and debris. They also help protect the eye from bacterial and other types of infections.

To help prevent dry eyes indoors, get a humidifier as well as an air cleaner to filter dust and other particles. Blinking or careful eye rubbing can spread the remaining tear film and provide some relief.

BOX 12.2

What Happens with Aging: A Deeper Dive

It takes longer for your eyes to adapt when entering bright or dark places.
With age, pupils are smaller and don't change size as quickly.

You need reading glasses.
You may need reading glasses in your forties, as the lens hardens and the muscles responsible for changing its shape weaken. This is called *presbyopia*, which is Greek for "old man's eye" (tells you a lot about how life expectancy has changed, doesn't it?). When you read or focus on close objects, the lens is no longer able to change shape to improve the sharpness of your vision.

Cataracts may form.
Cataracts develop from protein buildup in the normally clear lens, causing vision to blur and colors to fade.

It becomes harder to read in low lighting, or to tell the difference between similar colors.
These problems are caused by age-related changes in the cornea, lens, and the vitreous (gel like material of the eye), decreasing light transmission to the retina. Increasing the lighting level often helps.

Floaters increase.
Floaters are black filaments or blotches that drift through or on the edge of your vision. Floaters are usually annoying but not dangerous. They occur because with age the *vitreous*, which contains fibers that attach to the surface of the retina, slowly shrinks and liquefies, causing the fibers to break and the vitreous to separate from the retinal surface. Floaters tend to be more distracting to older people because they move faster and over a greater range in the liquified vitreous. Floaters also occur in *retinal detachment*—this is a medical emergency and *not* normal aging (see the Red Flags section below). Contact your medical care provider if there is a sudden increase in the number of floaters, light flashes, or a loss of peripheral vision.

Sensitivity to glare increases.
Age-related changes in the cornea, lens, vitreous, and retina cause greater light scattering, resulting in decreased vision and increased sensitivity to glare.

Eyelids change as you age.
Your eyelids may begin to droop because the tendons connected to them stretch out. This can irritate the eye and cause tearing and dry eye syndrome. Droopy eyelids can also block vision and may require surgical intervention for vision to improve.

Tear production may decrease.
As you get older, your eyes produce fewer tears and tear ducts narrow, which can cause dry eye and blurry vision, redness, foreign body sensations, and occasionally eye discomfort.

Over-the-counter artificial tears may help, but avoid preparations advertised to get the redness out, as these increase tearing by causing irritation to your eye, and the more you use them, the redder your eye will become. Also avoid preparations with preservatives if you need to use them repeatedly throughout the day.

If symptoms persist, see your eye doctor to determine whether medications or another disorder may be causing your dry eye, and what treatments may be available.

I love to read, but I'm finding it harder and harder to read the newspaper or a book. It's getting me depressed, especially since I expect that it will just get worse over time.

Start with increasing the intensity of the light where you're trying to read. As we age, our eyes need more light to see clearly. Reading in a well-lit area can help.

Increase the print size and contrast of your reading materials. Use magnifiers, or get large-print versions of books and newspapers (often available at your local library). E-readers like an iPad or Kindle allow you to control the type size and contrast. You can also increase the size of documents you view on your computer by using the zoom feature.

Try listening to an audiobook. Services like Audible offer many titles in audio form. Audiobooks may also be available for checkout at your local library. Computer and tablet applications that can read text aloud are another option.

My ophthalmologist has done his best, but I'm still limited in what I can do because of my vision. I'm afraid to go outdoors because I'm nervous that I may fall. Isn't there something else that can be done?

Low vision is when eyesight can't be corrected with glasses, contact lenses, medicine, or surgery, and interferes with everyday tasks like reading, cooking, or sewing, reading street signs, or recognizing familiar faces.

Vision rehabilitation helps people with low vision and those with central or peripheral visual field loss, reduced contrast sensitivity, glare sensitivity, and/or light-to-dark adaptation difficulties to better compensate and function in their environment. This includes teaching safer ways to navigate out-of-doors. *Ask your eye care professional about a referral to a low-vision center or vision rehabilitation in your area.* See the end of this chapter for information about low-vision resources.

Never Say Never

Keisha is a retired English teacher with macular degeneration who became depressed and irritable as her vision worsened. A few years ago, her niece Tamara bought her an e-reader for her birthday. Tamara taught Keisha to use it and how to make the print darker and larger.

Now, Keisha can't see using the e-reader, and Tamara wants her aunt to try audiobooks. Keisha's refusing. She thinks she won't be able to keep the characters straight. Tamara suggested that they both "read" the same book at the same time, and that Keisha write each character's name and distinguishing features in large print with a dark felt pen in a notebook that she could refer back to. Keisha finally agreed to try because she loved—and missed—discussing books with Tamara. They started their own book club for two, and Keisha has now started listening to books on her own as well.

What Isn't Normal Aging?

 Red Flags: Symptoms Needing Prompt Medical Attention

- Sudden loss of vision or onset of blurred vision.
- Flashes of light or bursts of new floaters may indicate a detached retina.
- Sudden eye pain—often red with blurred vision, severe headache, nausea, and vomiting—may indicate acute glaucoma (see pages 206–7).
- Double vision.
- Shingles with a painful blistering rash or pain on one side of the forehead, especially if it affects the side or tip of the nose. Shingles in this area of the body can involve the eye and cause vision loss; early diagnosis and treatment are critical.

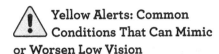 **Yellow Alerts: Common Conditions That Can Mimic or Worsen Low Vision**

Medications

Medications can affect your vision and even your eye health. For a list of drugs associated with eye symptoms and disease, see table 12.1.

Cataracts

Cataracts, a condition in which the lens of the eye becomes cloudy or yellow, cause blurry vision, faded colors, increased glare sensitivity, poor night vision, decreased contrast perception, and a decline in vision that glasses can't correct. People who have cataracts commonly describe glare, starbursts, or halos around lights when driving at night.

About 20 percent of people 65 years and older and 50 percent of those 75 years and older have cataracts. Risk factors for developing cataracts include advancing age, decreased vitamin intake, ultraviolet B light exposure, smoking, alcohol use, long-term steroid use, and diabetes.

Consider having your cataracts removed sooner rather than later. Cataract surgery is an outpatient procedure where the cloudy lens is removed and replaced with an artificial lens. Cataract surgery used to require hospitalization, and patients were advised to wait until the cataracts were "ripe" before they were removed. It's now a much quicker and safer procedure, and early removal significantly decreases your chance of having a fall and improves your vision, literally brightening your world. The good news is that cataracts do not grow back. The success rate of surgery is 98 percent, and it is usually well tolerated with a relatively short recovery time. Advanced age, however, can increase the risk of postoperative complications from cataract surgery.

Glaucoma

There are two types of glaucoma: open angle and closed angle. Both occur more often in older adults, and both, if left untreated, can lead to blindness.

Open-angle glaucoma is the most common type of glaucoma in older adults; in the United States, it affects 31 percent of people age 70–79. You may lose substantial vision before you're diagnosed with open-angle glaucoma because your *central vision*, which enables you to read and see what's in front of you, is not initially affected. Rather, your *peripheral vision*, or side vision, is slowly lost. This results in your having tunnel vision, where when you're looking straight ahead, you see less and less of what's on the side. A loss of peripheral vision can cause you to miss things outside your sight range, like a child entering the crosswalk when you're driving through an intersection. Open-angle glaucoma is due to a slow buildup of pressure in the eye, causing damage to the optic nerve and loss of peripheral vision. Treatment usually begins with eye drops to lower the eye's pressure, but eventually lasers or surgery may be required. If glaucoma is detected early, and treated, most people will not lose their vision.

Acute glaucoma (also called acute closed-angle glaucoma) is less common, but this condition is an ophthalmic emergency and requires immediate treatment. The eye suddenly becomes painful and red, and you can develop headache, blurred vision, nausea, vomiting, and the sudden appearance of halos around lights. This happens when there is a sudden blockage in the eye's drainage system, causing a dangerous rise in eye pressure.

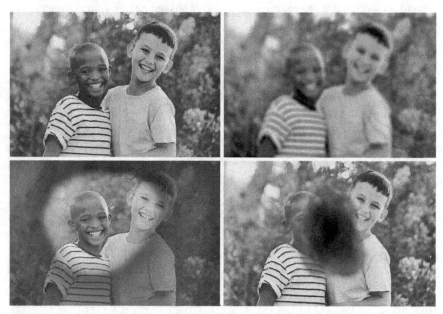

Common age-related eye diseases: *A*, normal vision; *B*, cataracts; *C*, glaucoma; *D*, age-related macular degeneration. Courtesy of the National Eye Institute, https://www.nei.nih.gov/learn-about-eye-health

Age-Related Macular Degeneration

Age-related macular degeneration, or AMD, damages the macula, the part of the retina that is responsible for central vision, the ability to see what's directly in front of you. Central vision is needed to read, see faces, and drive. AMD is the most common cause of irreversible vision impairment in older adults. It rarely causes total blindness because peripheral vision is usually spared. In the United States, 12.5 percent of people over age 60 and 33 percent of those over age 80 have AMD. The greatest risk factor is increasing age, but family history, smoking, obesity, and cardiovascular disease also contribute. Attending to these contributing factors may help reduce your risk of developing AMD.

There are two types of age-related macular degeneration: *wet and dry*. The usual symptoms of dry AMD include a blurry spot in your central vision and the sense that objects don't look as bright as they did previously. Wet AMD also leads to blurriness or even a blind spot in your central vision. Additionally, straight lines can look wavy. You may not notice these symptoms if you have AMD in one eye only, however, since your healthy eye tends to compensate for vision loss in the affected eye.

The dry form, found in 90 percent of people with AMD, progresses more slowly than the wet form. Light-sensitive cells at the back of the eye break down, leading to blurred central vision. There is no cure, but the National Eye Institute's Age-Related Eye Disease Studies (AREDS/AREDS2) found that combinations of vitamins and minerals can decrease the risk of vision loss for some people with intermediate to advanced dry AMD.

Wet AMD develops in about 10 percent of people with dry AMD. In wet AMD, abnormal blood vessels grow behind the retina. These new vessels are weak and can leak fluid, bleed, or form scar tissue. Treatment consists of medications that can be injected into the eye to stop the formation of new blood vessels and the leakage from existing vessels. Some people have regained vision with this procedure. Regular injections may be needed to keep wet AMD under control. Laser therapies are also used to destroy the new blood vessels.

TABLE 12.1
Medications Associated with Eye Symptoms and Disease

	Ocular Emergencies	Dry Eyes, Blurred Vision, or Light Sensitivity	Other
Blood pressure, cardiac, and diuretic medications			
Diuretics, alpha-blockers, and beta-blockers: hydrochlorothiazide (Microzide); metolazone (Zaroxolyn); furosemide (Lasix); doxazosin (Cardura); atenolol (Tenormin); carvedilol (Coreg)		X	
Antiarrhythmics			
Amiodarone (Cordarone)		X	Optic neuropathy* Colored halos
Digoxin (Lanoxin)		X	Decreased visual acuity; yellow colored vision
Statins: simvastatin (Zocor); atorvastatin (Lipitor); rosuvastatin (Crestor)		X	
Pain relief			
NSAIDs: indomethacin (Indocin); ibuprofen (Motrin, Advil); naproxen (Naprosyn, Aleve); piroxicam (Feldene)		X	
Triptans for migraines: sumatriptan (Imitrex); rizatriptan (Maxalt)	Acute glaucoma		
Anticholinergic medications			
Some antidepressants, antihistamines, antipsychotics, anti-Parkinsonian agents, antispasmodics, skeletal muscle relaxants, bladder relaxants, anti-dizziness medications (see table 3.2)	Acute glaucoma	X	

TABLE 12.1 *(continued)*

	Ocular Emergencies	Dry Eyes, Blurred Vision, or Light Sensitivity	Other
Endocrine medications			
Corticosteroids: prednisone; dexamethasone (Decadron); methylprednisolone (Solu-Medrol)			Open angle Glaucoma
			Cataracts
			Optic neuropathy*
Bisphosphonates: risedronate (Actonel); alendronate (Fosamax); ibandronate (Boniva); zoledronic acid (Reclast)		X	Conjunctivitis
Antiestrogen: tamoxifen	Vision loss within the first month (rare)		Cataracts
			Retinal changes*
			Decreased color vision
Erectile dysfunction			
Phosphodiesterase inhibitors: sildenafil (Viagra); tadalafil (Cialis, Adcirca); vardenafil (Levitra, Staxyn)		X	Optic neuropathy*
			Blue discoloration to the vision
Neurological and psychological medications			
Anticonvulsant: topiramate (Topama, Qudexy XR)	Acute glaucoma	X	
Antidepressants, including TCAs, SSRIs, SNRIs: mirtazapine (Remeron); vortioxetine (Trintellix); bupropion (Wellbutrin, Zyban); trazodone (Desyrel)	Acute glaucoma	X	
Benzodiazepine-type sleeping medications: zolpidem (Ambien); zaleplon (Sonata); temazepam (Restoril); triazolam (Halcion)	Acute glaucoma		

(continued)

TABLE 12.1 (*continued*)

	Ocular Emergencies	Dry Eyes, Blurred Vision, or Light Sensitivity	Other
Some antipsychotics, including: chlorpromazine (Thorazine); thioridazine (Mellaril); trifluoperazine (Stelazine)	Acute glaucoma	X	Cataracts Pigmentary retinal degeneration*
Cold, allergy, and itch medications			
Decongestants: phenylephrine (SudafedPE); pseudoephedrine (Sudafed Sinus)	Acute glaucoma		
First- and second-generation antihistamines: diphenhydramine (Benadryl); chlorpheniramine (Chlor-Trimeton); meclizine (Antivert, Bonine); loratadine (Claritin); cetirizine (Zyrtec)	Acute glaucoma	X	
Pulmonary medications			
Inhaled beta agonists and anticholinergics: albuterol (Proventil, Ventolin); ipratropium (Atrovent); tiotropium (Spiriva); ipratropium/albuterol (Combivent, Duoneb)	Acute glaucoma		
Gastrointestinal medications			
H_2 blockers: cimetidine (Tagamet); famotidine (Pepcid); nizatidine (Axid)	Acute glaucoma		
Antimicrobial agents			
Antimalarials: chloroquine; hydroxychloroquine (Plaquenil) (also used for some rheumatic diseases)			Macular disease*
Anti-tuberculosis: isoniazid; ethambutol (Myambutol)			Optic neuropathy*
Fluoroquinolone antibiotics: ciprofloxacin (Cipro); levofloxacin (Levaquin)	Acute retinal detachment		

TABLE 12.1 (*continued*)

	Ocular Emergencies	Dry Eyes, Blurred Vision, or Light Sensitivity	Other
Urinary medications			
BPH alpha-blockers: terazosin (Hytrin); alfuzosin (Uroxatral); tamsulosin (Flomax)		X	Floppy lens syndrome[†]
Other			
Sulfa medications: sulfamethoxazole/ trimethoprim (Bactrim, Septra); glyburide (Diabeta); sulfasalazine (Azulfidine); dapsone; sumatriptan (Imitrex); celecoxib (Celebrex)	Acute glaucoma		

Note: Abbreviations are as follows: BPH, benign prostatic hyperplasia; NSAID, nonsteroidal anti-inflammatory drug; SNRI, serotonin-norepinephrine reuptake inhibitor; SSRI, selective serotonin reuptake inhibitor, TCA, tricyclic antidepressants.

*Can cause vision loss that, depending on the medication, may be temporary or permanent.

†Can interfere with cataract surgery.

HEARING

For an overview of how we hear, what we hear, and how we measure hearing, see box 12.3.

What's Normal with Aging?

For a deeper dive into age-related changes in hearing and speech discrimination, see box 12.4.

Does everyone's hearing get worse with aging, or is this just another myth?

Hearing loss affects about one-quarter of people over age 65 and almost half of those over age 80. *Presbycusis*, loss of the ability to hear high frequencies, is the most common form.

Sounds that are high frequency include birds' chirps and clock or watch ticks. The consonants f, k, s, sh, th, and p can be particularly difficult to understand. This can lead to some interesting conversations—hearing "bitch" when the word "fish" is said, "dumb" for "thump," "why" for "wise," or "choose" for "shoes." Presbycusis can also lead to *mondegreens*, where we mishear one phrase and substitute a similar-sounding phrase. An example would be the song "Bad Moon Rising" by the Creedence Clearwater Revival, where a person with mondegreens may hear "There's a bathroom on the right" instead of "There's a bad moon on the rise."

Ear wax plugs are the next most common reason for hearing impairment in older adults. The plugs block sound from entering the inner ear. With age, earwax was becomes drier and harder. Once the earwax is removed, hearing will return.

Why is my husband having so much trouble hearing me? He hears his male friends just fine. Is he having "selective" hearing loss?

No. Women's voices are higher frequency, so all people with presbycusis have more difficulty hearing and understanding women. I learned this when I was an intern working at a US Department of Veterans Affairs (VA) hospital where 98 percent of the patients were male, as were the vast majority of doctors. The older male patients were ignoring me, but they clearly responded to my male colleagues when they repeated what I had just said. Initially, I thought this was pure sexism; after all, it wasn't uncommon at that time for VA patients to refuse care from a woman doctor. This may have been the case, but in reality they likely just couldn't, rather than wouldn't, hear me, because older people with presbycusis hear and understand men's voices better because they are low frequency. I finally got it, and when it was clear my patient couldn't hear me, I would ask my male colleague to repeat my words to the patient.

I saw an audiologist, and he said my hearing was fine. Yet I'm having a lot of trouble understanding what people are saying. Should I see another audiologist?

No. Even if your hearing is normal, you may find that you have more difficulty understanding speech, particularly when there is background noise. That's due to the competition of sounds in the room. Audiograms are done in sound-proof booths, so your hearing may have tested fine, but you still may have trouble in noisy environments or if the speech is rapid-fire or dense with information. Your problem is quite common. Around one-third of people 61–70 years old have problems understanding speech when there is background noise, and this figure rises to around 80 percent for those aged 85 years and over, even if they have normal or near-normal hearing levels. This can be even worse if you have tinnitus, which is when you hear sounds in your own head despite there being no external cause (see the Yellow Alerts section below).

BOX 12.3

Hearing 101

HOW WE HEAR

When we hear sound, our brain is actually interpreting vibrations made by objects like our vocal cords, a telephone, or a musical instrument. These objects cause air particles to vibrate and move away from the source of the sound in the form of a *sound wave*. The ears capture sound waves and convert them to electrical signals that are sent along nerves to the brain. But if your ears and brain don't work together, you won't hear or understand sounds.

The ear has three parts—the outer, the middle, and the inner ear—each of which plays a specific role in hearing. All the parts of the ear are designed to stimulate the auditory nerve to carry signals to the brain, which then interprets them as sound and speech.

The *outer ear* has two sections, the *pinna*, which is the part of the ear you see, and the *ear canal*. The pinna captures sound waves from the environment and directs them into the ear canal. This helps your brain locate where the sounds are coming from. The sound waves then travel down the ear canal to the eardrum.

The *middle ear* consists of the *eardrum* and a chain of three small bones, called *ossicles*, which act as a series of levers connected at one end to the eardrum and at the other end to the inner ear. Sound waves from the ear canal hit the eardrum, causing it and the ossicles to vibrate. Blockage of the *eustachian tube*, which carries air into the middle ear from the back of the nose, causes the eardrum to vibrate less efficiently and sound to become muffled. Swallowing, blowing your nose, or yawning can open the tube, often causing a popping sound, and improve your hearing.

(continued)

BOX 12.3 *(continued)*

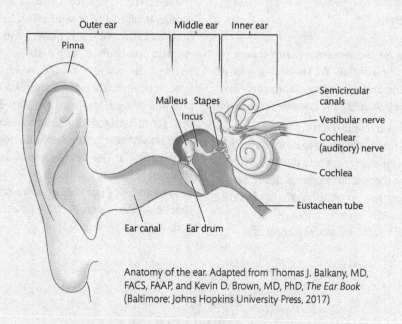

Anatomy of the ear. Adapted from Thomas J. Balkany, MD, FACS, FAAP, and Kevin D. Brown, MD, PhD, *The Ear Book* (Baltimore: Johns Hopkins University Press, 2017)

The *inner ear* consists of the *cochlea*, a fluid-filled snail-shaped bone, and the *vestibule*, which contains the *semicircular canals*. Vibrations from the ossicles in the middle ear cause the fluid in the cochlea to vibrate. The louder the sound, the greater the amplitude of the vibration. *Hair cells* inside the cochlea are arranged so that distinct cells vibrate in response to specific sound pitches, and these hair cells transform the vibrations into electrical signals that are relayed to the *auditory nerve*.

The *vestibule* with its *semicircular canals* comprises the other half of the inner ear. It is key to our sense of balance, direction, and spatial orientation. The auditory nerve is one branch of the eighth cranial nerve, and the other is the vestibular nerve. This is why vestibular problems, like vertigo and tinnitus, are often linked to hearing problems. Chapter 9 discusses the role of the ear in balance.

THE BRAIN

The ear is one factor in being able to hear and to understand speech. The auditory nerve carries impulses to the brain, which needs to process this information. In addition to the brain auditory pathways, other cognitive functions play a role in hearing and understanding speech. This includes your executive function, which is critical to your ability to pay selective attention, and short-term memory (or working memory), which is required for speech processing (see chapter 6). Anything that interferes with these functions can affect your ability to understand speech.

BOX 12.3 (*continued*)

WHAT WE HEAR

Whether we hear a sound depends both on the loudness as well as the frequency (or pitch) of the vibration. Frequency is measured in hertz (Hz), the number of vibrations per second. The higher the frequency, the higher the pitch. We are able to hear frequencies between about 60 and 16,000 Hz. Most speech is in the 1,000 to 4,000 Hz range.

The loudness of a sound is measured in decibels (dB). The higher the dB level, the louder the sound. To hear any sound, it has to be above 0 dB. A whisper is about 30 dB, normal conversation 60 dB, and traffic 80 dB. Sounds above 90 dB can lead to chronic hearing loss if you're exposed to them every day or all the time.

AUDIOGRAMS: MEASURING HEARING LOSS AND SPEECH DISCRIMINATION

An audiogram measures your sensitivity to sound throughout the entire hearing system, from ear to brain. It measures hearing levels and speech discrimination by having you respond when tones or words of differing intensity and frequency are played into each ear. This testing is done in a sound-proof booth, so the audiogram response is considered your *overall hearing ability*, not your ability to hear in every situation. Specialized hearing tests are required to accurately represent your ability to hear or discriminate speech in noisy environments. The pattern of overall hearing suggests the direction of change in your hearing loss and what further testing might be required.

Audiograms measure the softest sound you can hear at frequencies from 250 to 8,000 Hz. A hearing loss of 20 dB, meaning that the softest sounds you can hear are at 20 dB, is still considered normal. Losses of 25–40 dB are considered mild, 41–60 dB moderate, and 61–80 dB severe. Many people can use their own hearing to get along in the world if their hearing loss is less than 40 dB. Hearing impairment is considered to be a loss of more than 40 dB, while profound hearing loss or deafness is a hearing loss of more than 81 dB.

My family is constantly harping at me that I need hearing aids. I don't think I have a problem, but if they're right, what should be tipping me off?

Many people are unaware of their hearing loss, and many others are in denial. It is important to recognize that you may have a problem, as hearing loss can seriously affect memory, mood, cognition, social connections, and possibly balance and posture.

You should suspect that you have a significant hearing loss if any of the following applies to you.

- It seems as if everyone is mumbling. (This was me!)
- People complain that you have the television on too loud.
- You keep saying, "What?" "Can you repeat that?" and "I didn't hear you" when conversing with either individuals or in a group.

- You often misunderstand what's said.
- You cup your hand around an ear to better direct the sound.
- You give inappropriate answers to questions (because you misunderstood the question).
- You hear better when you see the person speaking.

BOX 12.4

What Happens with Aging: A Deeper Dive

Age-related hearing loss, or presbycusis.
With presbycusis, both ears are usually affected. Higher-range hearing frequencies are affected first, although over time the lower frequencies may also become impaired. The ability to understand speech is affected early in presbycusis, since the consonants f, k, s, sh, th, and p are high frequency. Presbycusis is due to damage to the hair cells of the inner ear. Hair cells do not regenerate, so this is a permanent hearing loss. The reasons for hair cell damage are not totally clear; however, smokers and those with family history of age-related hearing loss, repeated loud noise exposure, and certain medical conditions and medications are at higher risk.

Understanding speech.
This can be difficult for older adults, even when hearing is essentially normal. For those with hearing loss, speech discrimination is worse than would be expected from the degree of hearing loss alone. Speech that occurs in noisy environments, is rapid, or that is loaded with information can be particularly hard to understand. The competition of sounds for your hearing contributes greatly to this problem for all of us. Some of this may be due to age- and disease-related changes in the numbers of hair cells or nerve fibers in the auditory pathways of the brain, resulting in reduced clarity of understanding and distortion of hearing. Some is due to the normal age-related changes in executive function, and the inability to multitask or split attention. For example, when different words are played into each ear, older people have more trouble identifying each word than younger people.

Earwax buildup.
When the cells lining the ear canal slough off, they create wax that migrates into the canal to cleanse the ear. With aging, the wax gets drier and can create a ball that blocks sound waves from hitting the eardrum, impairing your hearing. Lower tones are blocked more than higher ones, and you can experience a muffling effect with a loss of up to 25 to 30 decibels. This hearing loss will improve when the wax is removed.

Adapting to Your New Normal

I don't have a hearing problem yet, although it seems like every older person I know does. Is there anything I can do to protect the hearing I currently have?

Quitting smoking, eating a healthy diet, and exercising are the best things you can do to protect your hearing.

Avoid prolonged noise. One way to do this is by lowering the volume when using earphones. When prolonged noise is unavoidable, such as at a construction site or on a firing range, use hearing protectors (special ear plugs or ear muffs). These devices can be purchased at sporting goods stores, and it's worth paying for good-quality ones that offer better protection.

Get your ears cleaned regularly. Wax buildup can interfere with your hearing. Ask your primary care provider if you have ear wax and, if so, how you can get it removed.

I'm having trouble hearing, especially when I'm talking with someone in person or on the telephone. What can I do to make it easier for me to hear what they're saying to me?

Position yourself correctly. You and the person you're speaking with should be at eye level, three to six feet apart, and the light should shine on them, not you, allowing you to see their lips. Lip, face, and tongue movements provide information in addition to sound to aid in comprehension. For me and some of my friends, using a mask during the COVID-19 pandemic was probably life-saving, but we had more difficulty understanding what others were saying.

Minimize background noise. Hard surfaces like windows and plaster walls exaggerate background sounds. Try to hold conversations where sound can be absorbed, such as in areas with drapes or upholstered furniture.

Embrace technology to improve your ability to hear the television or the telephone without having the people next door complain.

- *Telephone:* There are amplified, captioned, and hearing aid–compatible phones, as well as vibrating and flashing ringer alerts that indicate an incoming call. Most states have agencies that provide resources, services, and possibly financial assistance to help the hearing impaired use their phones.

- *Television:* A variety of amplifier systems and assisted listening devices allow hearing-impaired people to watch TV without the volume being too loud for others. Use closed captioning to help augment speech discrimination.

Replace high-pitched, hard-to-hear alarms with ones that vibrate or flash. Alarm clocks, smoke alarms, doorbell alerts, and motion sensors with these features can be added to your home. An alarm with a louder noise may also work; you might need the noise to awaken you in case of an emergency.

My hearing is definitely not what is was, but hearing aids are really expensive. Are there cheaper ways to amplify sound?

Personal amplifiers are small microphones that transmit sound directly into a receiver worn in the ear. They are cheaper than a hearing aid and don't require a prescription. They can resemble a Bluetooth receiver, an earbud, or headphones. They are particularly helpful in one-on-one conversations or in small group settings. I often have my patients try one of these devices in my office. Some reluctant patients concede that they have a hearing loss once they're able to hear better with the amplifier.

Hearing aids work best for people who have hearing loss but are able to understand most speech. Hearing aids fit behind the ear, in the ear, and in the ear canal. Your hearing, eyesight, and ability to manipulate small objects with your hands will help determine which is best for you. Ear, nose, and throat (ENT) doctors and audiologists can best help you understand the pros and cons of these different types. Having two hearing aids, one in each ear, has advantages. The first provides amplification, and the other helps with understanding speech and where sounds are coming from. But hearing aids are not cheap (see the Resources section at the end of this chapter), and they're not covered by Medicare, so you may want to start with one. Make sure you get at least a 30-day trial period, during which you can return the hearing aid and get your money back if you find it is not helping. The US Food and Drug Administration has approved over-the-counter hearing aids to treat mild to moderate hearing loss. These are starting to be available and cost considerably less than prescription ones.

Give hearing aids a chance. Hearing aids have a bad rep: less than half of older people who could benefit never try them, others give them up after a short trial, and only 20 percent actually use them. Why? Many people refuse to try a hearing aid because they remember how their parents reacted to them, or even more often, because they see it as a visible sign that they are getting old. The truth is that not hearing well makes you appear really out of it. You stop participating in conversations and can become isolated, depressed, and lose your self-esteem.

In the past, hearing aids amplified all sounds, those that you wanted to hear and those that you didn't. They were often cosmetically unappealing, leading to the concerns mentioned above about "looking old." Now there are many options for hearing aids, and newer ones are nearly invisible, but more importantly, they amplify more selectively, and some automatically adjust the volume. They are much better at improving hearing and the ability to understand speech. For a small additional price, you can get a built-in telecoil for use when talking on the phone or in auditoriums like theaters or places of worship that have public amplification systems.

Get over your resistance to hearing aids. I did, and now I can hear the birds chirp. I also have more energy because I'm expending less effort trying to understand what people are saying.

What amount of hearing loss means that I should be getting hearing aids?

There is no specific number, but there

are reasons to get a hearing aid earlier rather than waiting. Some studies suggest that uncorrected hearing may increase the rate of future hearing loss. Hearing aids can relieve symptoms of depression associated with hearing loss. Recent studies suggest that earlier use may improve memory, even if only because you are able to hear something and thus have a *chance* to remember it. People also seem to adjust better if they start using hearing aids early in the course of their hearing loss. If you have tinnitus, a good digital aid can compete with it to allow you to hear and also understand sounds in the room.

Will I benefit from cochlear implants?

Unlike hearing aids, which amplify sound, cochlear implants bypass damaged structures in the ear and transmit sound directly to the brain. Implants are recommended for those with severe hearing loss in both ears who are unable to understand 40 percent of words spoken in a quiet room while wearing hearing aids. The surgery takes about three hours and is done under general anesthesia. If you think you are a candidate, discuss this option with your ENT physician.

What Isn't Normal Aging?

 Red Flags: Symptoms Needing Prompt Medical Attention

- Sudden loss of hearing.
- Worsening inability to understand speech.
- Decreased hearing accompanied by a sense of the room spinning.
- Hearing loss with associated weakness of facial muscles.
- Onset of dull and gradually increasing ear pain and tenderness.
- Discharge from the ear.

⚠️ **Yellow Alerts: Common Conditions That Can Mimic or Worsen Hearing Loss**

Tinnitus

Tinnitus is hearing sounds in the absence of external sounds. When the auditory nerve is either damaged or wounded, you may hear sounds that aren't generated from your auditory system. Often described as a ringing in the ears, tinnitus may sound more like hissing, whooshing, pulsing, roaring, or buzzing. This "head noise" is heard by you alone, not by others. It is not part of normal aging, but it occurs more often in older adults. It is not a disease itself, but it can be a symptom of other disorders, such as hearing loss, middle ear obstruction (occasionally from ear wax), temporomandibular joint (TMJ) disease, sinus pressure after an infection, medication use (see table 12.2), or other metabolic or systemic medical conditions. It is important that you see an ENT doctor for evaluation and treatment, particularly when tinnitus first starts or if the quality of it changes.

Medications

Some medications can cause temporary or permanent hearing loss and tinnitus. For a list of drugs that are associated with hearing changes, see table 12.2.

Advice for Loved Ones

Problems with vision can make it much harder to do simple tasks like taking a walk, shopping in a store, or preparing meals, and can also cause falls or fears of falling. If your loved one has a visual impairment, encourage them to seek help and to try out new devices like magnifiers or e-readers. Family support has been found to be the most powerful predictor of continued use of devices that are prescribed for vision rehabilitation. Learning how to use these devices can also be an opportunity for bonding with tech-savvy grandchildren. Recognize that visually impaired people take longer to do things, like adapting to changes in lighting in their dark home when first entering. Give them time to adjust, and when appropriate, help them navigate. Have them hold your arm, and if the path isn't wide enough for both of you, have them hold your arm and walk behind you.

People often are not as patient with those living with hearing impairment as they are of those with vision impairment. Sometimes there's confusion as to whether there really is a problem or if it's a case of "selective hearing." This can lead to frustration on both sides as well as miscommunication from literal misunderstanding. Often, a hearing impaired person's response is totally appropriate for what they heard, even though it seems out of left field to you. Always consider a possible hearing loss when you think someone is depressed, developing dementia, or simply ignoring you.

Remember, the world is a playground for competing noises, which in combination with internal noises (tinnitus) make it both harder and more frustrating for you and your loved one. Patience really is a virtue in this situation.

What can you do to improve communication with a hearing-impaired person?

- Talk only when you're in the same room; don't try to be heard from another room.

- Make sure you get the listener's attention before speaking.

- Ask if one ear has better hearing, and position yourself so you can speak more directly to that ear.

- Keep your mouth visible when speaking; don't cover it, smoke, or chew.

- Speak slowly, and don't drop volume at the end of a sentence.

- Don't shout. Shouting can cause conflict and frustration; try rephrasing instead of repeating the same thing over and over again in a louder voice.

TABLE 12.2
Medications Associated with Hearing Changes

Temporary hearing loss improves after the medication is stopped. For each drug class, the specific medications noted are only those that have been reported in the literature to have the effect. It is unknown whether others in each drug class can cause the effect.

Medication Class	Temporary Hearing Loss	Permanent Hearing Loss	Tinnitus
Blood pressure, cardiovascular, and diuretic medications			
Loop diuretics: high-dose furosemide (Lasix); ethacrynic acid (Edecrin)	X		
Antiarrhythmics			
Quinidine, flecainide (Tambocor)			X
Amiodarone (Cordarone)	X		
Beta-blockers and calcium channel blockers: metoprolol (Toprol); timolol; amlodipine (Norvasc); nicardipine (Cardene)			X
Statins: atorvastatin (Lipitor)			X
Pain relief			
Aspirin: 12 or more daily	X		X
All NSAIDs: indomethacin (Indocin); ibuprofen (Motrin, Advil); naproxen (Naprosyn, Aleve)	X		X
GABA-ergic neurogenic pain medications: gabapentin (Neurontin)			X
Cold, allergy, and itch medications			
First-generation antihistamines: chlorpheniramine (Chlor-Trimeton); hydroxyzine (Atarax); promethazine hydrochloride (Phenergan)			X
Neurologic, psychological, and sleeping medications			
Benzodiazepine and benzodiazepine receptor agonists: diazepam (Valium); alprazolam (Xanax); lorazepam (Ativan); zolpidem (Ambien)			W
Antidepressants (TCAs, SSRIs, SNRIs): nortriptyline (Pamelor); amitriptyline (Elavil); citalopram (Celexa); sertraline (Zoloft); venlafaxine (Effexor)			X

(continued)

TABLE 12.2 (*continued*)

Medication Class	Temporary Hearing Loss	Permanent Hearing Loss	Tinnitus
Anticonvulsants: divalproex sodium (Depakote); valproic acid (Depakene); topiramate (Topamax)	X		topiramate
Anxiolytic: buspirone (Buspar)			X
Dementia cholinesterase inhibitors: galantamine (Razadyne)			X
Antimicrobials			
Antibiotics			
Aminoglycoside antibiotics (given intravenously): gentamicin; amikacin (Amikin)		X	X
Vancomycin (Vancocin)		X	X
High-dose erythromycin		X	
Others: clarithromycin (Biaxin); doxycycline (Periostat, Vibramycin)			X
Antifungals: amphotericin		X	
Antimalarials: chloroquine; hydroxychloroquine (Plaquenil)			X
Quinine (Qualaquin)	X		X
Other medications			
Cancer drugs: higher-dose vincristine (Vincasar PFS); vinblastine; cisplatin (PlatinolAQ); carboplatin (Paraplatin)		X	X
Corticosteroids: prednisone; dexamethasone (Decadron); methylprednisolone (Solu-Medrol)			X
Diabetes medications: Tolbutamide (Orinase)			X
Osteoporosis bisphosphonate: risedronate (Actonel, Atelvia)			X
BPH alpha-blockers: terazosin (Hytrin); alfuzosin (Uroxatral); tamsulosin (Flomax)			X

Note: X, may cause this condition; W, withdrawal symptoms occur when drug is abruptly stopped. Abbreviations are as follows: BPH, benign prostatic hyperplasia; GABA, gamma amino butyric acid; NSAID, nonsteroidal anti-inflammatory drug; SNRI, serotonin-norepinephrine reuptake inhibitor; SSRI, selective serotonin reuptake inhibitor; TCA, tricyclic antidepressant.

- If you're not sure the listener heard, have her repeat back what she heard you say.
- Eliminate noise exposure whenever possible.

- Be supportive, and explore and encourage the use of adaptive and assistive listening devices with your loved one. Have empathy for and patience with their frustration.

Bottom Line

Vision and hearing loss are common in older adults. Vision impairments increase your risk of falls or accidents and can compromise your ability to read, while high-frequency hearing loss, or presbycusis, can make it hard to hear or understand speech, especially in noisy environments. Hearing loss also affects memory and can cause depression. There's not a hard and fast rule for when you should get help with vision and hearing loss, but this chapter provides guidance on this often subjective question.

RESOURCES

Vision Impairment

National Eye Health Education Program
(https://www.nei.nih.gov/learn-about-eye
-health/resources-for-health-educators)
The NEHEP, which is an initiative from the National Eye Institute, provides information on eye conditions for patients and families.

See What I See App
(https://www.nei.nih.gov/learn-about-eye
-health/resources-for-health-educators
/see-what-i-see-virtual-reality-eye-disease
-experience)
The National Eye Institute offers this virtual reality app to allow you to experience what it's like to have different types of vision loss.

Turbert, David. "Resources and Links for People with Low Vision." American Academy of Ophthalmology. September 23, 2021. https://www.aao.org/eye-health/diseases
/low-vision-resources.

VisionAware
(https://visionaware.org/)
This website "provides timely information, step-by-step daily living techniques, a directory of national and local services, and a supportive online community."

Hearing Impairment

Better Hearing Institute of the Hearing Industries Association
(www.betterhearing.org)
Offers brochures and information about hearing loss, tinnitus, and hearing aids, as well as a directory of hearing care providers.

Hearing Loop
(hearingloop.org)
The Hearing Loop is a universal symbol that indicates accommodations for people with hearing loss. A service of the Hearing Loss Association of America, the Hearing Loop logo is a blue sign with a white ear and white slash through it.

In addition, if the specific accommodation uses a hearing aid's telecoil (t-coil or t-switch), the sign has a "T" in the bottom right corner.

Hearing Loss Association of America (https://www.hearingloss.org/chapters -state-orgs/)
The HLAA provides advocacy, information gathering and dissemination, referral to appropriate state agencies, interpretation services, statewide planning, job placement, and development. It also offers help in obtaining free or low-cost telephone equipment for people with hearing loss. For up-to-date information for each state, visit the Telecommunication Equipment Distribution Programs Association (TEDPA) at tedpa.org.

National Institute on Deafness and Other Communication Disorders (NIDCD) Information Clearinghouse (www.nidcd.nih.gov/; 800-241-1044)
Resource center for normal and abnormal hearing, balance, smell, taste, voice, speech, and language.

BIBLIOGRAPHY

Altissimi, G., A. Colizza, G. Cianfrone, et al. "Drugs Inducing Hearing Loss, Tinnitus, Dizziness and Vertigo: An Updated Guide." *European Review for Medical Pharmacological Sciences* 24, no. 15 (2020): 7946–52.

Dillon, C. F., Q. Gu, H. J. Hoffman, and C.-W. Ko. "Vision, Hearing, Balance, and Sensory Impairment in Americans Aged 70 Years and Over: United States, 1999–2006." *NCHS Data Brief* 31 (2010): http://www .cdc.gov/nchs/data/databriefs/db31.pdf.

Jain, N. S., C. W. Ruan, S. R. Dhanji, and R. J. Syme. "Psychotropic Drug-Induced Glaucoma: A Practical Guide to Diagnosis and Management" *CNS Drugs* 35 (2021): 283–89.

Li, J., R. C. Tripathi, and B. J. Tripathi. "Drug-Induced Ocular Disorders." *Drug Safety* 31, no. 2 (2008): 127–41.

Yang, M. C., and K. Y. Lin. "Drug-Induced Acute Angle-Closure Glaucoma: A Review." *Journal of Current Glaucoma Practice* 13, no. 3 (2019): 104–9.

CHAPTER 13

Aches and Pains

Pain and discomfort are not normal aging, but they certainly occur more often as you get older. Studies suggest that 60 to 70 percent of older people have had pain that lasted at least a year, and over 15 percent report daily pain. How pain affects you depends on where the pain is, the type of pain, and your response to it (see box 13.1).

Pain is a warning sign; it tells you something isn't right. Pain can be *acute*, caused by a specific event such as trauma (a fall, or a broken bone), infection, organ obstruction, or a paper cut. Acute pain improves and eventually resolves. *Persistent pain* (also called chronic pain) lasts longer than six months and can happen for myriad reasons, including tissue injury, nerve damage, or tumor growth. Any pain is difficult to live with, but persistent pain often causes depression, anxiety, agitation, irritability, and social isolation.

There are many misconceptions about pain, its prevention, and treatment. In this chapter we'll discuss the musculoskeletal system, which is responsible for 70 percent of pain in older adults, how age influences the musculoskeletal system and pain perception, how you can adapt to your new normal, when pain needs urgent evaluation, common painful conditions that occur mainly in older adults, and how to prepare for a pain evaluation, including how to describe the pain's location, characteristics, and how it's affecting you.

Box 13.2 describes the anatomy of the musculoskeletal system.

BOX 13.1

Pain 101

BIOLOGY OF PAIN

Physical pain is our body's response to injuries like severe pressure, heat, or chemicals, including molecules that are released from cells in response to tissue injury. *Nociceptors* are pain receptors present in the skin, muscles, joints, bones, and internal organs that send messages about the intensity and location of a painful stimulus to nerves, the spinal cord, and the brain. Glutamate is the primary neurotransmitter involved in the sensation of pain in the brain. When the brain receives the message that you're having pain, it activates emotional and

(continued)

BOX 13.1 (*continued*)

fight-or-flight responses, sending nerve impulses and pain-relieving substances like endogenous opioids back down the spinal cord to help alleviate the pain.

Even though there is great variability in how people respond to pain, the threshold at which a stimulus produces pain is similar for all. This is because pain response is modified by one's emotional state, expectations, previous experience of pain, and the context in which pain occurs. In the presence of persistent pain or nerve damage, the response of pain receptors and nerve, spinal cord, and brain cells may be modified.

Pain is classified by its duration. *Acute pain* has a clear onset, cause, and quality. It may cause a rapid heart rate, high blood pressure, or sweating. Acute pain ends when the cause has been addressed, like when a fracture or a cut heals. Acute pain, by definition, resolves in three to six months. *Persistent pain* (also called *chronic pain*) usually lasts more than six months. Causes include tissue injury, inflammation, nerve damage, tumor growth, and blood vessel occlusion.

Pain signals in persistent pain remain active in the nervous system for weeks, months, or years. Prolonged noxious stimuli, including inflammation and tissue injury, are thought to sensitize nociceptors so that they fire spontaneously or in response to weaker or non-pain stimuli. This results in a greater barrage of nerve impulses, causing hyperexcitability of the brain and spinal cord neurons. *Allodynia*, painful responses to non-painful stimuli, or *hyperalgesia*, a response that is more painful than expected, can result. For example, diabetes can damage nerves in the feet, leading to a condition known as diabetic neuropathy. For some people with diabetic neuropathy, simply covering a foot with a bedsheet can cause pain.

TYPES OF PAIN

Determining the type of pain helps clarify what's causing the pain and what may help relieve it. Pain is classified as either *nociceptive, neuropathic,* or *inflammatory.* Some pain may be due to more than one cause, like that which occurs when cancer that metastasizes to the spine (nociceptive pain) impinges on spinal nerves (neuropathic pain).

Nociceptive pain is stimulated by tissue injury and inflammation, and it is generally either *somatic* or *visceral*. It is protective, a warning that damage is occurring to your body.

- Somatic pain results from injury to soft tissues and bone, like touching a hot stove or breaking a hip. It is usually well localized and described as sharp, aching, or throbbing.

- Visceral pain results from injury to internal organs or their fibrous coverings. It is diffuse, more difficult to localize than somatic pain, and can cause nausea, cold sweats, and light-headedness. Some examples include the gnawing, crampy, or colicky pain that occurs when structures like the gall bladder, the ureter, or the

BOX 13.1 *(continued)*

colon are blocked by stones or hard feces. The discomfort of *angina*, a temporary decrease in blood flow to the heart, is often described as pressure, a deep
pain, or indigestion.

Visceral pain is often *referred pain*, felt at a site other than the site of injury. It is
achy and feels like it's close to the body's surface. For example, a heart attack may
cause pain in the left arm, or a gall bladder infection may cause right shoulder or
scapula pain. It's thought that this happens because the area of referred pain—the
left arm, for example—developed embryologically from the same structures as the
injured one, the heart. Another theory is that the sensory nerves from the heart
and the left arm overlap in the gray matter of the spinal cord, causing the brain to
interpret the visceral pain as coming from the skin of the arm.

Neuropathic pain results from nerve injury. The pain is described as numbness or
burning with sharp, shooting pains. Diabetic neuropathy, shingles, and sciatica
are examples. The damaged nerve causes nociceptors and nerves to fire without
a specific stimulus, causing pain and hypersensitivity without an obvious precipitating factor. Sometimes, neuropathic pain persists long after an injury heals, as
with shingles, where nerve pain can last, at times, for years.

Inflammatory pain is due to chemical mediators released in response to tissue
injury, whether from trauma, arthritis, infections, or surgery. The purpose of the
inflammatory response is not to cause pain but to eliminate the cause of injury
and the damaged tissue, and to start tissue repair. Immune cells in the injured
area release substances that lead to inflammation, including histamine, serotonin,
substance P, bradykinin, prostaglandins, and nitric oxide, which result in increased
blood flow to the area, bringing more immune cells, antibodies, and clotting proteins into the injured tissue. In addition to causing inflammation, these molecules
stimulate nerve endings and cause hypersensitivity to pain. Once the cause of the
injury is removed, the inflammation ceases.

HOW PAIN MEDICATIONS WORK

One of the key principles in pain management is that different classes of medications work in different ways, so pain relief may be enhanced by adding a medication with a different mechanism of action. For example, drugs like Percocet
(oxycodone and acetaminophen) provide greater pain relief than either drug
alone because the oxycodone works by binding to opioid receptors, inactivating
central pain pathways, whereas acetaminophen reduces pain through a different,
not fully understood, mechanism. Inflammatory molecules like histamine, bradykinin, and serotonin play a role in increasing pain hypersensitivity, so that drugs
that can deplete these or block their actions can be effective in pain relief. Other
drugs interrupt nerve conduction or prostaglandin production. The different
mechanisms of action of common pain medications are outlined in table 13.1,
and the side effects of these drugs are discussed in table 13.2.

BOX 13.2

Anatomy of the Musculoskeletal System

Over 70 percent of pain in older adults originates in the *musculoskeletal system*, which includes the joints, the spine, and the tissues involved in their stability and movement, including cartilage, ligaments, muscles, tendons, and bursa. Inflammation, trauma, and wear-and-tear deterioration can cause pain to these structures as well as to the nerves that are in the area. The anatomy of common pain hot spots in the musculoskeletal system follows.

JOINTS AND THEIR SUPPORTING STRUCTURES

A joint is the juncture of two bones. Joints provide stability and often allow movement. Some joints don't move at all, like those that fuse the bones of the skull. Others, like the intervertebral discs of the spine, have limited movement. Still others work with a gliding motion along a plane, such as the wrist. Condyloid joints like those in the finger and jaw permit movement with no rotation.

Most joints in the body are *synovial joints* and move more freely, like your shoulder and your knee (see the figures below). Synovial joints cushion the two opposing bones. Without this cushion, the bones would press on each other, causing pain, joint instability, and bone erosion. The cushions consist of smooth *articular cartilage* that covers the surfaces where the bones touch and a *joint capsule* between the bones that is filled with synovial fluid. This arrangement allows the bones to move over each other without friction, while synovial fluid lubricates and diffuses pressure on the joint's surfaces by acting as a shock absorber. The joint capsule has a fibrous outer layer that holds the bones together, creating an air-tight, sterile joint. Its inner layer is called the *synovial membrane*, or the *synovium*, which produces the synovial fluid and contains the joint's blood vessels, which provide nutrients to the joints and its nerves. The nerves supply the brain with information about the joint's position and whether it is painful.

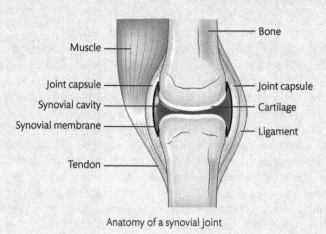

Anatomy of a synovial joint

BOX 13.2 (*continued*)

When a joint bears weight, the force is absorbed by the joint's muscle and cartilage. *Cartilage* is a specialized form of connective tissue composed of cells (chondrocytes) that produce an *extracellular matrix* made of collagen, proteoglycans, and elastin fibers. Damaged cartilage heals poorly because cartilage doesn't have blood vessels or nerves.

A joint's stability and range of motion depend on how the bones are held together. For the hip and shoulder, the bones are joined by a ball and socket, while the bones in the knee are held together like a hinge. The shoulder and hip can move in multiple directions, whereas the elbow and knee can only flex and extend. Although the shoulder has greater range of motion, it is a less stable joint than the hip. One often hears of shoulder dislocations, but rarely of hip dislocations. The figures below illustrate why.

In the shoulder joint, the ball (head of the humerus) is much larger than the socket that it fits into (glenoid fossa).

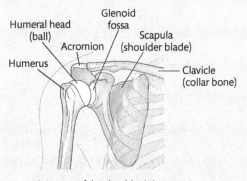

Anatomy of the shoulder joint

In the hip joint, in contrast, the ball (head of the femur) is completely surrounded by the socket (pelvic acetabulum).

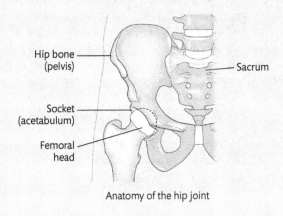

Anatomy of the hip joint

(*continued*)

BOX 13.2 *(continued)*

Strong ligaments and surrounding muscles, like the rotator cuff muscles of the shoulder, attach to the bones to help keep the joint stable. *Ligaments* are bands of fibrous tissue that hold bones together at joints, holding them in place and restricting their movement. *Muscles* cross over joints, allowing them to bend. *Tendons* connect muscle to bone. When a muscle contracts, it pulls on its tendon, which moves the bone to which it is attached.

Bursae are small sacs lined by synovium and filled with synovial fluid that are located between bones and muscles, tendons, ligaments, and skin. They reduce the rubbing and friction that occurs when these tissues glide over bones during joint movement. *Bursitis* occurs when bursae become inflamed from an infection or irritated by overuse of the joint.

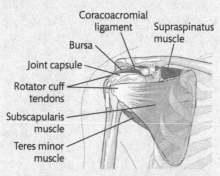

The shoulder and its supporting structures

THE SPINE AND ITS SUPPORTING STRUCTURES

The spine protects the spinal cord, supports body weight, and is integral to movement and posture.

Anatomy of the Spine

The spine consists of 24 vertebrae, 23 intervertebral discs, the fused vertebrae of the sacrum, and the tailbone (coccyx). Each vertebra is named by its region and where it is positioned. The cervical vertebrae are C1–7, thoracic T1–12, and lumbar L1–5. All vertebrae except for C1 and C2 look similar, with a large vertebral body at the front and a "spinous process" at the back (the spinous process is what you feel when you run your hand down a spine). Strong ligaments connect the vertebrae in front and back to keep the spinal column in position.

The *vertebral canal*, which contains the spinal cord, is formed by alignment of the vertebral cavities. These cavities are formed by the vertebral arches connecting the vertebral body and the spinous process. *Facet joints* are synovial joints connecting the bones of the spine that allow it to bend and twist, while limiting its motion to keep the vertebrae properly aligned. Each vertebra has two sets of these synovial joints, one pair facing upward and one downward. The 31 pairs

BOX 13.2 *(continued)*

of *spinal nerves* pass through these joints and go to specific areas of the arms, legs, and other parts of the body. The *spinal cord* ends in the lower back, around the first and second lumbar vertebrae, and the remaining nerve roots, called the *cauda equina*, Latin for "horse's tail," exit the vertebral canal through the facet joints of the remaining vertebrae.

Intervertebral discs sit between each vertebral body, providing a cushion and allowing slight movement of the vertebrae. Along with the facet joints, they facilitate the spine's movement by providing stability and support for bending forward, backward, sideways, and twisting. The discs are flat, about half an inch thick, and have *end plates* that are attached to the vertebrae and fused to the disc. Each disc has a flexible outer ring called the *annulus fibrosus*, which along with the vertebral end plates hold the jellylike center, the *nucleus pulposus*, in place. The nucleus pulposus is partly made of water and gives the disc flexibility and strength. When you stand or move, and especially when you run or jump, pressure is put on the spine, and the nucleus pulposus acts like a shock absorber, distributing the pressure in all directions.

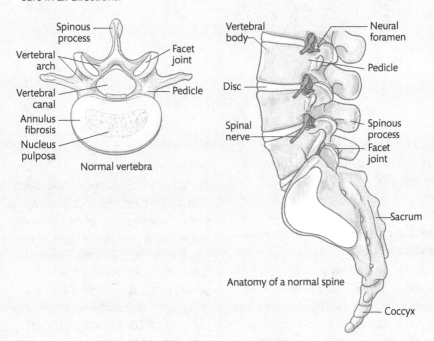

Normal vertebra

Anatomy of a normal spine

Spinal and Peripheral Nerves

The brain and spinal cord make up the central nervous system (CNS), while the spinal nerves and the peripheral nerves formed from them are the peripheral nervous system (PNS). Spinal nerves relay messages from the body to the CNS, and

(continued)

BOX 13.2 (*continued*)

vice versa. Each spinal nerve supplies a single area of skin, called a dermatome, as well as muscles and joints in a certain area. Symptoms that occur along a single dermatome can indicate what part of the spine may be affected. In general, the eight cervical nerves supply the arms, parts of the neck and chest, and some of the head. The twelve thoracic nerves supply the skin over the chest, some of the skin over the abdomen and armpit, and muscles in the thoracic and lumbar region. The five lumbar nerves mainly supply the muscles of the abdomen, pelvis, and some of the thigh, as well as some of the skin of the abdomen, back, groin, and thigh. The five sacral nerves supply the skin, muscles, and joints of the lower limbs and some pelvic muscles. The coccygeal nerve supplies the skin over the coccyx.

Peripheral nerves are formed from combinations of the spinal nerves. For example, in the pelvis, parts of two lumbar and three sacral nerves re-form into the *sciatic nerve*, which extends down the leg. In the armpit, parts of three cervical and one thoracic nerve re-form into the *median nerve*, the culprit in carpal tunnel syndrome.

What's Normal with Aging?

For a deeper dive into age-related changes in pain, joints, and the spine, see box 13.3.

You say aches and pains aren't normal aging, but they sure seem to be common. What causes them?

Most everyday pains are musculoskeletal, like arthritis, back soreness, muscle aches, repetitive-use injuries like carpal tunnel syndrome or tennis elbow, or misaligned postures or gait abnormalities that put additional stress on muscles and joints. Although they're not "normal," or due to age-related physiological changes, they're so common I discuss ways to prevent and alleviate them in the next section.

What aches and pains are due to osteoarthritis?

The common symptoms of osteoarthritis (OA) are pain, stiffness, tenderness, and decreased range of motion, most frequently affecting the joints of the hand, knee, hip, and spine. Activity makes the pain worse, while rest improves it. But too much rest, or inactivity, can cause stiffness. This is why people with OA feel most stiff in the morning, while they feel the greatest pain at the end of the day. OA can be progressive, and over time you may find that you're having more pain and difficulty using these joints.

BOX 13.3

What Happens with Aging: A Deeper Dive

PAIN

Pain severity may not reflect the severity of illness.
The sensation of visceral pain, which is caused by injury to internal organs or their coverings, often decreases with age. In fact, more than 50 percent of people 85 and older do not have chest pain when they have a heart attack (some have no symptoms, some get shortness of breath, lose consciousness, or experience confusion), and many people who have a raging abdominal organ infection or perforation have bellies that are soft and not particularly tender. Conversely, one's ability to perceive somatic pain (from injury of the external body or skin) and neuropathic (nerve-induced) pain doesn't change significantly with age.

Sensitivity to pain medications increases.
As discussed in chapter 3, there are many reasons why older people respond differently than younger people to medications. Such changes occur also with medications for pain. Some of this increased sensitivity is due to changes in the way older adults metabolize drugs, and some is due to changes in an organ's responsiveness to a given drug level. This can result in the need for lower doses of medication to relieve pain and the occurrence of more side effects even at these lower doses. See table 13.2 for precautions for older adults when using specific pain medications.

THE MUSCULOSKELETAL SYSTEM

Joints and Their Supporting Structures

Cartilage deteriorates with age, which can cause joint stiffness and pain.
Excessive mechanical force, sometimes referred to as "wear and tear," damages cartilage by degrading its extracellular matrix, releasing growth factors. Growth factors should stop matrix degradation, but aged chondrocytes don't respond to this process, so the matrix continues to be destroyed, releasing inflammatory mediators like cytokines. This degeneration wears away the articular cartilage (the cartilage at the ends of the bones). With aging, there is also a decrease in the volume of synovial fluid produced, decreasing lubrication and shock absorption. For these reasons, the bones of joints may come into direct contact with each other, causing scraping, pain, and inflammation in the surrounding joint tissues and the development of *bone spurs*, or *osteophytes*. The result is joints that are stiffer and less flexible.

Osteoarthritis is not normal aging, even though it's very common in older adults.
Osteoarthritis (OA) was long thought to be due to mechanical factors, the wear and tear of articular cartilage over decades of use. But it is now evident that there is more to OA than damaged cartilage. The entire arthritic joint is affected, including the synovium, cartilage, bone, and muscle.

(continued)

BOX 13.3 *(continued)*

Osteoarthritic cartilage differs from normal, aged cartilage. The bone underneath the cartilage thickens, and bone cysts develop even before articular cartilage is lost. Bone cysts release inflammatory molecules into the joint space. Inflammation causes joint injury and cartilage degradation. Joint injury, whether due to trauma or age-related changes to the cartilage, also produces inflammatory molecules. These molecules can cause *synovitis*, or inflammation of the synovial membrane. It is not currently known whether the primary trigger for age-associated OA is the change in cartilage or the presence of inflammation.

Bursitis is more common.
Bursitis is usually caused by repeated pressure on the bursa or by overusing a joint (see box 13.2). Anything that interferes with the usual function of a joint can put more stress on a bursa. This is exacerbated by the age-related decrease in tendon strength.

Joint range of motion declines, affecting flexibility.
With aging, you may have difficulty turning your neck to see when driving out of your driveway or bending over to pick objects off the floor. You may find that you are no longer able to reach items on a high shelf (losing height also contributes to this problem). A person's joint range of motion declines 20 to 25 percent with aging owing to decreased activity, diminished joint synovial fluid, increased cartilage deterioration, ligament shortening, and tight muscles.

Tendons and ligaments are more likely to tear or rupture.
The strength of tendons and ligaments decreases with aging, weakening their attachment to muscles and bones. This predisposes the tissue to injury after minor trauma. Tendons and ligaments take longer to heal because they have relatively few blood vessels, limiting the supply of inflammatory cells and nutrients reaching the tissue. A common example is the prevalence of chronic rotator cuff injuries in older adults due to tendon tears.

The Spine in Decline

Intervertebral discs degenerate with age, resulting in a back and neck that are stiffer and not as flexible.
The same process discussed above for joints occurs to the cartilage in intervertebral discs. The discs become drier, thinner, harder, and lose some of their cushioning ability. Most of the changes are in the nucleus pulposus, which dehydrates, becomes fibrotic, and develops fissures and cracks. The end plates calcify. As the cartilage thins, the bones start to rub together, causing friction that can result in the formation of bone spurs, or vertebral osteophytes. The loss of cartilage and the development of spurs make the spine stiffer and the back less flexible.

Degenerative changes in the intervertebral discs can cause spinal osteoarthritis, radicular pain, and spinal stenosis.
Intervertebral disc degeneration increases the load on the facet joints, degrading the cartilage and causing *facet joint arthritis* (also called spinal osteoarthritis)

BOX 13.3 (*continued*)

with facet hypertrophy and the formation of bone spurs or osteophytes. These changes are evident on x-rays but don't always cause symptoms. If the osteophytes compress a nerve root, *radicular pain* (a type of neuropathic pain) can occur along the course of the nerve. For example, pain from a lumbar spinal nerve may radiate into the buttock, leg, or foot. Compare the figure below to that of a normal spine in box 13.2.

   Spinal stenosis is caused by a narrowing of the vertebral canal, usually due to osteophytes, thickened ligaments, or extrusion of nucleus pulposus material from cracks in the disc's annulus. Symptoms occur when the narrowing causes pressure on the spinal cord or nerve roots. Compare the figure below to that of a normal vertebra in box 13.2.

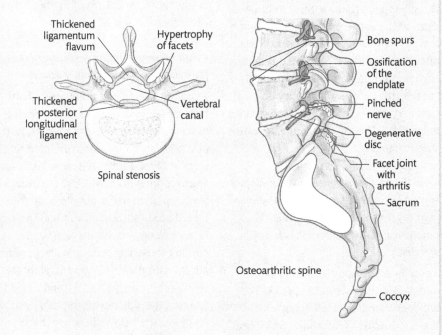

Spinal stenosis

Osteoarthritic spine

Herniated discs can occur but are less common in older adults.

Disc herniation occurs because we often use the spine to help carry excessive loads, such as recurrent lifting of heavy objects. This can cause tears in the annulus pulposus, squeezing the nucleus pulposus (*bulging disc*) and eventually pushing it through the annulus (*disc herniation* or a *slipped disc*). If the disc compresses the spinal cord, you may feel severe back pain and muscle spasms, and if it compresses a spinal nerve root, you may also have pain, numbness, and weakness in the area supplied by the nerve. Disc herniation occurs less commonly in older adults because a dehydrated nucleus pulposus is unlikely to move into or through the annulus.

I've been told that OA is a "wear-and-tear" arthritis. By the time you're my age, you've got a lot of miles on you. So, is OA inevitable as I age?

Not all older people have pain from OA, but almost everyone's joints show some radiological signs of degeneration. The "wear-and-tear" component usually refers to the thinning of the joint cartilage that covers the ends of bones, which can result in the bones rubbing directly against each other. The same thing happens to the intervertebral discs of the spine, causing stiffness and less flexibility. Osteoarthritis, however, affects not just the cartilage, but also the joint lining, bone, and muscle. Osteoarthritis causes joint injury and further cartilage degradation, as discussed in box 13.3. Normal aging doesn't cause these changes.

Over the past few months I've developed some hard, painful bumps on the joints near my fingernails. They're not like anything I've had before. Should I be worried?

These bumps are called Heberden's nodes, and they are a sign of OA. They are *bone spurs*, or *osteophytes*, which are outgrowths of new bone from local inflammation. As noted in box 13.3, osteophytes form not just on the fingers but on other areas like the vertebrae and heels. Pain from Heberden's nodes will get better over time, but the nodes themselves will remain.

You mentioned that OA can cause morning stiffness. I now wake up stiff and it takes at least an hour before I start to move normally. Is this OA, or do I need to be concerned about something else?

Morning stiffness from OA rarely lasts more than 30 minutes. In other types of inflammatory arthritis, particularly rheumatoid arthritis, morning stiffness can last up to 90 minutes. Prolonged morning stiffness also occurs in polymyalgia rheumatica, or PMR, a disorder that occurs almost entirely in people over the age of 50, and in those with Parkinson's disease. Morning stiffness is not prominent in statin muscle disorders. See the Yellow Alerts section below for more information about these disorders.

What nonprescription medication is best for aches and pains in older adults?

Acetaminophen and nonsteroidal anti-inflammatory drugs (NSAIDs) provide quick relief for many discomforts, but oral NSAIDs have significant adverse effects in older adults (see table 13.2). Acetaminophen is an effective treatment for OA pain in many people, although recent studies have found that OA pain often responds better to NSAIDs, including those applied topically. In older adults with painful OA, we usually start with acetaminophen or a topical NSAID to avoid the side effects of oral NSAIDs. As discussed below, there are many nonpharmacologic options for pain relief, including ice and exercise.

I keep seeing television ads for medications to treat nerve pain. The people in the ads are mostly old or have diabetes. What is nerve pain, and is it common in older people?

Nerve pain, sometimes referred to as neuropathic pain or neuropathy, is a burning sensation with sharp, shooting pains, numbness, or tingling that follows the course of an injured nerve. The injury can be caused by a disease like diabetes, inflammation as in shingles, or compression by bone spurs as in sciatica. Many of these disorders are common in older adults. The symptoms can originate in a different place than where you feel the discomfort, so it's important that you get a physical examination to diagnose the source of the problem. See the Yellow Alerts section below for specific information about the types of neuropathy common in older adults.

I've been having some shoulder discomfort and can't raise my arm to comb my hair. I went to Urgent Care, and they said I had a rotator cuff tear. I don't remember falling, so how could I have torn something?

With aging, tendons and ligaments fray. More than 50 percent of people over age 65 have rotator cuff tears. Many people are unaware of them until years later, when they develop pain, weakness, or decreased ability to move the joint. Simple movements like lifting a heavy package can cause the initial tear, which over time can get larger and impair function. Other joint pains that occur more commonly in older adults include bursitis and tendonitis, usually due to joint overuse. Joint range of motion also decreases with age.

Adapting to Your New Normal

Prevention along with early evaluation and treatment are the keys to avoiding severe pain. Ignoring pain is really not an option; it will only result in it taking more time, medication, or invasive treatments to make you feel better. Pain is an early warning sign that something's wrong in your body, like an infection or a muscle strain, and if you ignore it, the condition can get serious. If the pain is increasing, it's important to identify what's causing the pain. You also may develop new pain if you disregard the warning. For example, if you keep walking even though it causes left knee pain, you'll put additional stress on your right knee and hip, and eventually they may also cause you pain.

Prevention

Many of my friends have fallen, resulting in aches and pains and even broken bones or joints. How can I prevent falls and the injuries that may come with them?

See chapter 9 for information on fall prevention.

What other things can I do to prevent aches and pains, other than just stopping all my activities?

Actually, curtailing your activities is the worst thing you can do. You need to keep your muscles and joints in good shape to prevent discomfort or injury. To help prevent aches and pains, do the following.

Move around. Don't stay in any one position for too long. If you must sit for extended periods, whether on the couch or at a desk, take regular breaks to get up and get moving.

Stretch to increase your flexibility and range of motion. Routine stretching can decrease the stiffness in your neck, back, and shoulders.

Carefully strengthen your muscles to decrease joint pain and the likelihood of tendon and ligament tears. Avoid injury by having a trainer or physical therapist show you the proper techniques for doing exercises, whether aerobic, strength (using free weights, bands, or a machine), or stretching.

Pay attention to your posture. When you slouch, read while lying on your stomach, lift with your back, or hunch forward while driving or using the computer, you are leaving your spine, neck, and shoulders unsupported. This places greater tension and stress on your muscles, joints, and spine, resulting in aches and pains. If you pay attention to the times when your posture slips, you can change position or add the support of a cushion or the back of a chair to relieve the discomfort. If you don't work to improve your posture, your pain and stiffness could get worse and last longer.

Right-size your expectations. Recognize that if you try to do everything you used to be able to do, you're more likely to injure yourself. Shrinking, arthritis, decreased joint range of motion, and impaired balance are just some of the age-related conditions that can increase the possibility that older adults will injure themselves doing things they were able to do previously. Be smart, and ask for help or get adaptive equipment when needed.

What equipment might help?

If you have arthritis, use assistive devices to decrease joint pressure and pain when doing specific activities. Depending on the site of your arthritis, there are different tools that may help you. A fork, toothbrush, or pen with a larger-diameter handle will put less pressure on your hand joints. By switching the knob on your cabinet or front door to a lever, you won't have to twist your wrist to open it. Appendix 2 discusses assistive devices for mobility. See the Resources section at the end of this chapter for additional suggestions.

If your discomfort comes from repetitive motions, like texting or using a computer, make an appointment with an occupational therapist. In addition to providing occupational therapy, they can do work or home office evaluations to help configure your workspace for optimal ergonomics. Ergonomic equipment and voice recognition software may also be helpful.

Consider getting a new mattress. There's no clear expiration date for mattresses, but there are signs that it's time for a new one. Most mattresses last about eight to ten years. Your mattress and pillow need to keep your spine aligned, and if they don't, you may wake up tired, stiff, and achy. If your mattress is lumpy, sags an inch or two for a while after you get up, or if you find that you awaken with less pain after sleeping on a different bed—at a hotel, for example—it's time to for a new one.

What's the best way to treat pain? I don't want to be dependent on medications.

There are many approaches to pain relief. Which you choose depends to some extent on whether the pain is acute or persistent. You may see stars when you stub your toe, but you know it won't last long. You may find that using ice, staying off your foot for a short while, or taking acetaminophen provides adequate relief, especially since you know the pain will soon get better.

Persistent pain, on the other hand, can wear you out; interfere with your daily activities and sleep; precipitate depression, irritability, or anger; and decrease your interest in being with other people. It can be exacerbated by being overweight, doing repetitive movements, or assuming positions where your posture is unsupported. Managing persistent pain is usually not as simple as taking a pill. For these reasons, persistent pain is considered multifactorial, and addressing each of these factors can provide some relief. In fact, most pain clinics have an interprofessional team to address the contributing factors involved in pain. This book covers some of these factors, such as your sleep (chapter 10), mood (chapter 8), and weight (chapter 15). Consult these chapters for suggestions on what might work for you.

The specifics of pain management depend on the severity and persistence of the pain, and consists of nonpharmacologic and pharmacologic treatments. In general, nonpharmacologic and topical treatments are better tolerated and are good initial treatments for mild to moderately severe acute pain.

Once again, it's important to "right-size your expectations," as we discussed earlier. It'd be great if our pain management regimen could cause all of our physical pain to completely disappear. Unfortunately, that often doesn't happen because the underlying cause is still present, we're unable to change lifelong habits and behaviors, or we need to decide on a trade-off between pain relief and medication side effects. Most treatments, other than surgery and "tincture of time," decrease pain temporarily. But there are things that you can do on your own, or with the help of a trainer or other professional, that may greatly decrease the degree of pain and distress that you have.

Nonpharmacologic Pain Management

When and how should I use heat or cold to relieve pain?

The application of heat or cold can help in different situations, depending on what type of pain you have and where in the body it is occurring.

Heat for Muscle Pain and Stiffness

Heat works by increasing circulation and blood flow. You can apply a heating pad or moist heat to the painful area. Moist heat disseminates deeper into the tissue than dry heat. You should not apply heat to an area that is bruised, swollen, or that has an open wound.

Cold for Acute Injuries

Cold is particularly effective in injuries that develop inflammation and swelling. Cold works by decreasing circulation to the area. You can apply ice or a cold pack to the painful area, but do not apply cold to areas where your ability to feel is compromised, circulation is poor, or if your muscles or joints are already feeling stiff.

 Do not apply heat or cold therapy directly to the skin. Always wrap it in a thin cloth before applying.

What other nonpharmacologic pain-relief treatments are there, and how do they work?

Many pain-relief methods work by modifying circulation to the painful area, either increasing or decreasing blood flow. Some provide distraction, which can decrease your perception of the pain's severity. The relief provided may be temporary, especially if the pain is caused by positions or movements you're likely to do again, such as how you hold the steering wheel when driving or how you sit when watching TV. The results of clinical trials evaluating the effectiveness of many of these treatments are mixed, but you may find them worth trying either alone or in combination.

Exercise

Aerobic and resistance exercise, walking, tai chi, and yoga have been demonstrated to improve leg and hip pain from osteoarthritis, chronic low back pain, and chronic pain in general. By increasing muscle strength, flexibility, joint stability, and endurance, you'll decrease pain and improve function. Exercise also improves mood. Without exercise, persistent pain can result in even more pain and disability.

Pain is a major barrier to starting an exercise routine, and you will need

be cautious if you have certain injuries or types of arthritis. Ask your provider if there are contraindications or limitations to your exercising, if there is a pain medication you can take to decrease the pain prior to exercising, and if you qualify for physical therapy. If not, find a trainer at a gym, senior center, or through the Arthritis Foundation to help you develop a routine. There are many ways to decrease stress on painful areas when exercising, including aquatic programs (exercising in water reduces pressure on joints and increases their range of motion) or by using light weights or elastic bands for strengthening. It's normal to feel some pain when you first start working out, but you should begin to see some positive results in a week or two. If pain is progressively worsening, stop exercising and see your medical provider.

Regular Stretching

Stretching can be therapeutic as well as preventative. Stretching lengthens muscles, increases joint range of motion, and can relieve stiffness. Stretch slowly without bouncing to avoid tearing weak muscles.

Weight Loss

If you are overweight, weight loss is likely to improve pain due to hip or knee osteoarthritis.

Behavioral Health Techniques

Cognitive behavioral therapy, guided imagery, or mindfulness-based meditation can help decrease your response to pain (see the Resources section at the end of chapter 8). It often helps to work with a behavioral health professional who uses these techniques.

Muscle Relaxation

Muscle relaxation can help decrease muscle tightness or spasms that may be contributing to headaches or back pain. It may also help with falling asleep. For more information on muscle relaxation, see the Resources section at the end of chapter 10.

- *Progressive muscle relaxation* is an exercise you can do at home. Starting with one group of muscles at a time, breathe in and tense them, then breathe out and relax them. Go through all the muscles of the body in this way. See the Resources section at the end of chapter 10.

- *Biofeedback* can help you become aware of when you are tensing muscles by attaching electrodes to them. Biofeedback helped me with my temporomandibular joint (TMJ) pain, and I learned that when I was paying attention and concentrating, my TMJ muscles tightened up. Doing a "stupid, open mouth" look totally relaxed them. I've changed my facial expressions (and my beliefs about how I look when doing them), and as a result I have a lot less TMJ pain.

Music

At night, pain may worsen because there are fewer distractions. Some studies have shown that listening to music they enjoy while in bed can provide some people with nighttime pain relief.

Therapeutic Massage

Massage can relax muscles, tendons, and joints and has been found to be effective for back and neck pain. Massage does not have to be painful to help. As mentioned above, however, if you return to the activities that caused the discomfort, the pain will return. Massage should not be done in areas of inflammation or infection.

Acupuncture

Acupuncture has been found to be effective for some back, knee, shoulder, and neck pain. Needles are inserted and left in place for 10 to 30 minutes. Some people feel relief right away, others need several treatments, and others don't respond. The more severe and chronic your pain, the more treatments you will need before you feel relief.

Transcutaneous Electrical Nerve Stimulation

Transcutaneous electrical nerve stimulation, or TENS, can be effective for osteoarthritis, diabetic peripheral neuropathy, and other areas of chronic pain. It works by sending electrical pulses through the skin, releasing endorphins and other "natural" pain killers. It is most effective when used for at least 30 minutes during movement and activity; it is less effective when used at rest. Speak with your medical provider before using TENS, as there are important contraindications.

Physical and Occupational Therapy

Physical therapy (PT) and occupational therapy (OT) may help if pain is interfering with your ability to move, balance, or do your usual activities. PT typically focuses on movement and mobility by improving gait, balance, neck and shoulder mobility and pain, lower extremity and back discomfort, and by teaching fall prevention strategies. OT assists with your fine and gross motor skills to help you with everyday tasks like bathing, toileting, feeding, managing the household, or performing work-related activities. Some occupational therapists specialize in providing hand therapy. Physical and occupational therapists use similar strategies, including stretching, assisting with range-of-motion exercises, massage, and performing hands-on manipulation. They use hot and cold packs, massage, ultrasound, and electrical stimulation to target inflammation, stiffness, and soreness. Both will teach you about proper body mechanics, how to use adaptive equipment and/or special adaptive techniques, and how to use energy-conservation techniques to help prevent pain and promote function. They also can assist with the use of splints and braces, and suggest ergonomic equipment.

Osteopathic and Chiropractic Manipulation

Spine adjustments and manipulations are done by both chiropractors and osteopathic physicians (DOs), while peripheral joint manipulation is done only by DOs. Osteopathic medical schools teach techniques such as stretching, gentle pressure, and resistance to move muscles and joints. If you are considering seeing a DO for osteopathic manipulative treatment (OMT), call first, since not all DOs continue to practice

OMT after graduation. *High-velocity, low-amplitude (HVLA) manipulation techniques* may be used by either chiropractors or DOs on the spine and the joints. HVLA techniques should be used with caution in older adults and are contraindicated in people who have osteoporosis. If you are taking anticoagulants or high-dose steroids, spinal or joint manipulation may increase bruising or bleeding.

Pharmacologic Pain Management

I'm concerned about using medications to treat my pain. I keep hearing about addiction to pain pills as well as their side effects. What can I do to get relief but not get side effects or addicted?

Pain medication regimens can be tricky (see table 13.2). In older adults, pain medication should be started at a low dose. Pay attention to how long it takes for the medication to help, and how long the relief lasts. Work with your health care provider to increase the dose until you get good relief with minimal side effects. Ask if there are things you should be doing to prevent side effects. Keep a daily log of which medications you're taking, the dose, and what time you take them. Remember, adding nonpharmacologic modalities to your treatment regimen may lower the amount of medication you need to control your pain.

Make sure you know what medicines, at what doses, you should be taking. Ask your prescriber the following questions. Which medications should be taken regularly, and which should be taken only if the pain starts to get worse? Should you take this medication only when the pain is severe, or when you begin to feel the pain coming on? Most pain responds best to regularly scheduled doses, which don't allow the pain to become extreme. These doses can then be decreased as the problem improves. Have your health care provider write down the names of the medications, when to take them, and why you're taking them.

Many people are concerned about opioid addiction, for good reason. But if nothing else is helping and your pain is affecting your ability to function, a trial of opioids may make sense. Make sure your health care provider is aware of your concerns, and together discuss the pros and cons of a trial.

Topical Medications

Are creams and patches safer and as effective as oral medications?

Topical medications like creams, ointments, and patches are most effective if the pain is localized to one area. They should be applied to the area where you're having pain. Most topical treatments are minimally absorbed into the body, whereas oral and intravenous medications are absorbed and can produce unwanted, sometimes serious, side effects.

⟨CAUTION⟩ **Apply topical treatments using gloves, or wash hands thoroughly after using. Capsaicin can cause a burning sensation. Do not use a topical medication if your skin is not intact. Do not use with a heating pad or electric blanket.**

How do topical medications work?

Some are counterirritants, and some are pain killers.

Counterirritants include *menthol, camphor, eucalyptus, wintergreen,* and *capsaicin*. They irritate or cause mild inflammation of the skin, producing a feeling of warmth or cold that may relieve mild pain in muscles and joints. It's thought that the sensations of warmth and irritation distract attention from the pain. These agents may decrease the muscle soreness that occurs the day after exercise and increase a joint's range of motion. Some counterirritants also contain salicylates (such as Aspercreme or BENGAY), which may provide pain relief when absorbed. Capsaicin comes from chili peppers and causes a burning sensation. Although this burning sensation can stop pain, some people find it too painful to use.

Topical painkillers contain ingredients that dampen pain.

Topical NSAIDs are good initial pain-relieving agents for older adults who are at risk for adverse effects from oral NSAIDs. The topical version may not be as effective as the oral form but has far fewer side effects.

Lidocaine can be delivered through a gel or patch. It is similar to Novocain given by dentists, but it does not cause numbness. Little is absorbed into the body. At this time, 4 percent lidocaine patches and gel are available without prescription, while 5 percent patches require a prescription. Topical lidocaine works best on neuropathic pain, but it also relieves some other types of pain. The US Food and Drug Administration (FDA) has approved topical lidocaine by prescription only for the treatment of postherpetic neuralgia, and for temporary relief of pain associated with minor burns, including sunburn, abrasions of the skin, and insect bites.

Corticosteroids, when applied directly to the skin, reduce inflammation and irritation. Low doses are available without prescription for temporary relief of pain associated with minor burns, including sunburn, abrasions of the skin, and insect bites. Higher doses require a prescription and are used to treat inflammatory skin diseases.

Cannabidiol, commonly known as CBD, is a component of hemp and marijuana that does not cause a "high." There are few if any high-quality clinical trials of its use. A few trials suggest that topical CBD (oil or cream) may help with inflammatory and neuropathic pain. As with other supplements, there is no FDA oversight of its safety or purity, or whether the active ingredients are actually contained in the product (see the Dietary Supplements section in chapter 3). Some studies suggest that topical CBD is absorbed into the body and can interact with certain medications, so make sure you discuss the possibility of any interactions with your health care provider before you start using it.

Oral Medications

How do oral pain medications differ, and which can cause serious side effects in older adults?

The differences in how pain medications work are detailed in table 13.1, and special precautions for older adults in table 13.2.

Other Treatments

What can I try if neither the nonpharmacologic nor the pharmacologic treatments relieve my pain?

Localized Injections

Injections of corticosteroids and local anesthetics may be effective for temporary relief of joint pain or other musculoskeletal problems. Pain relief from an injection generally lasts about two months.

Surgical Treatments

Surgical treatment should be considered if you're unable to get relief and the pain is interfering with your ability to function. Speak with your primary care provider and a specialist to determine the optimal timing and the pros and cons of surgery for you. Pain doesn't have to be your new normal. If you are considering a knee or hip replacement, see the section on Severe Knee and Hip Osteoarthritis on page 148.

TABLE 13.1
Pain Medications and How They Work

Medication Class	Indications	Mechanism of Action	Examples
Acetaminophen	Mild to moderate pain	Unclear. Works centrally, through the brain. Little anti-inflammatory effect.	Tylenol

NSAIDs	Mild to moderate pain
	
	Inflammation
		Block prostaglandin synthesis by inhibiting the enzyme COX, which has two forms. Nonselective NSAIDs inhibit both forms, and selective NSAIDs inhibit only COX-2, resulting in different side effects for nonselective and selective NSAIDs.	Nonselective:
			  ibuprofen
			  (Motrin, Advil)
			  Naprosyn (Aleve)
			
			Selective:
			  celecoxib
			  (Celebrex)

Opioids	Moderate to severe pain	Bind to opioid receptors in the brain and spinal cord, inactivating the ascending pathways that alert the brain to pain, and activating the descending pathways that send pain relieving substances back down the spinal cord.	Oxycodone Morphine
Certain anticonvulsants	Neuropathic pain	Unclear. Reduces membrane excitability and suppresses abnormal neuronal discharges. Pain relief is not due to ability to suppress seizures.	Gabapentin (Neurontin) Pregabalin (Lyrica) Carbamazepine (Tegretol)
Certain antidepressants*	Neuropathic pain Chronic musculoskeletal pain	Block the reuptake of serotonin and norepinephrine, enhancing endogenous pain-modulating pathways. Pain relief is not due to antidepressant activity.	Tricyclic antidepressants (such as nortriptyline [Pamelor]) SNRIs (such as duloxetine [Cymbalta] and venlafaxine [Effexor])

(continued)

TABLE 13.1 (continued)

Medication Class	Indications	Mechanism of Action	Examples
Corticosteroids	Inflammatory pain	Inhibit formation of arachidonic acid, the precursor of prostaglandins.	Prednisone Solumedrol (Medrol)
Central muscle relaxants	Muscle spasms, spasticity	Each drug has different mechanism of action. Some decrease glutamate, and some increase GABA.	Tizanidine (Zanaflex) Methocarbamol (Robaxin)
Local anesthetics	Neuropathic pain	Inhibit the generation of abnormal impulses by damaged nerves by blocking sodium channels.	Lidoderm
		Depletes and prevents reaccumulation of substance P in peripheral sensory neurons.	Capsaicin
Medical marijuana	Neuropathic pain, cancer pain	Not known; studies conflict on effectiveness and mechanism of action.	

Note: Abbreviations are as follows: COX, cyclooxygenase; GABA, gamma amino butyric acid; NSAID, nonsteroidal anti-inflammatory drug; SNRI, serotonin-norepinephrine reuptake inhibitor; SSRI, selective serotonin reuptake inhibitor.

*SSRIs are not pain relievers.

TABLE 13.2
Pain Medication Precautions for Older Adults

Medication Class	Concerns for Older Adults
Acetaminophen	Can cause severe liver damage or impairment if one takes more than 3 grams daily (if robust, may be able to tolerate 4 grams).
	Dangerous with alcohol abuse.
	Large doses may also cause kidney damage.
	Check for the presence and amount of acetaminophen in all your other medications, and add the amounts together when you calculate your daily dose.
	Avoid Tylenol PM or any other "nighttime" medication that contains diphenhydramine (Benadryl, which can cause confusion).

TABLE 13.2 (*continued*)

Medication Class	Concerns for Older Adults
NSAIDs	If taken chronically, ask your PCP about the use of acid-suppressant medication to decrease the chances of peptic ulcer and/or GI bleeding. Also discuss use if you have kidney disease, heart disease, or history of peptic ulcers. NSAIDs can cause fluid retention, worsening blood pressure and heart failure.
Opioids	Start with lower doses because the brains of older adults are more sensitive to these medications.
	Take a laxative when starting opioids to avoid drug-induced constipation.
	Monitor acetaminophen dose if taking combination medications like Percocet or Vicodin.
	Codeine is often poorly tolerated in older adults (may cause nausea and vomiting).
	Side effects include falls, cognitive impairment, car accidents, and urinary retention (caution in men with BPH).
	Some side effects may improve over time: dry mouth, sedation, respiratory depression, nausea, confusion.
Certain anticonvulsants	Sedation, dizziness, confusion, and falls may occur. These medications have many interactions with other drugs, so check with your doctor or pharmacist.
Certain antidepressants	All antidepressants increase risk of falls in older adults.
	Try to avoid tricyclic antidepressants. These cause significant side effects, including sedation, confusion, dizziness, and abnormal heart rhythms. Duloxetine and venlafaxine have fewer side effects. Venlafaxine can increase blood pressure.
Corticosteroids	Oral corticosteroids should only be used to treat pain in a limited number of conditions. Adverse effects can be significant in older adults, including insomnia, psychosis, fluid retention, osteoporosis, and diabetes.
Skeletal muscle relaxants	Try to avoid. Very sedating and can cause confusion and falls. These drugs relax muscles throughout the body, not just the one that's causing you pain.
Medical marijuana	Little data in older adults. Can be abused. Can cause cognitive and mood changes, sleepiness, and dizziness.

Note: Abbreviations are as follows: BPH, benign prostatic hyperplasia; GI, gastrointestinal; PCP, primary care provider; NSAID, nonsteroidal anti-inflammatory drug.

What Isn't Normal Aging?

 Red Flags: Symptoms Needing Prompt Medical Attention

- Sudden onset of a warm, red, swollen joint that is especially painful with movement. This could be a joint infection, which might require drainage and/or intravenous antibiotics to avoid permanent joint damage.
- *Cauda equina syndrome* can present with *any* of the following symptoms: severe pain and weakness of one or both legs, increasing numbness between the legs and inner thighs, or loss of control of bowel or bladder. Cauda equina syndrome can be caused by spinal stenosis or a large herniated disc. *This is a medical emergency.* If left untreated, it can lead to permanent loss of bowel and bladder control, numbness and tingling, and paralysis of the legs.
- Pressure, pain, squeezing, or heaviness in the chest and/or neck, jaw, or arm may be a sign of a heart attack or that your heart is not getting enough blood.
- Back pain mainly at night can be a sign of an infection, tumor, or severe arthritis.
- Pain in the jaw muscles while chewing, sudden blurred vision, or headaches with tenderness along the temples (in front of the ears). These are symptoms of giant cell arteritis (see below). If not treated, GCA can cause blindness.
- Headaches that are persistent and worsening, especially if associated with loss of balance or visual changes.
- Inability to bear weight (stand up without pain) whether you have fallen or not. You may have a stress fracture that, if not recognized, could turn into a full fracture of the bone.

 Yellow Alerts: Common Conditions That Can Mimic or Worsen Aches and Pains in Older Adults

Medications and medication withdrawal, especially when certain drugs are stopped abruptly, can result in aches and pains. For a list of drugs that can cause pain, see table 13.3.

Statins can cause many muscle symptoms, including muscle discomfort, aches, soreness, or weakness in the shoulders, upper arms, and thighs. These symptoms usually occur within the first six months of taking statins. In rare cases, muscles may become inflamed or break down, impairing kidney function. The type of statin, the higher the dose, and interactions with other medications increase the likelihood of statin-associated muscle events. Risks are lower with fluvastatin and pravastatin, and higher with rosuvastatin, lovastatin, simvastatin, and atorvastatin. Stopping the medication or switching to one with lower risk will almost always alleviate the symptoms. When low levels of vitamin D or thyroid hormone are identified, replenishment reduces the likelihood of statin-related muscle symptoms.

TABLE 13.3
Medications That Can Cause Joint Pain, Muscle Pain and Cramps, and Peripheral Neuropathy

Drugs and Examples	Joint Pain	Muscle Pain	Muscle Cramps and Spasms	Peripheral Neurop-athy
Blood pressure, cardiac, and diuretic medications				
Loop and potassium-sparing diuretics: furosemide (Lasix); torsemide (Demadex); triamterene-hydrochlorothiazide (Dyazide); spironolactone (Aldactone)			X	
Thiazide and thiazide-like diuretics: hydrochlorothiazide (Microzide); chlorthalidone; metolazone (Zaroxolyn)			X	?
Antiarrhythmics: amiodarone (Cordarone); procainamide				X
Other antihypertensives: hydralazine				X
Statins: pravastatin (Pravachol); atorvastatin (Lipitor); rosuvastatin (Crestor)		X	X	X
Pain relief				
Opioid analgesics: morphine, oxyco-done (in Percocet); tramadol (Ultram)	W	W		
Neurological, psychological, and sleep medications				
Benzodiazepine-type medications: zolpidem (Ambien); estazolam (Prosom); temazepam (Restoril); triazolam (Halcion)	W	W		
Anticonvulsant medications: phenytoin (Dilantin); valproic acid (Depakote); lamotrigine (Lamictal); levetiracetam (Keppra)	W	W		Phenytoin (Dilantin)
All antidepressants	W	W		
Cholinesterase inhibitors: donepezil (Aricept); rivastigmine (Exelon); galantamine (Razadyne)			X	

(continued)

TABLE 13.3 (*continued*)

Drugs and Examples	Joint Pain	Muscle Pain	Muscle Cramps and Spasms	Peripheral Neurop-athy
Anti-Parkinsonian medications				
Decarboxylase inhibitors: carbidopa/ levodopa (Sinemet)		X	X	X
COMT inhibitors: tolcapone (Tasmar); entacapone (Comtan)		X	X	
Dopamine agonists: pramipexole (Mirapex); amantadine (Symmetrel); bromocriptine (Parlodel)			X	
Endocrine drugs				
Corticosteroids: prednisone, dexa-methasone (Decadron); methylpred-nisolone (Solu-Medrol)	W	W		
Estrogens	X		X	
Bisphosphonates: alendronate (Fosamax); ibandronate (Boniva); zoledronic acid (Reclast)		X		
Pulmonary medications				
Long- and short-acting beta-blockers: formoterol (Perforomist); salmeterol (Serevent); albuterol (Proventil, Ventolin); terbutaline	X	X	X	
Inhaled corticosteroids: fluticasone (ArmonAir); budesonide (Pulmicort); ciclesonide (Alvesco)	W	W		
Diabetes medications				
Thiazolidinediones: pioglitazone (Actos); rosiglitazone (Avandia)	X	X		
Meglitinide analog: pramlintide (SymlinPen); nateglinide (Starlix); repaglinide (Prandin)	X			
DPP-4 inhibitors: sitagliptin (Januvia); saxagliptin (Onglyz)	X	X		

TABLE 13.3 *(continued)*

Drugs and Examples	Joint Pain	Muscle Pain	Muscle Cramps and Spasms	Peripheral Neuropathy
Gastrointestinal medications				
Proton pump inhibitors: pantoprazole (Protonix); omeprazole (Prilosec); esomeprazole (Nexium)	X	X		omeprazole
Urinary medications				
Bladder relaxants: tolteradine (Detrol); oxybutinin (Ditropan); solifenacin (Vesicare)	X			
Beta-3 agonists: mirabegron (Myrbetriq)	X			
Autoimmune medications				
Disease modifiers: etanercept (Enbrel); infliximab (Remicade); leflunomide (Arava)				X
Antimicrobials				
Antibiotics: chloramphenicol; dapsone; metronidazole (Flagyl); nitrofurantoin (Macrodantin)				X
Fluoroquinolones: ciprofloxacin (Cipro); levofloxacin (Levaquin); moxifloxacin (Avelox)	X	Cipro		?
Tetracyclines: minocycline; doxycycline	X			
Antifungals: itraconazole (Onmel, Sporanox); voriconazole (Vfend); ketaconazole	voriconazole			X
Anti-tuberculosis: isoniazid; ethambutol (Myambutol)				X
Rifabutin (Mycobutin)	X			
HIV medications: zalcitabine/ddC (Hivid); didanosine/ddI (Videx); stavudine (Zerit)				X

(continued)

TABLE 13.3 (*continued*)

Drugs and Examples	Joint Pain	Muscle Pain	Muscle Cramps and Spasms	Peripheral Neurop- athy
Cancer drugs				
Vinca alkaloids: vincristine (Vincasar PFS); vinblastine; vinorelbine (Navelbine)	X	X		X
Platinum and taxanes: cisplatin (PlatinolAQ); carboplatin (Paraplatin); Paclitaxel (Taxol); docetaxel (Taxotere, Docefrez)	X			X
Aromatase inhibitors: anastrazole (Arimidex); exemestane (Aromasin); letrozole (Femara)	X	X		
Many other chemotherapeutic agents				X
Other				
Alcohol		X		X
Botulinum toxin type A: onabotuli- numtoxin A (Botox); abbotulinum- toxin A (Dysport)	X	X		

Note: If you're not sure whether a drug you're taking is in one of the drug classes listed, ask your pharmacist or health care provider. X, may cause this condition; W, withdrawal symptoms occur when drug is abruptly stopped; ?, studies conflict on whether these drugs cause this symptom. Abbreviations are as follows: COMT, catechol-O-methyltransferase; DPP, dipeptidyl-peptidase; HIV, human immunodeficiency virus.

Common Painful Conditions in Older Adults

Muscle Pain

Muscle Spasms

These are sudden, involuntary contractions of one or more muscles that are often painful. These may be acute, for example, when you haven't warmed up prior to exercise, or chronic. *Chronic muscle spasms* may have an underlying medical cause, like poor circulation, malnutrition, kidney or liver disease, neurological conditions, or dehydration, especially from sweating, diarrhea, or vomiting.

Muscle Sprains

Muscle sprains occur when ligaments overstretch or tear, usually from repeated stress or trauma. If severe, they can also cause damage to the attached bone.

Muscle Strains

When a tendon or a muscle over-stretches or tears, it is considered a strain. Tendons are strong but not very stretchy.

Inflammatory Disorders

Polymyalgia Rheumatica

Polymyalgia rheumatica is an inflammatory disorder that causes aching and stiffness of the shoulders, neck, hips, buttocks, and thighs. It comes on over days to weeks. The stiffness is worst in the morning and improves over the course of the day. People with PMR may have difficulty getting dressed or getting out of a car. Some people also have more general symptoms like fever, fatigue, or weight loss. PMR is a disease of people over 50, and the average age of onset is 70. It is treated with low-dose corticosteroids. About 10 percent of people with PMR develop giant cell arteritis, a condition that needs immediate medical attention (see below).

Giant Cell Arteritis

Formerly known as temporal arteritis, GCA is an inflammation of the medium to large arteries that, like PMR, rarely occurs under age 50. About 40 to 50 percent of people with GCA have PMR. Other symptoms are headache, pain or fatigue in the jaw muscles during chewing, scalp tenderness, and blurred vision. People with GCA may also have more general symptoms like fever, malaise, weight loss, and depression. Headaches may be a new occurrence in someone who rarely has a headache, whereas in people who often have headaches, the CGA headache has a

different feel to it. The headaches are often located over the temple, although they can occur in the front or back of the head. Blindness may occur if treatment with high-dose steroids is not started immediately.

Arthritis

The signs and symptoms of some types of arthritis differ in older adults.

Rheumatoid Arthritis

Rheumatoid arthritis (RA) is a chronic inflammatory disease. When it develops after age 65, the shoulder joints are more commonly affected, and the hand and wrist joints are less involved than those who have a younger onset. People also more often have fever, malaise, fatigue, weight loss, muscle aches, and symptoms of polymyalgia rheumatica.

Gout

Gout is the most common type of inflammatory arthritis in older adults. In younger people, men are most likely to develop gout, and it usually presents as an inflammation of the big toe. In older adults, women are equally affected, and inflammation can occur in several joints, particularly osteoarthritic finger joints. Gout can be painful. Fortunately, there are a variety of oral and injectable medications that are effective treatments, including colchicine, NSAIDs, and prednisone.

Hip Osteoarthritis

Surprisingly, pain over the outside of the hip is usually due to bursitis or a pinched nerve in the back, not arthritis. Hip osteoarthritis often presents as a deep pain in the groin, buttocks, thigh, knee, or anterior shin.

Nerve Pain

Pinched Nerves

A pinched nerve can be caused by compression or inflammation of a peripheral nerve or of a spinal nerve as it exits the spine (see figure on page 235). The pain feels deep, and it radiates along the area of distribution covered by the spinal nerve root. If the pain is accompanied by numbness and tingling or weakness, it is called a *radiculopathy*. Examples include the following.

Cervical radiculopathies are pinched nerves in the neck and usually cause shoulder blade or outer arm pain; shoulder, arm, or hand weakness; or numbness or tingling in the fingers or hands.

Sciatica causes numbness, tingling, or burning that starts in the lower back or buttocks and travels down the back or side of the leg to the foot or ankle. Coughing or sneezing can worsen the pain from sciatica, as can prolonged sitting. Sciatica is due to inflammation or compression of the sciatic nerve on one side of your body from bone spurs or degenerated discs, spinal stenosis, pyriformis muscle spasms, or a herniated disc.

Peripheral Neuropathy

Peripheral neuropathy causes symmetrical burning pain, numbness, tingling, or weakness, usually starting in the feet. Balance can be affected, and over time the hands may become involved. Causes include diabetes, vitamin deficiencies (B_1, B_{12}, E, and niacin), vitamin B_6 toxicity, hypothyroidism, autoimmune diseases, Lyme disease, alcohol overuse, medications, and certain protein abnormalities. About 7 percent of people over 65 years old are affected. A definitive cause is less likely to be found the older you are. Speak with your health care provider about causes of and treatments for peripheral neuropathy.

Spinal Stenosis

Spinal stenosis is a narrowing of the vertebral canal that is usually due to osteoarthritis (see figure on page 235). The cervical and lumbar areas of the spine are most often affected. Symptoms depend on which spinal nerves are involved, whether there is pressure on the spinal cord, and how quickly the symptoms developed. When spinal nerves are affected, a radiculopathy may occur (see above).

Cervical stenosis with pressure on the spinal cord can cause pain in the neck, shoulder, and arms; numbness and tingling in the arms; weakness in the arms, legs, or both; an abnormal gait with weakness or balance difficulties; and occasionally urinary incontinence.

Lumbar stenosis with pressure on the spinal cord can cause numbness and tingling, burning, back pain, and/or weakness in the foot or leg. People with lumbar stenosis may also develop pain or cramping in the legs upon standing or when walking. The pain improves with sitting or bending forward, which increases the diameter of the vertebral canal and relieves the pressure that causes the symptoms.

Cauda equina syndrome can be due to lumbar stenosis and is a medical emergency. See the Red Flags section above for more information.

Back Pain

Most persistent lower back pain is from mechanical spine, muscle, tendon, and ligament problems, including spinal stenosis (discussed above). Other common causes of back pain in older adults include the following (see also figures on page 235).

Spine (or Facet Joint) Osteoarthritis

This is a condition where pain is localized to the back, or if the nerve root is compressed, pain and symptoms can occur in the distribution of the nerve. The facet joints of the spine are located between and behind adjacent vertebrae.

Disc Herniation

A herniated disc can cause sudden severe back pain and muscle spasms, and if it compresses a spinal nerve root, you may also have pain, numbness, and weakness in the area supplied by the nerve.

Vertebral Compression Fractures

These can cause sudden, localized spine pain, or they may be asymptomatic and only identified on x-rays. They are more common with age, and they are seen on spinal x-rays of about 25 percent of all postmenopausal women and 40 per-cent of women 80 and over. Vertebral compression fractures are usually due to osteoporosis and mainly affect vertebral bodies in the thoracic or middle part of the spine. If osteoporosis is severe, simple movements like a forceful sneeze or lifting a light object can cause a collapse. If you have one fracture, you are at greater risk of having more. Compression fractures can lead to spine deformity, loss of height, and in some people, severe pain that increases with standing or walking. Speak with your health care provider about treatment for osteoporosis.

Leg Pain

Hip OA, knee OA, lumbar stenosis, sciatica, and intermittent claudication can all cause pain in the legs. For a comparison of the symptoms and the back, buttock, and leg pain that occurs with these disorders, see table 9.2.

Leg Cramps

Cramps felt in the legs are sudden, painful muscle contractions in the leg or foot where you can feel the muscle hardening. They are more common and severe in older people, and they tend to be worse at night. As described in chapter 10, routine daily stretching exercises decrease the frequency and intensity of cramps for some people. Once the cramp occurs, forcefully stretching the affected muscles can release the contraction and relieve pain.

Getting Evaluated for Aches and Pains

Aches and pains can be fleeting, acute, or persistent; have an obvious cause; or be a mystery. Many types of pain can be treated at home and don't require any additional diagnostic procedures or treatments. If pain is interfering with your function, however, making it difficult for you to carry out your usual activities or causing you distress, you should have it evaluated. Most aches and pains can be initially diagnosed and treated by your primary care provider.

Should I See a Specialist?

Depending on the condition, it may make sense for you to see a specialist early on for help with diagnosis or treatment (see table 9.3 on page 155). If pain is persistent or interferes with your mood, sleep, behavior, or function, consider seeing a behavioral health specialist (psychiatrist, psychologist, social worker), or ask for a referral to a pain clinic. For musculoskeletal concerns, physical medicine and rehabilitation physicians, physical and occupational therapists, chiropractors, and doctors of osteopathy may be able to help. For undiagnosed neuropathic pain, see a neurologist or a physical medicine and rehabilitation doctor.

Preparing for Your Visit

Fill out the pre-visit checklist for chapter 13 on page 382 in Appendix 3 to help your health care provider determine what's causing your aches and pains, and what might give you relief. Don't wait until just before the appointment to complete the pre-visit checklist. Start several days before your appointment, so that you can observe yourself and your pain characteristics and be able to answer all the questions. Eighty percent of all diagnoses are made based on the history alone, so taking the time to do this will make it more likely that your health care provider will be able to help you at your visit.

Advice for Loved Ones

Any pain is difficult to live with, but persistent pain often causes depression, anxiety, agitation, irritability, and social isolation. It can be difficult to be around someone in pain. Everyone is anxious (and often worried that there is something serious going on), tempers get short, depression can set in. Be open to alternative treatments, particularly those that focus on changing behaviors and positions that might trigger the pain. Adding a cushion to a chair, working on posture, or getting ergonomic equipment can help with prevention, or at least decrease the discomfort.

Getting pain under control can be the first step to improving mood and behavior, and allowing someone to resume doing what matters to them. Make sure that your loved one is clear about what medications to take, when, and why. Many people are afraid to take pain medications given the current opioid crisis in our country. I find it helpful to let people know that the vast majority of people who take these medications for pain relief are more than happy to get off them when the pain goes away. If you or your loved one is concerned about addiction, make sure you discuss it with their health care provider so they can take this concern into account when discussing treatments.

People living with dementia may not be able to tell you they're having pain, or they may tell you they're in pain at the time they have it but not be able to recall it when asked later. If someone tells you they had pain, even if they don't remember later, you should believe that they had the pain and make sure they are evaluated or monitored for recurrence. Physical expressions, grimaces, not eating or drinking, and agitation can also tell you that someone you care for is in pain. On occasion, I have given people with these symptoms a short trial of around-the-clock acetaminophen to see if their behaviors, grimaces, and the like improve. If so, we try to determine what's causing the pain and treat that.

Bottom Line

More than 70 percent of pain in older adults originates in the musculoskeletal system, which includes the joints, the spine, and tissues involved in their stability and movement, including cartilage, ligaments, muscles and tendons, and bursa. Any pain is a warning sign, however, telling you there is something wrong in your body. Don't ignore it. It can be as minor as sitting slouched on the couch for too long or holding tension in your shoulders—things that you can fix with mild treatments or a change in behavior. More seriously, it could be a warning that there's something major going on, such as a broken bone or an infected organ. Older adults may have fewer symptoms and distress, or may become confused or fall, when serious illnesses occur. You should persist in trying to find out if there's something seriously wrong with you or your loved one if unexplained pain persists.

RESORY

RESOURCES

General

Arthritis Foundation
(https://www.arthritis.org/home)
The Arthritis Foundation provides information on different types of arthritis and treatments, including complementary and alternative medicine.

Centers for Disease Control and Prevention
(https://www.cdc.gov/arthritis/)
The CDC provides information on different types of arthritis, physical activity, and self-management programs.

Geriatric Pain
(www.geriatricpain.org)
Housed at the University of Iowa, Geriatric Pain is a website developed by the John A. Hartford Centers of Geriatric Nursing Excellence. It contains separate sections for older adults and for family caregivers on communication with health care providers, pain assessment, and pain management, along with a comprehensive list of resources for coping with pain in general and in specific medical conditions.

Assistive Devices

Best Mobility Aides
(https://bestmobilityaids.com/)
Impartial advice on selecting the best mobility aids, including mobility scooters, rollators, walking frames, wheelchairs, and home aids to keep you active and help you lead a fulfilling and independent life, no matter your age.

Pain Relief Modalities

American Chronic Pain Association and the Stanford Medicine Division of Pain Medicine. *ACPA and Stanford Resource Guide to Chronic Pain Management: An Integrated Guide to Medical, Interventional, Behavioral, Pharmacologic and Rehabilitation Therapies.* Overland Park, KS: American Chronic Pain Association, 2021. https://www.theacpa.org/resources/acpa-resource-guide/.

This guide, written for people with chronic pain, describes in detail chronic pain and its nonpharmacologic and pharmacologic treatments.

For more information on muscle relaxation, see the Stress and Relaxation Resources section at the end of chapter 10.

For more details on how meditation can help manage pain, see the Resources section at the end of chapter 8.

Finding Practitioners
Acupuncture National Certification Commission for Acupuncture and Oriental Medicine
(www.nccaom.org)
NCCAOM is a national organization that provides professional certification for practitioners of acupuncture. Make sure your acupuncturist is certified.

American Massage Therapy Association
(https://www.amtamassage.org/find-massage-therapist/)
This organization for massage therapists has a national locator service to help consumers find a therapist in their area.

Biofeedback Certification International Alliance
(https://www.bcia.org/consumers)
The BCIA is an organization that certifies specialists in biofeedback and neurofeedback. Use the search tool available on their website to find a practitioner.

For information on how to find a behavioral health specialist, see the Resources section at the end of chapter 8.

258 WHAT REALLY MATTERS AS YOU GROW OLDER

BIBLIOGRAPHY

Adwan, M. H. "An Update on Drug-Induced Arthritis." *Rheumatology International* 36 (2016): 1089–97.

Davies, J., and J. Read. "A Systematic Review into the Incidence, Severity and Duration of Antidepressant Withdrawal Effects: Are Guidelines Evidence-Based?" *Addictive Behaviors* 10, no. 97 (2019): 111–21.

Department of Neurobiology and Anatomy, McGovern Medical School, University of Texas Health Science Center at Houston. *Neuroscience Online.* Section 2, chapters 6, 7, and 8. Accessed April 8, 2021. https://nba.uth.tmc.edu/neuroscience/toc.htm.

Jones, M. R., I. Urits, J. Wolf, D. Corrigan, L. Colburn, E. Petrson, A. Williamson, and O. Viswanath. "Drug-Induced Peripheral Neuropathy: A Narrative Review." *Current Clinical Pharmacology* 15 (2020): 38–48.

Staff, N. P., and A. J. Windebank. "Peripheral Neuropathy Due to Vitamin Deficiency, Toxins, and Medications." *Continuum* 20, no. 5 (2014): 1293–306.

CHAPTER 14

Gut Feelings

One of the things I enjoy about aging is that I find I can trust my gut feelings more. This may be true when I'm referring to my instincts, but not so much when I'm talking about my gastrointestinal (GI) system. My patients seem to agree. Constipation, gas, liquids going down the wrong pipe, and occasionally a stool leak can cause discomfort and at times embarrassment.

For most of our lives, we haven't had to think about how we digest our food—it's on automatic pilot. The figure on page 261 shows the organs of the GI system. For a summary of the digestive process, see box 14.1. As we age, there are some physiological changes that increase our likelihood of developing certain GI disorders, but many of the GI symptoms we experience are due more to diseases, medications, or changes in our behaviors than to aging itself. Gut concerns include some about weight and nutrition, topics covered in chapter 15.

In this chapter we'll discuss what is "normal" and how to adapt your diet, medications, and activities to this new normal. We will also cover "red flag" signs and symptoms as well as conditions that commonly cause GI symptoms in older adults.

What's Normal with Aging?

For a deeper dive into age-related changes that affect your gut's response to medical conditions, foods, behaviors, and medications, increasing your risk of having GI problems, see box 14.2.

What about constipation? This isn't due to aging? I can count on one hand the number of my older friends who don't have problems with constipation.

Constipation is a common concern for older adults, but age-related physiologic effects on the GI system itself are not always to blame. The word *constipation* means different things to different people. Medically, it's defined as having two or fewer bowel movements a week along with at least one of the following: straining to pass stools, lumpy or hard stools, sensation of incomplete emptying, obstruction or blockage in the rectum or anus, or the need for manual maneuvers to facilitate bowel movement. True constipation is most often due to non-GI-tract causes, such as medication side effects or not drinking

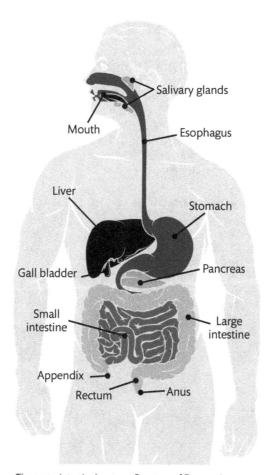

The gastrointestinal system. Courtesy of Dreamstime.com

enough fluid, eating enough fiber, or getting enough exercise (see the Adapting to Your New Normal section below for specifics).

As I've gotten older, my mouth has gotten drier, making it harder to swallow and causing me to wake up at night to drink more fluids, which then exacerbates my urinary incontinence. Is this normal aging?

Dry mouth is not a part of normal aging; however, it is a common concern of many older adults. Our production of saliva can decrease from medications, certain diseases such as diabetes, Parkinson's and Sjogren's syndrome, and having had treatments for cancer, including radiation therapy. Environmental conditions, like dry heat, can also cause it. Dry mouth is not just uncomfortable, it also increases the risk of tooth decay and other oral infections because one of saliva's primary jobs is to kill bacteria. For this reason, it's important to see your doctor or dentist to determine the cause.

BOX 14.1

Digestion 101

Food is composed of large molecules of proteins, fats, and carbohydrates, each of which must be broken down into its building blocks before being absorbed into the body. For proteins, these building blocks are amino acids; for fats, fatty acids; and for carbohydrates, simple sugars. This feat of digestion is accomplished by a combination of mechanical and chemical processes that occur in different parts of the gut, starting with the mouth.

FROM THE MOUTH TO THE STOMACH

Swallowing

The phases of swallowing. Courtesy of Dreamstime.com

Chewing stimulates saliva secretion from the salivary glands in the mouth. Saliva coats food particles with enzymes that initiate the breakdown of carbohydrates into smaller molecules. It also moistens and softens food, making it easier to swallow. After being swallowed, it passes through the esophagus into the stomach. Swallowing has three phases, the oral, pharyngeal, and esophageal (see the figure above). In the oral phase, chewed food is mixed with saliva to form a bolus, or "food packet," that the tongue moves toward the back of the mouth. In the pharyngeal phase, the tongue propels the food bolus into the pharynx, the back of the throat. This triggers a series of reflexes that move it through the pharynx and the *upper esophageal sphincter (UES)*, opening the esophagus and initiating the esophageal phase, where the food bolus is propelled through to the stomach by wavelike esophageal muscle contractions, or *peristalsis*. Other reflexes occur to protect the airway from food.

The *lower esophageal sphincter (LES)* is a ring-shaped valve at the point where the esophagus and stomach meet. The LES is usually closed; however, the presence of food in the esophagus causes the valve to open, allowing food to pass into the stomach. The proper functioning of the LES is critical to sealing off the

BOX 14.1 (*continued*)

esophagus and preventing stomach acid from flowing back into the esophagus, which can lead to gastroesophageal reflux disease and esophageal ulcers.

STOMACH TO SMALL INTESTINE

Once in the stomach, food is stored, mixed with digestive enzymes, and slowly emptied into the small intestine. The muscles in the upper stomach relax when large volumes of food need to be stored, and then contract to break food down into smaller particles and mix up the contents.

The insides of the esophagus, stomach, small intestine, and large intestine are lined by a layer of cells that secrete substances that help with digestion. These include hydrochloric acid and the enzyme pepsin, which breaks down protein, both of which are secreted from the stomach lining. Pepsin aids in the breakdown of protein from foods such as meat, eggs, and beans into amino acids. Hydrochloric acid provides the proper environment for pepsin to begin breaking down proteins. Hydrochloric acid can be corrosive, however. Prostaglandins and the mucus coating the lining of the stomach protect it from acid injury. If the lining wears away from bacterial infection or certain medications, the hydrochloric acid in the stomach can cause open sores called *ulcers*.

Food passes from the stomach into the small intestine, where further digestion takes place and nutrients are absorbed into the body's circulatory system. The small intestine is an exceptionally long organ—about 22 feet in length—and is coiled up inside the abdomen. This length is necessary to accomplish the task of absorbing all the nutrients you consume. Food enters the first section of the small intestine, the duodenum, where enzymes secreted by the pancreas, plus bile from the gallbladder and liver, mix with food. Microorganisms called gut microbiota, which are present in the intestinal tract, also help in the digestive process.

Most of the absorption of the digested molecules of food takes place in the rest of the small intestine. The now-small molecules of sugars, amino acids, and fatty acids are absorbed through the walls of the intestine and into blood vessels and lacteals (thin-walled lymphatic vessels that transport fats) that carry them to other parts of the body, where they provide energy and help build, repair, and maintain body tissues.

SMALL INTESTINE TO LARGE INTESTINE

Food molecules that aren't absorbed must be eliminated from the body. This is the job of the large intestine. Liquid waste material enters the pouchlike cecum from the small intestine, and peristalsis moves it though the colon, which absorbs the water and creates a solid stool. The stool then passes into the rectum, where it is held by contraction of the internal and external anal sphincters and the pelvic floor muscles. A reflex relaxes your internal sphincter when it's time to defecate and tells your brain to voluntarily relax the external anal sphincter and pelvic floor muscles, resulting in a bowel movement.

BOX 14.2

What Happens with Aging: A Deeper Dive

Normal aging alone doesn't have much effect on gastrointestinal (GI) function, but it does change your gut's response to other medical conditions, foods, behaviors, and medications, increasing your risk of having GI problems such as constipation or difficulty swallowing. The symptoms and complications of these problems are discussed further in the Yellow Alerts section of this chapter.

You're more likely to cough or clear your throat when eating and drinking.
Swallowing is a complex activity (see box 14.1). Eating and breathing share space in the back of the throat (the pharynx), and on occasion, food ends up in the lungs and air in the stomach. Food enters the esophagus by traveling through the pharynx, while air follows a similar path into the trachea and lungs. The trachea is directly in front of the esophagus. Intact neuromuscular reflexes are needed to tilt the epiglottis back and close the vocal cords to prevent food from entering the larynx (voice box) and trachea. With aging, some of these reflexes become less effective, and food or fluid may penetrate into the area above the larynx, making your voice sound wet while eating. *Aspiration* occurs when food or liquid enter the trachea and lungs. Coughing and clearing your throat are initial ways to clear your voice and airway.

Gastroesophageal reflux disease (GERD) may go unrecognized, causing more severe esophageal complications or anemia.
GERD is a condition in which stomach acid flows backward through the lower esophageal sphincter (LES) into the esophagus, irritating its lining. Heartburn and chest pain are the typical symptoms of GERD. Some older adults may not feel these symptoms, however, because the older esophagus is less able to feel pain. Additionally, the esophagus of an older person with GERD may be exposed to more acid than that of a younger person. There are a number of reasons for this: saliva, which contains bicarbonate that neutralizes acid, is produced in lower amounts; there is a small decrease in LES pressure, allowing more acid to enter the esophagus; and esophageal peristalsis is impaired, allowing acid to remain in contact with the esophagus for a longer period of time. If not recognized or treated, the acid irritation can cause serious esophageal conditions.

Peptic ulcers are more likely to develop, especially when taking nonsteroidal anti-inflammatory drugs to treat pain.
Most peptic (stomach and duodenal) ulcers are caused by the bacteria *H. pylori*, NSAIDs, or both. Natural factors including enzymes, mucus, and prostaglandins protect the stomach lining from the acid it produces. *H. pylori* are bacteria that often infect the stomach of older adults. *H. pylori* can burrow deep into the thick layer of mucus coating the stomach lining and damage it, allowing acid to irritate and inflame the sensitive tissue underneath. Continued irritation from acid and bacteria can lead to the formation of an ulcer. NSAIDs alleviate pain by

BOX 14.2 (*continued*)

deactivating an enzyme called cyclooxygenase (COX), which is responsible for generating the products of inflammation that are sensed as pain. COX also has a role in protecting the stomach's lining. When NSAIDs deactivate COX, pain is relieved, but the enzyme's protective effect on the stomach is lost. Older age is a major risk factor for developing ulcers from NSAIDs; the exact reason is not known. The combination of having *H. pylori* and taking an NSAID is even more likely to cause ulcerations and bleeding.

Gallstones are more common.

Gallstones occur in about 35 percent of women and 20 percent of men 70 years or older. Why? Bile is produced in the liver and stored in the gallbladder until the body needs it to digest fats. When you eat a high-fat meal, the gallbladder contracts and sends bile through a system of tubes (ducts) into the small intestine. Bile is composed of several substances, including bile acids and cholesterol. With aging, the proportion of cholesterol increases and may saturate the bile, causing solid crystals to form in the gallbladder and clump together into gallstones. Gallstones can vary in size, from as small as a grain of sand to as large as a golf ball. Most people live peacefully with their gallstones. Problems only occur when a gallstone is large enough to block the normal flow of bile through the ducts. Gallstones can cause pain, inflammation, or infection.

After age 80, almost everyone has diverticulosis, NOT diverticulitis!

Diverticula are small pouches about the size of large peas that bulge outward from the colon. They are thought to result from eating a low-fiber diet. Fiber helps keep stools soft, so they pass easily through the colon. Hard stools cause constipation, and straining to expel hard stools puts pressure on the colon. This pressure causes the inner layer of the intestine to push through weak spots in the outer lining, where blood vessels pass through, creating diverticula. Most people with diverticulosis have no symptoms, but some develop an infection or bleeding from the diverticula.

Constipation begets worse constipation.

Constipation increases with age, but it's not mainly due to age-related changes in the large intestine (see the Adapting to Your New Normal section in this chapter). The frequency of bowel movements considered normal ranges from three times a day to three times a week. In general, it takes about three days for food to move through the digestive tract in both old and young adults; this is called the *transit time*. But if you have chronic constipation, the transit time can increase to four to nine days, and if bedridden, up to two weeks. This increase in transit time is due to a decline in propulsive activity in the colon. After the undigested fiber and other waste passes into the colon, the water it contains is absorbed, leaving a solid waste product (stool) that will be eliminated. If peristalsis becomes sluggish, however, the stool will move too slowly, allowing more water to be absorbed and

(continued)

BOX 14.2 *(continued)*

resulting in a hard, dry stool that causes constipation. In general, the bulkier the bowel movement, the greater the stimulus for peristalsis to occur.

Gas and stool leakage may increase.
With older age, the tone of the internal anal sphincter and the strength of the external anal sphincter and pelvic floor muscles decline, increasing the likelihood of stool leakage and flatulence. There are exercises that may help to decrease leakage and dietary changes to decrease gas production (see the Adapting to Your New Normal section in this chapter).

The urge to have a bowel movement may weaken, which can cause constipation and/or leakage.
This is not normal aging, but the result of medical conditions as well as years of disregarding the urge to defecate. When this happens, stools need to be bulkier to trigger the reflex that relaxes the internal sphincter and allows stool to begin to leave the rectum. Depending on the strength of the external sphincter and pelvic muscles, the result may be soiling oneself or difficulty having a bowel movement.

I've read that that older people with gastroesophageal reflux disease often don't have heartburn. But my heartburn is getting worse as I get older. What's going on with me?

If you have heartburn, you most likely have gastroesophageal reflux disease (GERD) and should take this as a warning sign to get evaluated and treated before complications set in. People who have GERD but no heartburn don't have this option and are more susceptible to developing serious esophageal complications (see the Yellow Alerts on page 274) and painless blood loss, causing anemia. If your heartburn is getting worse, you should speak with your medical provider.

I almost died from a recent gallbladder infection. The Internet says it's people with the four F's who develop gallstones: Female, Fertile, Fat, and Forty, and that

when a stone causes an obstruction or an infection, there's severe pain or rigidity in the right upper abdomen. I'm 70, in good shape, and although I'm female, I'm not fertile, fat, or forty. Why did I even develop gallstones? And when I was sick, I had a high fever and a low blood pressure, but no problems with my right upper abdomen, even when the doctors pushed on it. I think this is why it took so long for them to figure out what was going on. Is this normal?*

As with so many things we discuss in this book, what's "typical" in medicine is often only typical for middle-aged adults, not older people. At 70, you may not consider yourself "older," but your body's physiology and responses differ from those who are 40 or 50. Gallstones are more common in older adults because their bile composition is more likely to form stones. As discussed in chapter 2, traumatic abdominal events like infections, obstructions, or even organ perforations may not produce the same signs and symptoms in older adults as younger adults. There may be little nausea, vomiting, or abdominal pain, and on physical exam the belly can appear "normal." That's why it's important for medical providers to strongly consider an abdominal problem as the source of an illness when an older person feels sick but there's no obvious cause.

I'm 75 years old and have chronic diarrhea and lots of gas. My doctor is trying to figure out what's going on and is ordering test after test. Haven't I "aged out" of the possibility of developing lactase insufficiency, celiac disease, irritable bowel syndrome, or inflammatory bowel disease (like Crohn's or ulcerative colitis)? Do I really need all these tests?

You're looking for something that can be treated to improve your symptoms and quality of life, so this is a good question to ask. It's uncommon for irritable bowel syndrome (IBS) to be diagnosed for the first time at age 65 or older, so if you're given this diagnosis, it's important to be sure there's not another explanation for your symptoms. Confirming the diagnosis may require blood or stool tests and/or a colonoscopy. Conversely, about one-third of people with celiac disease (or gluten-sensitive enteropathy) are not diagnosed until after age 65. *Lactase insufficiency* causes decreased ability to break down lactose, the sugar in milk and milk products. In children, lactase insufficiency is genetic, but in older adults, it's usually due to small intestinal diseases. Only about 5 percent of new cases of inflammatory bowel disease (IBD) occur in older adults, but IBD can cause pain, bleeding, and other significant complications, so it needs to be diagnosed. There is effective treatment for IBD, and both gluten intolerance and lactase insufficiency can be treated with diet and/or enzymes, so it's probably worth finding out if these are the cause of your symptoms. These conditions are discussed more in the Yellow Alerts section below.

Adapting to Your New Normal

I take a lot of medications, and occasionally I feel like they get stuck in my chest, causing pressure and actual pain. What can I do to ensure this doesn't happen?

Always take your medications with a full glass of water and while sitting up to avoid this problem. *Pill esophagitis*, which is when drugs get "stuck" in the esophagus, is a condition that occurs more often in older adults and can cause inflammation, injury, and pain. Avoid lying down for 30 minutes after taking pills, especially tetracycline, doxycycline, nonsteroidal anti-inflammatory drugs, potassium chloride, iron sulfate, and bisphosphonates (for osteoporosis). Gelatin capsules are of particular concern and tend to get stuck more often than coated tablets. Liquids don't get stuck in the esophagus, so if you keep having a problem even after sitting up and taking a full glass of water, ask your medical provider if the medication is still needed, and if so, whether it comes in liquid form or if there is an alternative less likely to get stuck. If you have severe pain or if you continue to have a problem, you may need to have a study to evaluate your esophagus.

Everyone I know complains about constipation. I know you say it's not normal aging, but what can I do to prevent it?

There are a few rules to follow to make it less likely that constipation will develop:

Whenever you have the urge to move your bowels, go to the bathroom. Ignoring the urge allows stool to stay longer in the colon, where more water is absorbed from it, resulting in a hard stool that is more difficult to expel.

Try to have a bowel movement after you've eaten a meal. After you eat, your stomach stretches, triggering what is known as the *gastrocolic reflex* to increase the movement of ingested food toward the rectum, increasing rectal pressure and stimulating a bowel movement. This reflex works just as well in older as younger people, so take advantage of it.

Drink fluid. Water and other liquids help make stools softer and easier to pass.

Exercise more. Sitting and being sedentary can cause constipation, while being physically active can prevent it. Any type of exercise can prevent constipation; even walking can be helpful.

Review all your medications. Both prescription and over-the-counter (OTC) medications can cause constipation. Calcium, iron, and aluminum (found commonly in antacids) don't require a prescription but often cause constipation (see table 14.1). Review any drugs you take with your medical provider.

Speak with your medical provider to see if you have a condition that can increase constipation. If so, work with your provider to develop a regimen for constipation before there's a problem. Sometimes this will include taking laxatives, which work prophylactically to prevent constipation as well as to treat it. For example, laxatives should always be prescribed when an opioid is prescribed. Conditions that increase constipation include stroke, untreated thyroid disease, and neurological conditions like Parkinson's disease, as well as taking constipating medications like opioids or some antihypertensives.

I keep being told to eat more fiber, but I'm not sure what that means. Is all fiber the same?

Fiber is found in plant foods, such as grains, vegetables, and fruits. The average American consumes only 15 grams of fiber a day, much less than the recommended intake of 25 grams per day for women, and 38 grams per day for men, so most of us actually need to increase our fiber intake.

Fiber comes in two forms. *Insoluble fiber* is not digested but adds bulk to stools. It's found in wheat bran, whole grains, and whole-grain products, along with the skins of apples, cucumbers, and grapes. *Soluble fiber* attracts water as it passes through the large intestine, resulting in soft stools. It's found in beans, fruit, oats and oat bran, nuts, seeds, and many vegetables, as well as psyllium.

There are a few ways to increase your fiber intake:

Add fiber slowly over time. Soluble fiber has the potential to produce gas, so you may notice more gas or bloating when you suddenly increase your fiber intake. But if you start low and progressively increase the amount, your GI tract will adjust. If one type or source of fiber causes more gas, try another.

Drink more fluids if you're increasing fiber. Try to drink eight glasses of liquids (water, soup, broth, juices) a day. If you don't drink enough fluid, the fiber may get stuck in your intestines.

Consider these dietary changes. Easy ways to increase your fiber intake is by eating 2–3 cups of vegetables and 2 cups of fruit every day; three servings of beans, lentils, or peas every week; whole-grain bread instead of white bread; whole-grain cereals and bran cereal; and brown rice instead of white rice.

When I go to the pharmacy to get a laxative, there are shelves and shelves of products. I have no idea which one I should be taking. What are the differences among them?

There are four major types of laxatives that are mostly available without a prescription. If lifestyle changes don't work, ask your medical provider which laxative would be best for you and whether you need additional GI evaluation. Each type of laxative has its own precautions, particularly for people with certain medical conditions or who are unlikely to be able to drink enough fluid.

Bulk or fiber agents work by holding water in the colon, making stools softer, larger, and easier to pass. You can use these daily. You should drink at least six to eight glasses of fluid a day to avoid side effects. Examples include Metamucil, Citrucel, Konsyl, Serutan, Fibercon, and Benefiber.

Osmotic laxatives cause water secretion into the colon, which can help keep the stools soft and moving along. You can use these daily. These laxatives also require drinking at least six to eight glasses of fluid a day. Examples include Milk of Magnesia, lactulose, MiraLAX, and sorbitol.

Stool softeners such as Colace and Surfak are not actually laxatives, but they provide moisture to hard stools, making them easier to move. You can use these daily if needed.

Stimulant laxatives move stool more quickly by causing muscle contractions in the colon. Don't use these more than two to three times a week without discussing with your provider. Examples include Correctol, Dulcolax, Purge, and Senokot.

I have acid reflux that can be bothersome. What can I do to get it under control, other than taking medications?

Minimize pressure in or on the stomach by doing the following.

- Wear loose-fitting clothing or belts. Wearing tight garments affects your stomach like squeezing a toothpaste tube, increasing reflux.

- Try to lose weight if you are over-weight or obese and have increased belly fat, which places pressure on the stomach.
- Eat small meals frequently, rather than large ones less often. An overly full stomach may push some of the acidic contents back up into the esophagus.
- Try the Mediterranean diet, which has been shown to decrease symptoms from stomach acid or food refluxing into the throat. The Mediterranean diet includes high amounts of fruits and vegetables, whole grains, nuts, and healthy oils like olive oil, and limits red meat, full-fat dairy, and processed, fried, and fatty foods.

Identify other factors that may be exacerbating your symptoms. The following factors may be contributing to your acid reflux.

- Foods like chocolate, peppermint, acidic foods like orange juice or tomato sauce, fatty foods, and caffeine can increase GERD. If you have GERD, eliminating these foods from your diet should decrease the symptoms.
- Medications that can worsen GERD include beta-agonists (used for treating asthma), calcium channel blockers (for treating high blood pressure), some antihistamines (such as Benadryl), and sedatives. Review your medications with your medical providers (see table 14.1).
- Smoking and alcohol increase your risk of heartburn and GERD.

My GERD keeps me up at night. Is there anything I can do besides taking medications that can help me get a better night's sleep?

When lying down, acid is more likely to flow from the stomach into the esophagus, especially if the lower esophageal sphincter (LES), which separates the esophagus from the stomach, loses tone or doesn't properly close. This is why many people have their worst pain during the night. To alleviate nighttime discomfort:

- Don't lie down for at least an hour after eating.
- Don't eat or drink anything after 7:00 p.m.
- Avoid exercises that increase abdominal pressure, such as sit-ups, at night.
- Elevate the head of your bed on 6- to 8-inch blocks, or put a foam rubber wedge below the mattress under your shoulders and upper back.

Sometimes my GERD gets really bad, and I feel I need a medication. There are several available at the pharmacy that don't need a prescription. Can you tell me which I should take, if any, and what to watch for?

For a comparison of the medications used to treat GERD, see box 14.3.

BOX 14.3

Medications for Gastroesophageal Reflux Disease

GERD medications fall into three categories: antacids, H_2 blockers, and proton pump inhibitors (PPIs). Antacids and lower doses of the H_2 blockers and PPIs are available over the counter; higher doses require a prescription. Each has its pros and cons and are fine to take for occasional heartburn; however, if you're taking them regularly (see below), you should discuss this with your medical provider to make sure the GERD isn't due to a serious underlying condition.

Antacids

Antacids contain calcium carbonate, aluminum hydroxide, and magnesium hydroxide, all of which neutralize stomach acid. Examples include Maalox, Mylanta, and Tums. Antacids start working rapidly but the effects last only two hours or less. You can take them after a meal or at any time you are having symptoms. Keep in mind that long-term use of antacids can cause side effects; for example, magnesium salts can lead to diarrhea, and aluminum salts and calcium carbonate can cause constipation. *If you need antacids more than twice weekly for more than one month, and/or you have trouble swallowing or notice you are losing weight, see your doctor.*

H_2 Blockers

These drugs decrease the production of stomach acid, preventing heartburn for up to eight hours. Examples of H_2 blockers include cimetidine (Tagamet), famotidine (Pepcid), nizatidine (Axid), and ranitidine (Zantac). H_2 blockers require about 30 minutes to two hours to take effect, so you should take them before symptoms appear. They are effective in about half of people with GERD symptoms who take prescription doses. If reflux persists or worsens, you should see your medical provider.

Some older adults will develop confusion at higher doses of H_2 blockers, and cimetidine in particular has many interactions with other drugs, but in general these drugs are well tolerated. H_2 blockers have fewer long-term side effects than PPIs. Absorption of B_{12} can be impaired because stomach acid is needed to remove it from food. Additionally, H_2 blockers have been associated on rare occasions with decreased production of blood cells.

Proton Pump Inhibitors

PPIs are more potent than H_2 blockers and work by blocking an enzyme necessary for acid secretion. Examples include omeprazole (Prilosec), lansoprazole (Prevacid), pantoprazole (Protonix), and esomeprazole (Nexium). PPIs are effective for most people who have GERD, particularly when they are taken 30 to 60 minutes before the first meal of the day. Nonprescription PPIs are intended for a 14-day course of treatment up to three times per year. See your doctor if you're taking these medications more often.

PPIs block almost all stomach acid. Use for more than a year reduces the absorption not only of B_{12} but also iron, calcium carbonate, and magnesium. Other

(continued)

BOX 14.3 *(continued)*

sources of calcium, calcium citrate, and the calcium found in dairy products are normally absorbed. But an association has been found between PPIs and increased risk of fractures of the hip, wrist, and spine. Speak with your medical provider about whether you should be taking oral B_{12} or and magnesium. Low levels of magnesium can cause tremor, convulsions, weakness, and apathy.

Long-term use of PPIs has also been associated with an increased risk of C. *difficile* colitis, even in the absence of antibiotic use, microscopic colitis (another form of chronic diarrhea in older people discussed on page 282), and pneumonia. This risk is greater than with H_2 blockers.

Some studies have found an association between use of PPIs and dementia; others have not. An association does not mean that the PPIs cause the problem. Further study is needed to find this out.

It's embarrassing, but I seem to have a lot of gas that lets loose at the most inopportune moments. What can I do about this?

Increased flatulence can come from eating gas-producing food, the malabsorption of certain dietary components like gluten or lactose, or it can be a symptom of GI diseases like irritable bowel syndrome. You're also more likely to emit gas if your external anal sphincter is weak (see below).

What foods can cause gas?

FODMAPs (fermentable oligosaccharides, disaccharides, monosaccharides, and polyols) are poorly absorbed short-chain carbohydrates (saccharides) that are rapidly fermented by bacteria in the GI tract. This produces gas that makes the bowel distend and can cause diarrhea, bloating, flatulence, and pain as well as the feeling of urgently needing to evacuate your bowels.

FODMAPs include:

- *Oligosaccharides*, including fructans, which are found in wheat, onions, and garlic, and galactans, which are found in beans, lentils, and soybeans.

- *Disaccharides* such as lactose, which is found in milk and other dairy products.

- *Monosaccharides* like fructose, which is found in apples and honey.

- *Polyols* such as sorbitol and mannitol, which are found in fruits and vegetables as well as artificial sweeteners. *Note:* sorbitol, fructose, and mannitol are often found in chewing gum, hard candy, and carbonated beverages.

Not everyone reacts the same to FODMAPs, and some people can tolerate a small amount of a FODMAP without experiencing symptoms. For example, people who are lactose intolerant often can tolerate one cup of milk, which contains the recommended daily intake of calcium, or small amounts of yogurt or hard cheese throughout the day. A diet in which all FODMAPs are eliminated for two to four weeks, then slowly re-introduced one by one over six to eight weeks, can reveal which foods trigger the reaction. The good news is that avoiding the offending food can improve symptoms and restore quality of life.

Sometimes when I pass gas, stool also comes out. And sometimes I just leak stool. I need help.

There are some things you can do, but you also need to discuss this problem with your medical provider, since it may be due to an underlying medical condition.

- The more completely you empty your bowels, the less there will be to leak.
- Take your time when having a bowel movement. Don't rush.

- Raising your feet 8–12 inches on a chair or pile of books while going to the bathroom helps some people empty more completely.
- Strengthen your external anal sphincter. Remember the Kegel exercises to reduce urinary incontinence we discussed in chapter 11? These exercises are similar but target the external anal sphincter (see the Resources section at the end of this chapter). A good time to do these is after a bowel movement, before you wipe. Also discuss therapy and/or biofeedback with your medical provider.
- Try reducing your intake of caffeine, lactose, and artificial sweeteners, as they can make your stools looser.

If the above suggestions don't work, discuss medications, surgery, and alternative treatments (such as an anal plug or nerve stimulation) with your provider.

What Isn't Normal Aging?

 Red Flags: Symptoms Needing Prompt Medical Attention

- Symptoms that may indicate GI tract blockage, bleeding, perforation, or ischemia (lack of blood supply):
  1. Sharp, sudden, persistent, and severe abdominal pain.
  2. Abdominal pain followed by vomiting.
  3. Vomit that is bloody or looks like coffee grounds.
  4. Tarry, bloody, or black stools.

  5. Significant changes in bowel habits (if you're regular and suddenly become constipated, or if you develop persistent diarrhea).
- Urinary retention (may be due to stool being impacted, or stuck, in the bowel).
- Inability to keep fluids down because of vomiting, resulting in dehydration.
- Watery diarrhea (three or more loose stools in 24 hours) within two to four weeks of antibiotic treatment, often accompanied by lower abdominal

pain and cramping, low-grade fever, nausea, and loss of appetite. (These symptoms may indicate *C. difficile* colitis.)

- Recurrent coughing when drinking liquids or eating (see the Aspiration section below).
- Fever or pneumonia in a person who aspirates. Make sure to tell medical personnel about the aspiration, as this may influence their evaluation and treatment.
- Itchy skin, yellow eyes, or dark urine (these symptoms suggest hepatitis or another liver or blood problem).
- Iron-deficiency anemia (which may be due to GI tract bleeding or celiac disease).

⚠️ **Yellow Alerts: Common Conditions That Can Mimic or Worsen GI Symptoms**

Medications and Medication Withdrawal

Certain medications and the abrupt discontinuation of some medications can cause GI symptoms (see table 14.1).

Swallowing Problems

Aspiration

Swallowing is a complicated process (see box 14.1). With aging, food and fluids may occasionally get diverted into the lungs rather than entering the esophagus, causing coughing or a wet voice with eating or drinking. Aspiration can cause inflammation of the lungs (pneumonitis), actual pneumonia, choking, or, if long-standing, dehydration and malnutrition. Aspiration may

be provoked by eating too quickly, not chewing well, by taking medications that cause inattention, sedation, or dry mouth. Aspiration can also be caused by certain diseases like stroke, dementia, or Parkinson's disease. During a serious illness, swallow function may rapidly deteriorate. This is common in hospitalized patients, and with therapy, function usually recovers over time.

People who aspirate need to be evaluated by an ear, nose, and throat doctor along with a speech-language pathologist to determine why this is happening and what can be done to decrease aspiration and its complications. Interventions include exercises, diet modification, or positioning during eating to decrease aspiration.

Gastroesophageal Reflux Disease (GERD)

As discussed in box 14.2, older adults may have severe GERD without symptoms, or they may develop heartburn, chest pain, pain with swallowing, difficulty keeping food down after meals, the taste of stomach acid in the back of the mouth, a dry cough at night, a sore throat, hoarseness, or a repeated need to clear one's throat, particularly upon awakening. Complications of untreated GERD include esophageal narrowing, inflammation, and ulcers (see the discussion of esophageal dysphagia on page 280); *painless blood loss*, causing anemia; or *Barrett's esophagus*, a condition that alters the cells lining the lower esophagus. By itself, Barrett's does not cause symptoms or problems; however, in a small percentage of people it is a precursor to esophageal cancer.

TABLE 14.1
Gut Feelings

Drugs and Examples	Nausea and/or Vomiting	Diarrhea	Constipation	Heartburn and GERD
Blood pressure, cardiac, and diuretic medications				
All diuretics: furosemide (Lasix); triamterene-hydrochlorothiazide (Dyazide); spironolactone (Aldactone); hydrochlorothiazide (Microzide); metolazone (Zaroxolyn)	X	X	X	
ACE inhibitors: enalapril (Vasotec); lisinopril (Prinivil, Zestril)		X		X
ARBs: losartan (Cozaar); valsartan (Diovan); candesartan (Atacand)	X	X		
Olmesartan (Benicar)		X*		
Antiarrhythmics: quinidine; digoxin (Lanoxin)	X	X		X
Alpha-blockers: doxazosin (Cardura); terazosin (Hytrin); prazosin (Minipress)				X
Beta-blockers: atenolol (Tenormin); metoprolol (Lopressor); propranolol (Inderal)	X	X		X
Nitrates: nitroglycerin (Nitrostat); isosorbide dinitrate (Isordil); isosorbide mononitrate				X
Calcium channel blockers: amlodipine (Norvasc); diltiazem (Cardizem); verapamil (Calan)	X		X	X
Statins: simvastatin (Zocor); atorvastatin (Lipitor); rosuvastatin (Crestor)		X and MC		X
Pain relief				
Opioid analgesics: morphine, oxycodone (in Percocet); tramadol (Ultram)	X and W	W	X	
NSAIDs: aspirin; ibuprofen (Motrin, Advil); naproxen (Naprosyn, Aleve)	X	X and MC	X	X
Muscle relaxants: carisoprodol (Soma); metaxalone (Skelaxin)			X	

(*continued*)

TABLE 14.1 *(continued)*

Drugs and Examples	Nausea and/or Vomiting	Diarrhea	Constipation	Heartburn and GERD
Neurological, psychological, and sleep medications				
Benzodiazepine-type medications: zolpidem (Ambien); estazolam (Prosom); temazepam (Restoril); triazolam (Halcion)	W			X
Anticonvulsants: phenytoin (Dilantin); valproic acid (Depakote); lamotrigine (Lamictal); carbamazepine (Tegretol, Carbatrol); levetiracetam (Keppra); gabapentin (Neurontin)	X	X MC (carbamazepine)	X	X
SSRI antidepressants: escitalopram (Lexapro); fluoxetine (Prozac); sertraline (Zoloft)	X and W	X, MC, and W	X	X
Tricyclic antidepressants: amitriptyline (Elavil); imipramine (Tofranil); nortriptyline (Pamelor)	X and W	W	X	X
SNRI antidepressants: venlafaxine (Effexor); duloxetine (Cymbalta)	X and W	X, MC, and W	X	
Other antidepressants: mirtazapine (Remeron); vortioxetine (Trintellix); bupropion (Wellbutrin, Zyban); trazodone (Desyrel)	X and W	X and W	X	
Some antipsychotics (also used for nausea): chlorpromazine (Thorazine); prochlorperazine maleate (Compazine)			X	X
Anti-dizziness: meclizine (Antivert, Bonine); dimenhydrinate (Dramamine); scopolamine (Trans-scop)			X	X
Cholinesterase inhibitors for dementia: donepezil (Aricept); rivastigmine (Exelon); galantamine (Razadyne)	X	X		
Anti-Parkinsonian medications				
Decarboxylase inhibitors: carbidopa/levodopa (Sinemet)	X	MC?	X	
COMT inhibitors: tolcapone (Tasmar); entacapone (Comtan)	X	X and MC	X	

TABLE 14.1 *(continued)*

Drugs and Examples	Nausea and/or Vomiting	Diarrhea	Constipation	Heartburn and GERD
Dopamine agonists: pramipexole (Mirapex); amantadine (Symmetrel); bromocriptine (Parlodel)	X		X	
Anticholinergic Anti-Parkinson medications: benztropine (Cogentin); trihexyphenidyl (Artane)			X	X
Endocrine drugs				
Corticosteroids: prednisone; methylprednisolone (Solu-Medrol)	W	W		
Estrogens				X
Bisphosphonates: risedronate (Actonel); alendronate (Fosamax); ibandronate (Boniva)				X
Progesterone				X
Pulmonary medications				
Long- and short-acting beta agonists: formoterol (Perforomist); salmeterol (Serevent); albuterol (Proventil, Ventolin); terbutaline				X
Aminophylline, theophylline		X		X
Diabetes medications				
Biguanides and GLP-1 agonists: metformin (Glucophage, Glumetza); albiglutide (Tanzeum); dulaglutide (Trulicity); exenatide (Bydureon, Byetta)	X	X		X
DPP-4 inhibitors and meglitinide analogs: sitagliptin (Januvia); repaglinide (Prandin)	X	X		
Alpha-glucosidase inhibitors: acarbose (Precose); miglitol (Glyset)		X and MC		

(continued)

TABLE 14.1 (*continued*)

Drugs and Examples	Nausea and/or Vomiting	Diarrhea	Constipation	Heartburn and GERD
Gastrointestinal medications				
H₂ blockers and PPIs: cimetidine (Tagamet); famotidine (Pepcid); pantoprazole (Protonix); esomeprazole (Nexium)		X and MC	X	
GI antispasmodics: clidinium-chlordiazepoxide (Librax); dicyclomine (Bentyl); propantheline			X	X
5HT3 antagonists, antinausea, and vomiting: dolasetron (Anzemet); ondansetron (Zofran)	X	X		
Calcium and/or aluminum antacids: calcium supplements; Tums; Amphojel			X	
Magnesium antacids: Mylanta; Maalox; Gaviscon		X		
Genitourinary medications				
Bladder relaxants: tolteradine (Detrol); oxybutinin (Ditropan); solifenacin (Vesicare)			X	X
BPH alpha-blockers: terazosin (Hytrin); alfuzosin (Uroxatral); tamsulosin (Flomax)				X
Erectile dysfunction: sildenafil (Viagra); tadalafil (Cialis)				X
Cold, allergy, and itch medications				
First-generation antihistamines: diphenhydramine (Benadryl); chlorpheniramine (Aller-Chlor, Chlor-Trimeton); hydroxyzine (Atarax); meclizine (Antivert, Bonine)			X	X
Antimicrobials†				
Amoxicillin (Amoxil, Augmentin); ampicillin; cephalosporins cephalexin (Keflex); cefaclor (Ceclor); clindamycin (Cleocin); tetracycline	X	X		Clindamycin
Fluoroquinolones: ciprofloxacin (Cipro); levofloxacin (Levaquin); moxifloxacin (Avelox); ofloxacin (Floxin)	X	X		X

TABLE 14.1 (*continued*)

Drugs and Examples	Nausea and/or Vomiting	Diarrhea	Constipation	Heartburn and GERD
Tetracyclines: tetracycline, minocycline, doxycycline	X			X
Antifungals: itraconazole (Onmel, Sporanox, Tolsura); voriconazole (Vfend); ketaconazole	X	X		
Antivirals: acyclovir (Zovirax)	X			
Anti-tuberculosis: isoniazid; ethambutol (Myambutol); rifabutin (Mycobutin)	X			
HIV medications: didanosine/ddI (Videx); zidovudine/AZT (Retrovir)	X			
Most cancer chemotherapy drugs	X			X
Minerals and vitamins				
Iron sulfate or gluconate			X	X
Ascorbic acid (vitamin C)		X		X
Potassium				X
Calcium supplements			X	
Other				
Alcohol	X and W	X		X
Colchicine	X	X		

Note: If you're not sure whether a drug you're taking is in one of the drug classes listed, ask your pharmacist or health care provider. X, may cause this condition; W, withdrawal symptoms occur when drug is abruptly stopped; ?, studies conflict as to whether these drugs cause this symptom. Abbreviations are as follows: ACE, angiotensin-converting enzyme; ARB, angiotensin receptor blockers; BPH, benign prostatic hyperplasia; COMT, catechol-O-methyltransferase; DPP, dipeptidyl-peptidase; GERD, gastroesophageal reflux disease; GI, gastrointestinal; GLP, glucagon-like peptide; MC, microscopic colitis; NSAID, nonsteroidal anti-inflammatory drug; PPI, proton pump inhibitor; SNRI, serotonin-norepinephrine reuptake inhibitor; SSRI, selective serotonin reuptake inhibitor.

*Olmesartan has been associated with sprue-like enteropathy (similar to celiac).

†Most antibiotics have been associated with diarrhea. See discussion in the What Isn't Normal Aging? section of chapter 14.

Esophageal Dysphagia

Esophageal dysphagia, or the feeling that food is getting stuck after swallowing, has many possible causes. It may be due to an esophageal *stricture*, scarring that narrows the diameter of the esophagus; *esophagitis*, a severe inflammation or infection of the esophagus; *ulceration* or *pill esophageal injury*; or tumors or other disorders within or around the esophagus. If you have this feeling of food becoming lodged in your throat, you need to be evaluated.

Abdominal Pain or GI Bleeding

Peptic Ulcer Disease

Ulcers often cause a burning sensation in the upper to middle abdomen one to two hours after a meal; the pain improves after eating. The pain can feel like a dull, gnawing ache and is intermittent or constant, lasts for days to weeks at a time, and can strike in the middle of the night (or any other time that the stomach is empty). Nausea and vomiting, weight loss, a poor appetite, bloating, and frequent burping also are common symptoms. However, up to 60 percent of those who develop NSAID-related erosion, ulceration, or hemorrhage have no warning signs or symptoms (see box 14.2 for more information).

Gallbladder Disease

Most people coexist with their gallstones. Problems only occur when a gallstone is large enough to block the normal flow of bile through the *cystic duct*, which carries bile from the gallbladder, or the *common bile duct*, which carries bile from the liver and gallbladder into the small intestine. *Biliary colic* is when spasms of pain in the right upper abdomen occur after eating a fatty meal, when the gallbladder tries to push the bile through the obstructed cystic duct. If not successful, bile becomes trapped in the gallbladder, causing *cholecystitis*, gallbladder inflammation. Stones that obstruct the common bile duct can cause a blood infection or pancreatitis. Remember, older adults with gall bladder disease may not experience pain or fever, so problems with the gall bladder need to be considered when an older adult is quite ill, newly confused, or hypotensive, and no reason for these findings is apparent.

Diverticular Disease

Diverticulosis is the presence of many small pouches called *diverticula* that bulge outward from the colon. They are common in older adults and those who have had significant constipation. Most people with diverticulosis have no symptoms, but 10 percent will, on at least one occasion, bleed bright red blood briskly from the rectum. This can cause significant anemia and needs to be evaluated.

Diverticulitis is an infection that develops in 5 to 25 percent of those with diverticula and often requires antibiotic treatment. The reason diverticulitis develops is unclear, but it may occur when stool or bacteria get caught in the pouches. In the past, people with diverticular disease were advised to avoid eating hard-to-digest foods like nuts, seeds, and corn. Newer research, however, has put this recommendation into question. It appears that eating a high-fiber diet may be preventative.

This includes whole-grain pastas and cereals, beans, fruits, and vegetables.

Irritable Bowel Syndrome

IBS is an unusual new diagnosis for people age 65 and older, so it should only be made after a full GI evaluation. Symptoms include three to six months of cramping pain in the left lower abdomen. There is often a sense of urgency to have a bowel movement and a feeling that the bowels don't completely empty. Mucus discharge with stools is common, and symptoms increase with stress. Nighttime diarrhea is uncommon.

IBS is often suspected when at least two of the following three features are present:

- The abdominal pain is relieved by having a bowel movement.
- The frequency of bowel movements has changed.
- The form or appearance of the stool has changed, such as new diarrhea or constipation, or alternating diarrhea and constipation.

Inflammatory Bowel Disease

IBD includes Crohn's disease and ulcerative colitis. Only about 5 percent of new cases of inflammatory bowel disease occur in older adults. The main symptoms of ulcerative colitis are cramp-like abdominal pain, especially on the lower-left side of the abdomen, and bloody diarrhea. Loss of appetite, weight loss, nausea, anemia, and fatigue also are common. Crohn's disease symptoms vary depending on which part of the intestine is affected and the severity of the disease, but usually include abdominal pain, diarrhea, and

bloating. People with either type of IBD also can have symptoms outside the digestive system that may include joint inflammation (arthritis), eye pain, ulcers or rashes on the skin, or liver and kidney problems. Diagnosis is made by a biopsy during colonoscopy.

Bowel Concerns

Intractable Constipation

Most constipation, although uncomfortable, can be alleviated with lifestyle changes or, if needed, laxatives. It can be difficult to treat if there is an underlying metabolic disorder like too much calcium or too little thyroid or potassium in the blood, or when a person has certain diseases such as diabetes, kidney failure, or Parkinson's disease. When constipation can't be relieved, it can cause serious pain and other symptoms. *Fecal impaction* occurs when the stool blocks the rectum or colon and can cause nausea, vomiting, and pain. Impaction can also result a decrease in internal anal sphincter tone, allowing liquid stool to leak around the impaction, a condition called *overflow fecal incontinence*. Fecal impaction can also impair blood flow to the rectum, resulting in *rectal ulceration* or *perforation*. *Urinary retention* can occur if the impacted stool obstructs the neck of the urinary bladder.

Incomplete Stool Evacuation during a Bowel Movement

Incomplete evacuation is a concern for one-third of people with chronic constipation. It usually occurs when the muscles responsible for moving stools out of the anus do not relax sufficiently during defecation, or the pelvic floor muscles are too weak to contract to move the stool. Biofeedback pelvic floor retraining can teach you to increase pelvic floor pressures and to relax the anal sphincter during push maneuvers.

Fecal Incontinence

Fecal incontinence is the leakage of solid, liquid, or mucus stool. Fecal incontinence can occur for several reasons, including anomalies of the anal sphincter, rectum, pelvic floor muscles, and specific nerves; fecal incontinence; food intolerances; diarrhea; medications; and inability to get to the toilet on time. As mentioned above, fecal overflow incontinence can be caused by fecal impaction.

Diarrhea

Most diarrhea is due to mild food poisoning or a viral infection and lasts a day or two. Some antibiotics can cause diarrhea that stops when the antibiotic is stopped. Other infectious diarrheas can last longer, leading to dehydration and loss of vital blood salts and acids. See the Red Flags section above for symptoms of diarrhea due to a toxin produced by *C. difficile*, a bacterium that can overgrow and infect people who have been treated with specific antibiotics. *C. difficile* colitis occurs most commonly in older adults.

Chronic diarrhea may be caused by medications, parasitic infections, malabsorption (difficulty absorbing nutrients from food), intestinal diseases, and dietary factors such as artificial sweeteners like sorbitol and xylitol, caffeine, alcohol, or licorice. In older adults, the most common causes of chronic diarrhea are medications, intestinal diseases (including IBS and IBD, discussed on page 281), and malabsorption.

Microscopic colitis (MC) is an intestinal disease that causes between four and nine non-bloody watery stools per day, and on occasion many more. Patients may have a sense of urgency or nighttime diarrhea, and about half have abdominal pain. Diagnosis is made by biopsy of the colon.

Malabsorption in older adults is generally due to either lactose intolerance and celiac disease.

- *Lactose intolerance* is due to a deficiency of lactase, the enzyme that metabolizes lactose, the sugar in milk and milk products. Symptoms include gas, abdominal cramping, bloating, nausea, and/or diarrhea when more milk products are ingested than the person's lactase can handle. Importantly, low-fat and nonfat (or skim) milk contain the same amount of lactose as regular milk, so switching to these doesn't improve the symptoms. In older adults, lactose intolerance is usually due to a disease that destroys the lining of the small intestine where lactase lives, or to gluten intolerance, Crohn's disease, small intestinal bacterial overgrowth, or viral and non-viral infections.

- *Celiac disease* is caused by an intolerance to gluten, a protein found in wheat, rye, and barley. In people with celiac disease, the body's autoimmune system treats gluten as a dangerous invader, attacking it and triggering small-intestinal inflammation that impairs nutrients from being properly absorbed, causing malnutrition. Common symptoms are pale, foul-smelling, and difficult-to-flush stools that contain excess fat. Other common symptoms are gas, abdominal bloating, and anemia, which occurs in up to 80 percent of older adults with the condition. Celiac disease may also cause deficiencies of calcium, iron, and vitamin D.

Getting Evaluated for Digestive Concerns

See your primary care provider (PCP) if you have any of the symptoms discussed in this chapter. He will be able to help narrow down the causes and can usually provide suggestions for lifestyle changes and relief of your symptoms. Tell the office if you have any of the Red Flag symptoms at the time that you make an appointment; this will help them decide where and how quickly you should be seen by a provider.

Should I See a Specialist?

You should always discuss your symptoms with your PCP before seeing a specialist. See a GI specialist if the diagnosis is inconclusive, or if you have suspected inflammatory bowel disease, bloody diarrhea, GERD that doesn't respond to therapy, or are over 65 and have received a new diagnosis of irritable bowel syndrome. If aspiration is a concern (coughing or having a wet voice when eating, especially liquids, or occasionally choking), see an ear, nose, and throat doctor.

Preparing for Your Visit

The most important information to provide to your medical provider is a clear description of your symptoms. Complete the chapter 14 pre-visit checklist on page 384 in Appendix 3, bring it with you to your visit, and share it with your provider. Begin filling out the checklist as soon as you decide to see a provider, so that you have the time to recognize important patterns. You may feel uncomfortable discussing bowel habits, gas, vomit, and the like with your provider, but believe me, we're used to it.

Advice for Loved Ones

When I was growing up, my grandmother came to live with us after having colon cancer surgery. She had a colostomy, a hole in the colon through which feces passed into a removeable bag. But at that time the bags weren't very good, and accidents would happen or the smell of feces would linger long after she left the bathroom. I was told never to mention this to her, but one day I did, and we talked about what it was like for her to live with this condition—her real gut feelings. I think our talk helped both of us live better with this reality.

Conversations like these can be difficult, but these issues can interfere with quality of life and of relationships. Acting like there's not a problem can cause more distress, and stress makes many GI conditions worse. Gut problems can be scary or embarrassing not just to the older adult, but to you as well. If you notice something, or get a clue that there may be a problem, like when you're asked to pick up an antacid or laxative when you go shopping, take this as an opportunity to probe a bit to better understand what's going on. Be aware of the Red Flags and Yellow Alerts discussed in this chapter, and encourage a visit with a medical provider to determine if there's a serious condition that needs to be addressed or whether there are lifestyle changes or treatments that may help.

Bottom Line

Many gut problems affect one's comfort and ability to be with others. As a result, most people are amenable to changes in diet, medications, and lifestyle, including increasing movement or exercising. Swallowing difficulties may cause significant harm and need to be evaluated and treated to avoid complications. Be aware of your gut feelings, and when something unusual happens, pay attention and get help sooner rather than later.

RESOURCES

Health Information and Exercises

National Institute of Diabetes and Digestive and Kidney Diseases
(https://www.niddk.nih.gov/health-information)
Provides health information on diseases, symptoms, and testing.

Strengthening the Anal Sphincter
(https://www.wsh.nhs.uk/CMS-Documents/Patient-leaflets/Physiotherapy/6394-1-Exercises-to-strengthen-the-external-anal-sphincter-for-people-with-leakage-from-the-bowel.pdf)
This resource from the UK National Health Service West Suffolk provides exercise to help strengthen the anal sphincter.

Food Lists

Constipation: https://www.niddk.nih.gov/health-information/digestive-diseases/constipation/eating-diet-nutrition

FODMAPs: https://www.ibsdiets.org/fodmap-diet/fodmap-food-list/

GERD: https://www.hopkinsmedicine.org/health/wellness-and-prevention/gerd-diet-foods-that-help-with-acid-reflux-heartburn

Gluten-free: https://celiac.org/gluten-free-living/gluten-free-foods/

High fiber: https://www.med.umich.edu/mott/pdf/mott-fiber-chart.pdf

Lactose-free: https://www.drugs.com/cg/lactose-free-diet.html

BIBLIOGRAPHY

Christensen, L. *Digestive Diseases and Disorders: Symptoms, Diagnosis and Treatment.* Edited by Brijen Shah. Norwalk, CT: Belvoir Media Group, 2021.

Du, Y. T., C. K. Rayner, K. L. Jones, N. J. Talley, and M. Horowitz. "Gastrointestinal Symptoms in Diabetes: Prevalence, Assessment, Pathogenesis, and Management." *Diabetes Care* 41 (2018): 627–37, https://doi.org/10.2337/dc17-1536.

Holt, P. R. "Diarrhea and Malabsorption in the Elderly." *Gastroenterology Clinics of North America* 30 (2001): 427.

Münch, A., D. Aust, J. Bohr, et al., "Microscopic Colitis: Current Status, Present and Future Challenges. Statements of the European Microscopic Colitis Group," *Journal of Crohn's and Colitis* 6 (2012): 932.

Ratnaike, R. N., and T. E. Jones. "Mechanisms of Drug-Induced Diarrhoea in the Elderly." *Drugs and Aging* 13 (1998): 245.

CHAPTER 15

Weighing In

Other than having clothes that fit, does your weight matter when you're older? Does it affect how long you'll live or what you'll be able to do? The Duchess of Windsor was famous for saying, "You can never be too rich or too thin." Well, she was wrong. I won't speak about being too rich (at least in this book), but you certainly can be too thin. Being too thin increases your risk for becoming frail. Interestingly, being very obese can also cause frailty. This is another time to use the Goldilocks approach. Your weight should be enough to allow you to accomplish what you want to each day without adversely affecting your health. In other words, not too much, not too little, but "just right."

In this chapter we'll discuss how the body's composition, weight, metabolism, and nutritional needs change with age and how these changes affect longevity, health, energy, and strength. We will also cover the foods that are most beneficial, how to combat malnutrition, if it makes sense to take vitamins or supplements, whether you need to lose weight, what's not normal aging, and common conditions and medications that can affect your weight and nutritional state.

For an overview of weight, metabolism, and nutrition, see box 15.1.

What's Normal with Aging?

For a deeper dive into age-related changes in weight, body composition, and appearance, and nutrition, see box 15.2.

I'm 72, and my doctor recently retired. I just saw my new doctor for the first time. He says I'm overweight and that I need to go on a diet because my BMI (body mass index) is 29, and the higher it is, the greater my risk of developing diabetes, heart disease, or even dying sooner.

My previous doctor always said my weight was fine, but I don't know what my BMI was before.

The answer is simple: don't worry about your BMI being in the overweight range. Older people who are overweight (BMI of 25–29) or even mildly to moderately obese (BMI of 30–35) tend to live longer than those whose BMI is "normal" (BMI of 18.5–24.99), whereas for younger people, the higher the BMI, the greater the risk of death. BMI increases for some older people because their height decreases. There's a debate on whether to use one's adult height or their current height when calculating an older person's BMI. If the latter, BMI will increase.

Are you saying that now that I'm older there's no reason to lose weight?

No. If your weight is exacerbating medical conditions or interfering in what you're able to do, weight loss should be on your agenda. Obesity with a BMI of 35 or greater can decrease your walking speed, your reserves, and increase your risk of developing disability and frailty. Other conditions associated with a BMI of 30 or higher are high blood pressure, cardiovascular disease, diabetes, back pain, pain from arthritis, sleep apnea, gall bladder disease, some cancers, and urinary incontinence.

I'm 83 and having a lot of knee pain when I walk. My orthopedist says that I'm a poor surgical candidate (I have heart and lung disease) but that if I lose weight, I might have less pain and be able to walk farther. Any tips for how to lose weight when you're in your early eighties? Do I just need to decrease portion size and calories?

Cutting down is a start, but if you don't also exercise and increase your daily protein, you could further decrease your muscle and bone strength. A physical therapy referral will help you start an exercise program, and your medical provider may advise you to take a pain killer like acetaminophen a half hour before doing your exercises. See the next section for more specifics on ensuring you're taking enough protein to build muscle, and enough calcium and vitamin D to protect your bones. The amount of weight you lose probably doesn't need to be massive; even a loss of 5 to 10 percent of your body weight may improve your mobility.

Is bariatric surgery even an option for older people?

Bariatric surgery makes the stomach smaller in order to limit the amount of food eaten, and it may be an option if you haven't been able to lose weight with lifestyle changes. In properly screened older adults, it is as safe as in younger people. It's usually suggested for those whose BMI is 40 or greater or whose health is being adversely affected by their weight. But bariatric surgery is not a free pass—you'll need to change your eating habits and physical activity. Overeating after bariatric surgery increases the risk of complications and can eventually increase the size of your stomach, defeating the purpose of the surgery.

My weight hasn't changed, but I've developed a new potbelly. How do I get rid of it?

This is one of my patients' most common questions. As you age, more of your weight is made up of body fat. Muscle mass decreases, and new body fat is deposited centrally, explaining why your upper arms flap and your belly gets bigger. This is particularly true for women, because estrogen plays a role in where fat gets deposited. The rapid decrease in estrogen that accompanies menopause results in a rapid increase in abdominal fat. Exercising and eating more protein can decrease abdominal fat, but it won't eliminate your potbelly.

BOX 15.1

Weight, Metabolism, and Nutrition 101

WEIGHT

Your *weight* is based on the amount and types of food you eat, your physical activity, and your current size and muscularity. Food provides the fuel for your body, and you need to take in enough to keep the engine running—breathing, making new proteins and cells, circulating blood, and digesting and storing food—as well as to do your daily activities—moving around, working, and playing. This is called your *total energy expenditure*. You'll maintain your weight if you produce the same amount of energy that your body expends. Energy production is not just dependent on the calories, types, and portions of the food you eat, but also your body composition. The body is composed of *lean body mass (LBM)*, which is made up of the muscles, bones, ligaments, tendons, internal organs, and blood, and *fat body mass*. Lean body mass is usually 60 to 90 percent of total body weight, and men usually have a higher percentage of LBM than women. Lean body mass burns more calories even at rest than fat body mass, so having more LBM results in the production of more energy.

The *body mass index (BMI)* estimates your body's fat mass. Several diseases are more likely to occur in people with high body fat, including high blood pressure, heart disease, type 2 diabetes, obstructive sleep apnea, and certain cancers. Your BMI is calculated from your weight and height. In the metric system the measure is kg/m^2, and in the US customary system it is $(lb/inch^2) \times 703$. The BMI is used to classify people as follows: *normal weight*, BMI 18.5–24.9; *overweight*, BMI 25.0–29.9; *obese*, BMI 30 and above; and *underweight*, BMI below 18.5.

Note that these BMI classifications may not be appropriate for older adults (see box 15.2)

METABOLISM

Your *metabolism* converts what you eat and drink into the energy that fuels your activities and the raw materials needed to build, repair, and maintain body tissues. In the gastrointestinal tract, protein is digested into amino acids, carbohydrates into simple sugars like glucose, and fats into fatty acids. Depending on your body's needs, the sugars, fats, and amino acids are absorbed into the circulation and either metabolized or stored. The body, especially the brain and muscles, prefers sugar to fat or protein as an energy source. In response to your blood glucose levels, the pancreas releases insulin into the blood, where it increases glucose uptake into muscles, fat, and liver cells, and where it can be used for energy. When glucose uptake is inadequate, the body adapts by using fat as the primary fuel to conserve protein and muscle.

Whether you eat too much fat, protein, or carbohydrates, in the absence of specific weight loss programs or regular exercise, your body fat mass will eventually increase. Extra dietary fat is immediately stored in your adipose, or fat, cells. Carbohydrates are stored in the liver and muscles as glycogen, which if needed

BOX 15.1 (*continued*)

can be rapidly broken down into glucose for energy. The liver is limited in how much glycogen it can store, however, so if it is overloaded, the liver converts glucose into fat that is eventually stored in your adipose tissue. There is no place for excess protein to be stored. The liver breaks it down into amino acids that are excreted in the urine, and it recycles the rest into triglycerides that eventually are also stored in your adipose tissue.

NUTRITION

Nutrition recommendations are developed by many sources, but the US Department of Health and Human Services (DHHS) guidelines are most commonly used in this country (and well worth a read; see the Resources section at the end of this chapter). Calorie needs are estimated by age, sex, and physical activity level. Each age has a suggested dietary range, with the lower range appropriate for those who are sedentary, and the upper range for those who are quite active. The recommendations for how to divide up these calories are essentially the same by sex for all adults age 51 and older, with a few exceptions.

Nutrients are classified into *macronutrients* (protein, carbohydrates, fiber, and fats), which need to be consumed in large amounts, and *micronutrients*, which are needed in much lower amounts. The ways in which each of these contributes to digestion and nutrition follows:

Protein

The amino acids that are created from dietary protein are absorbed and reassembled to build and repair tissues, as well as to make enzymes, hormones, and other body chemicals. Proteins are made from 20 different amino acids, nine of which are the *essential amino acids* that must be part of the diet because the body can't produce them. Protein that contains all the essential amino acids is called *high-quality, or complete, protein.*

Carbohydrates

Carbohydrates are the sugars, starches, and fibers found in foods. They are the primary source of energy, particularly for the brain, enabling fat metabolism, and preventing the need for protein to breakdown to provide energy. *Simple carbohydrates* consist of one or two sugars, which are quickly digested and absorbed, leading to bursts of energy from spikes in blood sugar levels. *Complex carbohydrates*, which have three or more sugars, are absorbed and digested more slowly, providing more sustained energy.

Fiber

Although dietary fiber is a form of carbohydrate, it is not digested or broken down into sugar. It does, however, decrease the rate of sugar absorption and increase the sense of fullness. It also helps keep stools soft, so they pass easily through the colon.

(*continued*)

BOX 15.1 (*continued*)

Fats

Fat is an energy source, and one's diet needs to contain at least 10 percent fat to allow absorption of fat-soluble vitamins (A, D, E, and K). Just as there are essential amino acids, there are *essential fatty acids* that cannot be produced by the body and must be taken in as food. These include linoleic acid, which is an omega-6 fatty acid, and α-linolenic acid, an omega-3 fatty acid.

Micronutrients

Micronutrients are essential vitamins and minerals not produced in the body that are needed in small amounts for normal growth and development. There are many micronutrients, most of which are contained in a well-balanced diet.

A simple guide to the US DHHS daily goals for intake of macronutrients and certain micronutrients can be found in the table below.

BOX TABLE 15.1

Macro- and Micronutrients: Daily Goals and Average Intake for Americans 70 and Older

Macronutrients

	Women		Men	
	Daily Goal*	Average Intake	Daily Goal*	Average Intake
Calories (kcal)	1,600–2,000	1,662	2,000–2,600	2,159
Dietary fiber (g)	21	16	30	17.9
		(24% below goal)		(40% below goal)
Percentage of daily calories				
Protein	10–35	15	10–35	15
Carbohydrates	45–65	49	45–65	47
Total fat	20–35	36	20–35	37
Saturated fat	<10	12	<10	12

BOX 15.1 (*continued*)

BOX TABLE 15.1 (*continued*)

Micronutrients

	Women			Men		
	Daily Goal*	Average Intake	% of Daily Goal	Daily Goal*	Average Intake	% of Daily Goal
Calcium (mg)	1,200	784	65	1,200	968	81
Sodium (mg)	2,300	2,723	118	2,300	3,451	150
Vitamin D (µg)	20 (800 IU)	4.2	21	20 (800 IU)	6.2	31
Vitamin B$_6$ (µg)	1.5	1.7	113	1.7	2.09	123
Vitamin B$_{12}$ (µg)	2.4	3.88	162	2.4	4.97	207
Potassium (mg)	2,600	2,329	90	3,400	2,981	88
Iron (mg)	8	12.8	160	8	15.4	193
Magnesium (mg)	320	265	83	429	319	74

Sources: US Department of Agriculture, *Dietary Guidelines for Americans, 2020–2025*, 9th ed. (Washington, DC: US Department of Agriculture and US Department of Health and Human Services, 2020), https://www.dietaryguidelines.gov/; US Department of Agriculture, Agricultural Research Service, *Usual Nutrient Intake from Food and Beverages, by Gender and Age, What We Eat in America, NHANES 2015–2018* (Washington, DC: US Department of Agriculture, Agricultural Research Service, January 2021), https://www.ars.usda.gov/ARSUserFiles/80400530/pdf/usual/Usual_Intake_gender_WWEIA_2015_2018.

Note: These tables provide average nutrient intakes for older adults in the United States. There is wide variation in dietary intakes among Americans. Some eat much more, some much less. Abbreviations are as follows: IU, international units; kcal, kilocalories; g, grams mg, milligrams; µg, micrograms.

*Daily goals are recommendations from US Department of Agriculture.

BOX 15.2

What Happens with Aging: A Deeper Dive

WEIGHT

Weight increases until age 60–70, and then begins to decrease.
From age 30 to 60, we gain about one pound a year. After age 60 or so, weight usually stabilizes and then begins to decline. Both food intake and total energy expenditure decrease with older age. In general, we decrease our intake more than we decrease the amount of energy we use, resulting in weight loss. When we lose weight, we lose muscle as well as fat.

Appetite and food intake decline.
Older adults report that they are less likely to snack between meals, don't enjoy food as much as they once did, and that their meals have less variety. Compared with 20-year-olds eating the same restricted amount of food, healthy 70-year-olds feel less hungry, and after eating, they feel fuller. This loss of appetite and decrease in food intake result in weight loss and undernutrition, and it is known as the *anorexia of aging*.

The desire for food declines partly because of the age-related decline in taste and smell, both of which whet our appetite. Around age 50, the number of taste buds decreases, and the remaining taste buds begin to atrophy, further reducing the sense of taste. Salty and sweet are usually lost first; later, the perception of bitter and sour declines. The sense of smell is impaired in about 50 percent of people over 65 and 80 percent of people over 80.

There are multiple nonbiological reasons an older adult might eat less. Many older adults live and eat alone, and studies show that less energy is eaten at meals taken alone than when eating with others. Less food variety along with difficulties obtaining and preparing food can cause a decrease in the intake of certain foods, particularly high-quality protein.

Energy requirements decline.
Total energy expenditure and energy requirements decrease as much as 33 percent between one's twenties and eighties. This happens even to healthy adults because of age-related changes in body composition. With aging, body fat increases, and lean body mass, especially muscle, decreases. Muscle is much more metabolically active than adipose tissue, so as a person ages, fewer calories are burned. For most older adults, there's also a decline in physical activity, which further decreases energy expenditure.

It's harder to maintain your weight as you age.
During midlife, you may find that it's harder to lose weight than when you were younger. When you're over 60 or 70 years old, intentionally losing or gaining weight becomes even more difficult. In studies where healthy old and young men were overfed and gained weight, the young men were able to lose it all, whereas

BOX 15.2 *(continued)*

the older men could only lose about a third of the weight gained. When underfed, the older men lost more weight, yet they felt less hungry, and after eating, they felt more satiated than younger men. They only gained back two-thirds of what they lost, while the younger men overcompensated and gained back even more than they lost. In other studies, undernourished older adults, during and after a fast, felt even less hungry and more full than healthy older and young adults. It seems that the less one eats, the less one wants to eat. Weight maintenance becomes especially difficult in the advanced years of life.

Being underweight is a greater risk than being overweight (except for those who have been slender all their lives).
Being underweight (BMI ≤18.5), or having an unintended weight loss of 5 percent or more of your baseline body weight over 6–12 months, is associated with increased mortality as well as an increased risk of malnutrition, osteoporosis, fractures from falls, and frailty.

Waist circumference is better to estimate mortality and health risks than high BMI in older adults.
Compared with young adults, older adults who are overweight (BMI of 25–29) or even mildly to moderately obese (BMI of 30–35) have a lower risk of mortality, even cardiovascular mortality, than if their weight were "normal." This is called the *obesity paradox*. Waist circumference is a better measure of the health risks that come with obesity. High abdominal fat is associated with higher all-cause mortality, cardiovascular mortality and morbidity, cancer, diabetes and insulin resistance, high blood pressure, lipid abnormalities, and impaired physical function and quality of life. It's also associated with increased bone mineral density (a good thing!). These outcomes become much more common when a woman's waist size is greater than 35 inches or a man's is greater than 40 inches. Older adults with increased waist circumference are more likely to become frail. *To correctly measure your waist circumference*, stand and place a tape measure around your middle, just above your hipbones. Measure your waist just after you breathe out.

This is not to say that a high BMI doesn't matter. A BMI > 30 may exacerbate medical conditions associated with obesity, like pain from osteoarthritis, type 2 diabetes, or heart disease, and can exacerbate functional decline and frailty. BMI ≥ 35 in older adults is associated with difficulties walking, stair climbing, and rising from a chair. Risk of frailty increases further in those with an increased waist circumference if their BMI ≥ 30.

(continued)

BOX 15.2 (continued)

BODY COMPOSITION AND APPEARANCE

Whether your weight increases, decreases, or stays constant, as you age, your potbelly will get bigger while your muscles and your height will shrink.
With age, your body composition changes. Muscle mass decreases, especially in the arms and legs, as does the amount of fat underneath the skin of the arms and legs. Skeletal muscle oxidizes, or creates energy from, fat. A decrease in skeletal muscle causes less dietary fat to be oxidized, increasing overall fat mass. The body then stores this nonoxidized dietary fat as new fat in the adipose tissue of the belly (hence the potbelly), as well as in organs and muscles. Skeletal muscle infiltrated by fat is weaker and less able to support movement and exercise. After age 70, height decreases one to three inches from the drying out and shortening of the spine's vertebral discs.

Insulin resistance increases with aging.
Insulin resistance occurs when the pancreas releases insulin as usual in response to blood glucose, but the insulin causes less glucose to be taken into the cells. Muscle, an insulin-responsive tissue, decreases in mass and glucose uptake with aging, increasing blood glucose and its transformation into abdominal fat. The greater the amount of abdominal fat, the more severe the insulin resistance. The pancreas responds by releasing more insulin to keep the blood glucose in a healthy range. When the pancreas can't make or release enough insulin, blood glucose levels increase, and diabetes develops. Losing weight decreases adiposity and can reduce insulin resistance.

Both obese and underweight older adults are at risk for sarcopenia, a lower-than-expected muscle mass that can lead to frailty.
The combination of an inadequate diet and inactivity can lead to an even greater loss of muscle mass and strength than aging alone. It makes sense that underweight people would be prone to sarcopenia; however, obese people with the same risk factors can have an accelerated loss of muscle that is not appreciated because of a parallel increase in fat mass. Adiposity plays an important role in the inflammatory process and possibly the onset of sarcopenia. Illness can greatly exacerbate sarcopenia. Low muscle mass and strength further decrease the body's ability to produce and use energy, resulting in greater loss of strength, exercise ability, and endurance. Feelings of fatigue and exhaustion follow, gait slows, and physical activity further decreases, causing a cycle of increasing sarcopenia, weakness, and eventually frailty (see box 7.3). Adequate protein and energy intake along with physical exercise are the most effective strategies to manage sarcopenia.

BOX 15.2 (*continued*)

NUTRITION

Many older adults eat more fat and less protein and fiber than the recommended amounts.
The table in box 15.1 shows the average intake of macronutrients for older adults. On average, older adults' diets contain more fat than needed, including saturated fat, but only two-thirds of the daily recommended amount of fiber. Many older adults consume less than the daily recommended amount of dietary protein (0.36 grams per pound or 0.8 grams per kilogram of body weight), which would be about 58 grams for a 160-pound person. For many reasons, intake of high-quality protein like meat, eggs, and fish is decreased in older adults.

Losing weight requires attention to maintaining skeletal muscle and bone.
Decreasing calories (by going on a diet, for example) causes weight loss, but it also causes loss of skeletal muscle and bone. Physical activity alone doesn't cause weight loss, but the combination of regular aerobic exercise along with decreased calories and increased protein (see below) decreases weight, total body fat, and abdominal fat, increasing strength while limiting skeletal muscle loss. Bone health can be maintained by doing weight-bearing exercises and consuming adequate amounts of vitamin D and calcium daily.

Increased protein along with regular exercise can help attenuate age-related declines in muscle strength.
Regular aerobic physical activity and resistance exercises reduce intramuscular fat and maintain total lean body mass. To stimulate muscle synthesis, older people need more high-quality protein than the recommended daily allowance. The essential amino acids found in high-quality protein stimulate muscle protein synthesis. Higher-than-recommended daily amounts of protein (about 0.5 grams per pound, or 1.1 grams per kilogram of body weight) are needed to stimulate muscle synthesis in conjunction with exercise in the absence of liver or kidney disease. So, a 160-pound person would need to increase their daily protein from 58 to 80 grams. Increased dietary protein intake can improve physical performance, but to increase muscle mass and strength, it needs to be done along with resistance exercises. If you are overweight or obese, you should use lean body weight to calculate your exercise protein requirements (https://www.calculator.net/lean-body-mass-calculator.html).

Many older adults eat lower-than-recommended amounts of some micronutrients.
The table in box 15.1 shows that the average intake of *vitamin D, calcium,* and *potassium* is low in older adults. This may be from a lack of foods intrinsically high or supplemented with these micronutrients, like milk, orange juice, and other fortified foods, and fresh fruits and vegetables. For some older adults, selecting

(*continued*)

BOX 15.2 *(continued)*

foods with the right micronutrients is a matter of taste, while for others, fresh fruits and vegetables can be difficult to access, afford, or chew.

Micronutrient deficiencies can also be caused by certain medications. Table 15.1 points out some drugs that can cause nutrient deficiencies.

Older adults are less able to absorb calcium, vitamin B_{12}, and iron.
Adequate dietary intake of calcium is just one piece of the puzzle when it comes to calcium absorption, *vitamin D* is the other. Vitamin D increases calcium absorption from the intestine. In older adults, vitamin D levels decline steadily owing to inadequate dietary intake, reduced ability of the skin to synthesize vitamin D when exposed to unfiltered sunlight, and less exposure to sunshine without sunscreen. In many parts of the United States, the skin makes little vitamin D during winter. This seasonal decline, along with one's insufficient dietary intake of calcium, can result in a decrease in calcium absorption with age.

Vitamin B_{12} and *iron* require stomach acid for maximal absorption. Iron needs to be in the ferrous state to be absorbed, a task accomplished by gastric acid. Vitamin B_{12} binds to protein in food, and gastric acid releases it from food so that it can be absorbed. Acid production can be impaired by diseases like atrophic gastritis, an autoimmune disease of the stomach, as well as by medications used to treat acid reflux, like proton pump inhibitors and H_2 blockers. Although the average intake of vitamin B_{12} in the United States is above the recommended amounts, many older adults are B_{12} deficient because of their inability to free it from food. These people can take oral vitamin B_{12} supplements, which are easily absorbed regardless of acid-blocking medications or atrophic gastritis. Don't take extra iron or vitamin B_{12} unless your medical provider finds that you are deficient in them.

TABLE 15.1

Drugs That Can Cause Nutrient Deficiencies

Drugs and Examples	Vitamin B_{12}	Vitamin B_6	Vitamin D	Calcium	Potassium	Magnesium
Blood pressure, cardiac, and diuretic medications						
Loop diuretics: furosemide (Lasix); bumetanide (Bumex); ethacrynic acid (Edecrin)				X	X	X (rare)
Thiazide and thiazide-like diuretics: hydrochlorothiazide (Microzide); chlorthalidone, metolazone (Zaroxolyn)					X	X
Antiarrhythmic: digoxin (Lanoxin)						X
Antihypertensives: hydralazine (Apresoline)		X				

TABLE 15.1 (*continued*)

Drugs and Examples	Vitamin B$_{12}$	Vitamin B$_6$	Vitamin D	Calcium	Potassium	Magnesium
Pulmonary and cold medications						
Decongestants: phenylephrine (SudafedPE); pseudoephedrine (Sudafed Sinus)					X	
Inhaled beta agonists: albuterol (Proventil, Ventolin)					X	
Diabetes medications						
Biguanides: metformin (Glucophage, Glumetza)	X					
Gastrointestinal medications						
H₂ blockers: cimetidine (Tagamet); famotidine (Pepcid); nizatidine (Axid)	X					
Proton pump inhibitors: pantoprazole (Protonix); lansoprazole (Prevacid); esomeprazole (Nexium)	X					X
Stimulant laxatives: bisacodyl (Dulcolax); castor oil (Purge); and senna (Senokot)				X		
Antiseizure medications						
Phenytoin (Dilantin); carbamazepine (Tegretol, Carbatrol); primidone (Mysoline); phenobarbital			X phe-nytoin			
Antimicrobials						
Antibiotics						
Neomycin	X					
Aminoglycosides: gentamycin, amikacin, tobramycin						X
Anti-tuberculosis: isoniazid		X				
rifampin (Rifadin)			X			
Antifungal: amphotericin B					X	X
Endocrine medications						
Osteoporosis medications: calcitonin (Miacalcin); denosumab (Prolia, Xgeva), *Bisphosphonates*: alendronate (Fosamax); ibandronate (Boniva); zoledronic acid (Reclast)				X		
Corticosteroids: prednisone; dexamethasone (Decadron); methylprednisolone (Solu-Medrol)				X		
Cancer medications						
Platinum: cisplatin (Platinol AQ); oxaliplatin (Eloxatin); carboplatin (Paraplatin)				X		X
Antimetabolites: fluorouracil (Adrucil); leucovorin				X		

I've always loved to eat—my family calls me a "foodie." Recently, though, I've just not been as interested in eating. My appetite is down, and I'm even losing weight. Do I have cancer?

Most likely you have what is called the *anorexia of aging*, not cancer. Many older adults need to eat less to maintain their weight because they're less active. Aging also affects one's ability to smell and taste, decreasing the desire for food. The next section contains tips on how to improve your appetite. Medical conditions and medications can also affect appetite, so be sure to discuss any worrisome symptoms with your medical provider (see the Yellow Alerts section below).

You said there is such a thing as being too thin. How do I know if I am?

About 15 percent of older adults who live in the community (not in nursing homes) are malnourished or undernourished. Being underweight may leave you with diminished energy reserves to tap into should you become ill. An unintended weight loss of 5 percent or more of your baseline body weight over 6–12 months is associated with increased morbidity and mortality. Similarly, a BMI of 18.5 or less, assuming it has not been lifelong, is associated with increased frailty, falls and fractures, and mortality.

How about vitamins and supplements? Should I be taking any?

People who eat a truly healthy diet with fruits, vegetables, and the recommended amounts of protein, fiber, and fats don't need to take a multivitamin.

That being said, many older adults do not consume adequate amounts of several micronutrients (see box 15.1) and may benefit from taking a multivitamin made for seniors. These have higher levels of vitamin D and calcium but don't contain iron. Some concern has been raised about the cardiovascular effects of calcium supplements, so the best way to get calcium is through food sources. See the Resources section at the end of this chapter for sources of vitamin D and calcium, including fortified foods. Some people are unable to release vitamin B_{12} from food; discuss whether you need a B_{12} supplement with your medical provider.

I see aisle after aisle of nutritional supplements containing protein, minerals, and vitamins at my pharmacy and grocery store, and their labels all show a picture of an older person. Do you recommend nutritional supplements for older adults?

The best way to get protein and calories is by eating the proper foods, but if someone is having difficulty consuming adequate nutrition, oral supplements can help fill the gap. Nutritional supplements should be high-protein and high-calorie (often designated as PLUS on the label), to minimize the volume that needs to be swallowed to get the benefits. Supplements should be taken between, not instead of, meals. In those who are poorly nourished or have sarcopenia, drinking these supplements twice daily for six months has been shown to improve strength, muscle quality, and gait speed.

How do I know if I'm B₁₂ deficient? Is this something my primary care provider regularly checks?

Vitamin B_{12} is responsible for red blood cell development and for intact neurological function. Deficiencies can cause anemia, numbness and tingling of feet, lightheadedness when standing, and other neuropsychiatric symptoms like

dementia. Although oral B_{12} supplements will generally alleviate the deficiency, if the deficiency is long-standing or if the signs and symptoms are severe, it may be too late to reverse the symptoms. For this reason, many physicians recommend that all older adults be screened for B_{12} deficiency.

Adapting to Your New Normal

With aging, lots of physical, medical, environmental, and psychosocial changes result in a decrease in energy and muscle strength and an increase in abdominal fat. How much muscle mass is lost depends on the quality and quantity of your diet as well as your level of physical activity.

I think I eat a reasonable diet, but there seems to be endless debate about what's healthy, what's not, and what's the best diet to restore my youth and vigor. What should I be eating?

The first thing for you to do is to figure out what you are currently eating. Compare what you eat to the guidelines in box 15.1. If you want daily nutrient recommendations tailored to your age, height, weight, and activity level, use the National Academies of Sciences, Engineering and Medicine's calculator at https://www.nal.usda.gov/legacy/fnic /dri-calculator/. Most older adults' diets contain too little protein and fiber and too much fat. Eat lean meats and low-fat milk and cheese to limit saturated and trans-fat intake with your protein. The

recommended daily amount for protein is the minimum amount of protein to stop the loss of lean muscle. Try to make this high-quality, or complete, protein (see below).

Depending on your current diet, consider making the following changes.

Increase Your High-Quality Protein

High-quality proteins contain all nine essential amino acids. These include meat, poultry, fish, eggs, dairy foods, quinoa, and chia seeds. Many plant-based foods such as fruits, vegetables, grains, nuts, and seeds are missing one or more essential amino acids. If you are vegan, make sure you vary your foods so that you get all of the essential amino acids. Many foods are high in protein and low in fat, such as seafood, poultry without the skin, low-fat milk, cheese, yogurt, tofu, and soy products.

You can increase high-quality protein in your diet by replacing processed carbohydrates like cookies, cakes, pasta, and potato chips with fish, beans, nuts, seeds, peas, chicken, dairy, soy, and tofu products. Limiting processed carbohydrates can reduce your risk for heart disease and stroke, and the high-quality protein will make you feel full longer.

Increase Your Fiber Intake

Some foods are high in protein and fiber, like beans, nuts, and seeds. See pages 268–69 for tips on different types of fiber and how to increase your intake without increasing gas or abdominal pain.

Replace Saturated and Trans-Fat Intake with Mono- and Poly-Unsaturated Fats

Fat is an essential part of your diet, but there are "good fats" and "bad fats." Saturated and trans-fats increase your risk of cardiovascular disease and stroke, so they should be limited to less than 10 percent of your caloric intake (ideally 5% to 6%). Saturated fats are found in many fatty meats, poultry skin, butter, cheese, and whole or reduced-fat (2%) milk, as well as in palm oil, palm kernel oil, and coconut oil. These last three oils are known as tropical oils and are typically found in cakes, cookies, baked goods, and snack foods. Unsaturated fats are found in avocados; olives; peanut butter; sunflower, corn, or canola oils; fatty fish like salmon and mackerel; and nuts and seeds.

That's a lot to think about! Is there a one-size-fits-all diet that can ensure I eat all the right things?

The *Mediterranean diet* covers all the above. It's also been found that older adults who eat a Mediterranean diet are less likely to become frail. The basics of the diet are:

- Eating mostly plant-based foods, such as fruits and vegetables, whole grains, legumes, and nuts.
- Using olive oil and canola oil instead of butter.
- Flavoring your food with herbs and spices instead of salt.
- Eating red meat no more than a few times a month.
- Eating fish and poultry at least twice a week.
- Drinking red wine in moderation (optional).

I've been losing weight lately, and I am not eating as much as I used to. My provider has checked me out, and there doesn't seem to be a medical condition underlying my lack of appetite. Any suggestions for what I might do to maintain my weight, if not actually put some on?

It's not uncommon for older people to have smaller appetites and to feel full after eating less food. One thing that may help you take in more calories is to eat frequent small meals and snacks. Another thing you can do is to *liberalize your diet*. Many older people who are underweight or even malnourished are still restricting their diets either because they believe some foods are not good for them (sweets, carbohydrates) or because their medical provider told them to years ago. It is not known if fat- and cholesterol-restricted diets have any beneficial effects in reducing cardiovascular events when you're older, but being underweight certainly has adverse effects. Many of my patients gain weight and function when they start eating their favorite foods again, whether it's pizza, French fries, chocolate (in any form), ice cream, or a steak. Fats have twice the energy content per gram as carbohydrates or protein (9 calories vs. 4 calories for each). A diet high in fat may be necessary for frail older individuals to meet their maintenance energy requirements or to replete deficits.

Food no longer tastes good to me. Is it normal to lose the sense of taste with aging? Is there anything I can do to get it back?

Yes and yes. Some of this is due to loss of your sense of smell and taste, but not all. If you're still smoking, quit. It worked for me! If your nose feels stuffy frequently or during certain seasons, you may have allergies. Discuss allergy symptoms with your medical provider, since anti-allergy medications or other treatments may improve your sense of smell and therefore taste. Make sure you see your dentist at least once a year for a cleaning and exam, since poor oral hygiene can also affect taste.

In addition to the suggestions above, it helps to use flavor enhancers, including sauces, and to diversify your seasonings. Consider trying garlic, basil, oregano, turmeric, and cumin, for example. Use herbs and spices liberally without increasing your salt intake. By mixing up your foods, you'll enhance the contrast in taste and flavor, so don't wait to finish one type of food before starting another that's on your plate. Another way to improve your sense of taste is by taking smaller bites and chewing longer. Eating slowly allows the food to have greater contact with the taste and smell receptors, maximiz-

ing taste. Whenever possible, eat with others. It's been shown that you'll eat more than when you're alone.

Salt helps bring out the taste in food, and restricting it can make food bland and less enticing. If you've been told to restrict your salt and find low-salt food tasteless, discuss what's most important to you with your doctor. Salt restriction can lower systolic blood pressure by 4 to 8 mm Hg, but there are many other ways to lower blood pressure. If you need salt restriction to treat other medical problems, you can cook without salt but add a little to the finished product, producing a better-tasting meal containing far less salt.

I just got dentures, and I'm finding that foods don't taste the same; in fact, they sometimes taste like plastic. Do dentures affect taste? Is this only when they're new, or does it continue?

New dentures affect taste. Upper plate dentures cover the taste buds on the palate, decreasing your sense of taste. Meanwhile, the tongue taste buds are in constant contact with the denture, resulting in a taste of plastic. Your brain will adapt to this is short order, allowing you to again taste what you're eating.

Residual food on dentures can cause a bad taste or interfere with food's flavor, however, so make sure you properly clean them. Also, use as little denture cream as possible by having dentures that fit well. Excess denture cream can impact taste. Keep your dentures out of your mouth for at least four hours a day. If you still have denture-related loss of taste, ask your dentist about dentures supported by dental implants, eliminating the need for an upper plate. Note, though, that dental implants can be expensive.

I'm losing muscle mass and strength as I age, just like you said I would. Will eating more protein slow this process down?

Maintaining muscle and functional capacity requires doing moderate aerobic physical activity or resistance (strengthening) exercises regularly. By eating more high-quality protein prior to doing resistance exercises, however, your muscle strength and functional capacity will increase while your fat mass will decrease slightly. As discussed in box 15.2, you should eat at least 0.36 grams of high-quality protein per pound of body weight daily. To build muscle during exercise, increase this to about 0.5 grams per pound. Eat about one-third of this daily amount at each meal.

How much food is this? I'm not used to counting grams.

It depends on what you're eating. The number of grams of protein contained in an ounce of a protein-containing food is not the same for all types of protein. For example, a 3-ounce serving of skinless chicken contains 28 grams, salmon or tuna 22 grams, and ham 14 grams of protein. Half a cup of Greek yogurt contains 18 grams, ½ cup of cottage cheese 13 grams, lentils or edamame 9 grams, a cup of milk 8 grams, and cooked spinach 3 grams. See the Resources section at the end of this chapter for more information on the protein levels for different foods.

⟨CAUTION⟩ **People with liver or kidney disease should not increase protein intake without the approval of their medical provider.**

I've been a little heavy my whole life, and I think it's time to finally lose weight. Is there a best way to do this at my age?

First, decide whether you really need to lose weight (see box 15.2). If you do, fewer calories (smaller portion sizes help) and a combination of regular aerobic exercise along with increased protein intake works to decrease weight while limiting skeletal muscle loss and increasing strength. Make sure you're taking at least 800 IU of vitamin D and 1,200 mg of calcium daily. Try to get your calcium from food or fortified products rather than as supplements.

What Isn't Normal Aging?

 Red Flags: Symptoms Needing Prompt Medical Attention

- Unexpected weight gain
- Unintentional weight loss of 5 percent or more within the prior six months

- Difficulty swallowing
- Feeling full after eating a small amount

⚠️ **Yellow Alerts: Common Conditions That Can Mimic or Worsen Weight or Nutrition Problems**

Medications

Certain drugs can interfere with micronutrient absorption. See table 15.1 for information on which medications can cause nutrient deficiencies. For a list of drugs associated with weight change as well as taste and smell impairment, see table 15.2.

Difficulty Swallowing

Having trouble swallowing can be a sign of a serious medical problem. See the Yellow Alerts section on page 274 for more information.

Oral Health Problems

Poor dentition, poor oral hygiene, or gum disease can interfere with your ability to eat well. See your dentist regularly, at least once or twice a year.

Loss of Smell

Loss of smell can be part of normal aging, but it also can occur from sinus disease, growths in the nasal passages, hormonal disturbances, dental problems, prolonged exposure to certain chemicals such as insecticides, some medications, and, uncommonly, a brain tumor. It is rare for loss of smell to be the only symptom of these disorders, however. In addition, we now know that loss of smell is an early sign of COVID-19.

Unintentional Weight Loss

Weight loss that is not attributed to cancer can be caused by endocrine diseases like diabetes, hyperthyroidism, adrenal insufficiency, chronic infections (including dental infections), inflammatory and autoimmune disorders, and gastrointestinal problems that affect the esophagus and stomach, including their ability to empty. It can also be a result of malabsorption (like lactase insufficiency or gluten intolerance), depression, stress and anxiety, dementia (a common problem in its later stages), alcoholism, and severe heart, pulmonary, kidney or liver failure.

Difficulty Obtaining, Preparing, or Affording Food

Each of us is different. Some love to cook, others can't even boil water. Some hate to shop, some can't get to the store. Cooking for one may be fun, others enjoy the company of having a meal at a senior center. You may find yourself in several of these categories, or none. If you are having trouble obtaining or preparing healthy meals, there are services to help you get the nourishment you need. Such services include help with shopping or meal preparation, senior centers or Meals on Wheels, and actual or online grocery stores that deliver. Each state in the United States has an aging ombudsman, Department of Aging, or a Division of Aging that can usually direct you to local resources. Local places of worship also are good resources. They may provide the food or can tell you about local programs that do. See the Resources section at the end of this chapter for more information.

TABLE 15.2
Drugs That Can Cause Weight Gain, Loss, or Taste/Smell Impairment

Drugs and Examples	Weight Gain	Weight Loss*	Taste and Smell Impairment
Blood pressure, cardiac, and diuretic medications			
Diuretics: hydrochlorothiazide (Microzide); chlorthalidone; metolazone (Zaroxolyn); furosemide (Lasix); amiloride (Midamor)		X	X
Central adrenergic agonists: methyldopa; clonidine (Catapres)	X		X
ACE inhibitors and ARBs: lisinopril (Zestril); ramipril (Altace); candesartan (Atacand); Losartan (Cozaar)			Especially captopril
Calcium channel blockers: amlodipine (Norvasc); diltiazem (Cardizem); verapamil (Calan)			X
Antiarrhythmics		Digoxin (Lanoxin)	Amiodarone (Cordarone)
Alpha-blockers: doxazosin (Cardura); Terazosin (Hytrin); Prazosin (Minipress)	Especially terazosin		
Beta-blockers: carvedilol (Coreg); metoprolol (Lopressor); propranolol (Inderal)	Especially propranolol		X
Nitrates: nitroglycerin (Nitrostat); isosorbide dinitrate (Isordil, Dilatrate-SR); isosorbide mononitrate			X
Statins: simvastatin (Zocor); atorvastatin (Lipitor); rosuvastatin (Crestor)			X
Pain relief			
Opioid analgesics: morphine; oxycodone (in Percocet); hydromorphone (Dilaudid); tramadol (Ultram)		X	X
NSAIDs: indomethacin (Indocin); ibuprofen (Motrin, Advil); naproxen (Naprosyn, Aleve)	X†	X	X

TABLE 15.2 (*continued*)

Drugs and Examples	Weight Gain	Weight Loss*	Taste and Smell Impairment
GABA-ergic neurogenic pain medications: gabapentin (Neurontin); pregabalin (Lyrica)	X		
Neurological, psychological, and sleep			
Benzodiazepine-type medications: zolpidem (Ambien); eszopiclone (Lunesta); temazepam (Restoril); triazolam (Halcion)		X	X
Anticonvulsant medications			
Valproic acid (Depakote, Divalproex)	X		X
Carbamazepine (Tegretol, Carbatrol)	X		
Topiramate (Topamax)		X	X
Phenytoin (Dilantin); lamotrigine (Lamictal)			X
Antidepressants			
Amitriptyline (Elavil); citalopram (Celexa); mirtazapine (Remeron); nortriptyline (Pamelor); paroxetine (Paxil)	X		
Bupropion (Wellbutrin); fluoxetine (Prozac)		X	
Antipsychotics: olanzapine (Zyprexa); quetiapine (Seroquel); risperidone (Risperdal)			X
CNS stimulants: dexamphetamine (Dexedrine, Zenzedi); methylphenidate (Ritalin, Concerta); modafinil (Provigil); lisdexamfetamine (Vyvanse)		X	X
Cholinesterase inhibitors for dementia: donepezil (Aricept); rivastigmine (Exelon); galantamine (Razadyne)		X	X
Anti-Parkinsonian medications			
Decarboxylase inhibitors: carbidopa/levodopa (Sinemet)	X		X

(*continued*)

TABLE 15.2 (*continued*)

Drugs and Examples	Weight Gain	Weight Loss*	Taste and Smell Impairment
COMT inhibitors: tolcapone (Tasmar); entacapone (Comtan)		X	X
Dopamine agonists: pramipexole (Mirapex); amantadine (Symmetrel); bromocriptine (Parlodel)	X		X
Anticholinergic anti-Parkinsonian drugs: benztropine (Cogentin); trihexyphenidyl (Artane)		X	X
Endocrine drugs			
Corticosteroids: prednisone; dexamethasone (Decadron); methylprednisolone (Solu-Medrol)	X†		
Thyroid and anti-thyroid: levothyroxine (Synthroid); methimazole (Tapizole); propylthiouracil			X
Progestins: medroxyprogesterone	X		
Gastrointestinal medications			
GI antispasmodics: Atropine; clidinium-chlordiazepoxide (Librax); dicyclomine (Bentyl); propantheline			X
H₂ blockers and PPIs: famotidine (Pepcid); nizatidine (Axid); pantoprazole (Protonix); omeprazole (Prilosec); lansoprazole (Prevacid)			X
Pulmonary medications			
Inhaled corticosteroids: beclomethasone (Qvar); budesonide (Pulmicort); ciclesonide (Alvesco)	X		
Diabetes medications			
Insulin and sulfonylureas: glimepiride (Amaryl); glyburide (Glynase); glipizide (Glucotrol); tolbutamide	X		X
Thiazolidinediones: pioglitazone (Actos); rosiglitazone (Avandia)	X		

TABLE 15.2 *(continued)*

Drugs and Examples	Weight Gain	Weight Loss*	Taste and Smell Impairment
GLP-1 agonists: dulaglutide (Trulicity); exenatide (Bydureon, Byetta)		X	
DPP-4 inhibitors and *meglitinide analogs*: sitagliptin (Januvia); linagliptin (Tradjenta); repaglinide (Prandin)	X		
Biguanides and alpha-glucosidase inhibitors: metformin (Glucophage, Glumetza); acarbose (Precose); miglitol (Glyset)		X	X
SGLT2 inhibitors: canagliflozin (Invokana); dapagliflozin (Farxiga); empagliflozin (Jardiance)		X	
Antimicrobials			
Fluoroquinolone, penicillin, and cephalosporin antibiotics: levofloxacin (Levaquin); ciprofloxacin (Cipro); amoxicillin (Amoxil, Augmentin) ampicillin; cephalexin (Keflex); cefazolin (Kefzol, Ancef)			X
Other antibiotics: sulfamethoxazole/ trimethoprim (Bactrim, Septra); tetracycline; metronidazole (Flagyl); azithromycin (Zithromax); clarithromycin (Biaxin)			X
Antivirals: acyclovir (Zovirax); amantadine (Symmetrel); rimantadine (Flumadine)			X
HIV/AIDS drugs: didanosine/ddl (Videx); stavudine (Zerit)			X
Other drugs			
First-generation antihistamines: diphenhydramine (Benadryl); chlor-pheniramine (Aller-Chlor); hydroxyzine (Atarax); meclizine (Antivert, Bonine)	X		
Alcohol		X	

(continued)

TABLE 15.2 *(continued)*

Drugs and Examples	Weight Gain	Weight Loss*	Taste and Smell Impairment
Rheumatologics: colchicine; hydroxy-chloroquine (Plaquenil); allopurinol (Zyloprim)		X	X
Herbal and other supplements: herbal diuretics or tea; St. John's wart; nicotine; cascara; aloe		X	
Glaucoma medication: acetazolamide (Diamox)			X
Anticholinergics (see table 3.2)			X

Note: Abbreviations are as follows: ACE, angiotensin-converting enzyme; AIDS, acquired immunodeficiency syndrome; ARB, angiotensin receptor blocker; CNS, central nervous system; COMT, catechol-O-methyltransferase; DPP, dipeptidyl-peptidase; GI, gastrointestinal; GLP, glucagon-like peptide; HIV, human immunodeficiency virus; NSAID, nonsteroidal anti-inflammatory drug; PPI, proton pump inhibitor; SGLT2, sodium-glucose cotransporter 2.

*Any medication that causes dry mouth, nausea, vomiting, or difficulty swallowing can cause weight loss.

†Can increase water retention.

Getting Evaluated for Weight Concerns

As discussed throughout this chapter, the ability to maintain weight tends to be a greater problem for older adults than the need to lose it. Before going on a diet, discuss with your medical provider whether your weight is interfering with any of your medical conditions or impairing your physical function, and if you should even try to lose weight. If you've lost your appetite for food or you're losing weight, you do need an evaluation. As you can see from the Yellow Alerts above, there's a long list of possibilities for unintentional weight loss, many of which can be treated. Remember, you can be too thin, and this will affect your energy level, your bone density, and your strength. At the evaluation, your medical provider will check your weight and height, ask several questions about your eating, activity, whether you have any symptoms, perform a physical examination, and do some initial blood work.

Should I See a Specialist?

Not initially, unless you have specific symptoms other than loss of appetite or weight. Depending on what your primary care provider finds, you may be referred to a medical specialist, nutritionist, or physical therapist, among others.

Preparing for Your Visit

The most important things for your medical provider to know include a realistic sense of how much you eat each day, what your activities are, and what your weight has been over the past several years. Complete the chapter 15 pre-visit checklist on page 387 in Appendix 3, bring it with you to the visit, and review it with your provider.

Advice for Loved Ones

Eating is one of those areas we tend to focus on in those we care about: Are they eating enough, too much, the right things? In my experience, it's far more common for loved ones to be concerned that an older adult is not eating enough, and there's good reason for this. There are several reasons one's intake may decrease. Discuss your concerns with the older adult, and remind them that being underweight or undernourished can cause feelings of energy loss and difficulty getting around. Is the problem with their appetite, that food is no longer appealing, or that they don't want to cook? Or are they having difficulty shopping for and preparing food?

Depending on their answer, there are ways to help (see the Adapting to Your New Normal section above). If they're on a restricted diet, have them speak to their medical provider to see if this still makes sense, considering that they're having trouble maintaining their weight. Plan to eat with them when you're visiting. Remember, people eat more if they're eating with others. If they're not getting enough calories, protein, minerals, or vitamins, consider nutritional and protein supplements as well as a multivitamin.

If the problem is too much weight and it is interfering with their function, find out what they're eating. Oftentimes it's a lot easier to get and eat carbohydrates, especially simple ones like chocolate, than to get a balanced meal. See if you can help them get healthier food that they like into the house. Increasing their protein intake and their exercise, even walking, while doing some portion control can make a serious difference in losing weight that will help them function better.

When someone is near the end of life, it's a different story if they no longer want to eat or drink. This can be hard for us loved ones, since we often think of eating and drinking as providing comfort, and withholding this comfort may seem like we're starving someone we love. In reality this isn't the case. Nurses report that dying patients who are not eating or drinking seem more comfortable than those who are given IVs or forced to eat or take fluids. The body is shutting down, and nourishment can cause bloating, swelling, vomiting, gas, and choking. Hospice can be helpful in guiding families through decisions about feeding and other care at the end of life.

Bottom Line

For the most part, what older adults eat is more important than their weight or BMI. Food is fuel, and many older adults are not getting enough high-quality protein, fiber, calcium, or vitamin D. They may be trying to lose weight based on a number, not on whether their weight is exacerbating a medical condition or interfering with their daily functions. Some may still be restricting their diets for medical reasons even though they're losing weight. To be fit, it helps to increase body protein and exercise to help build muscle and decrease abdominal fat, which is associated with insulin resistance and mortality. Access to healthy food and help preparing it can improve nutrition. See the Resources section below for services that may be available in your area.

RESOURCES

What to Eat

EatRight.org
This website from the Academy of Nutrition and Dietetics contains information for older adults who are interested in learning more about nutrition.

MyPlate for Older Adults
(https://hnrca.tufts.edu/myplate/)
This service from Tufts University provides examples of foods that fit into a healthy, well-balanced diet.

US Department of Agriculture. *Dietary Guidelines for Americans, 2020–2025*. 9th ed. Washington, DC: US Department of Agriculture and US Department of Health and Human Services, 2020. https://www.dietaryguidelines.gov/resources/2020-2025-dietary-guidelines-online-materials. Contains food sources for calcium, dietary fiber, potassium, vitamin D, and iron.

US Food and Drug Administration. *Food Safety: For Older Adults and People with Cancer, Diabetes, HIV/AIDS, Organ Transplants, and Autoimmune Diseases*. Washington, DC: FDA, 2020. http://www.fda.gov/media/83744/download.

This booklet includes information about handling and preparing food, safe shopping, and foodborne illnesses.

Access to Food and Meals

Commodity Supplemental Food Program (https://www.fns.usda.gov/csfp/commodity-supplemental-food-program)
The CSFP supplements the diets of low-income older adults by providing nutritious food packaged by the US Department of Agriculture to support a healthy dietary pattern. The CSFP is federally funded, and private and nonprofit institutions facilitate the distribution of monthly CSFP packages to eligible older adults.

Congregate Nutrition Services
Congregate meals authorized by the Older Americans Act are available to any person age 60 and older and their spouse of any age. These are typically provided in senior centers, schools, churches, or other community settings. Check your state's website for more information on how to access congregate nutrition services.

Senior Nutrition Services
(https://acl.gov/programs/health-wellness
/nutrition-services)
The Older Americans Act authorizes meals
and related services in a person's home
for individuals ages 60 and older and
their spouse of any age. Older adults who
experience difficulty leaving the home
due to frailty, health concerns, or certain
medical conditions may benefit from
home-delivered meals offered under the
Older Americans Act. This program is also
known as Meals on Wheels.

Supplemental Nutrition Assistance Program
(https://www.fns.usda.gov/snap
/supplemental-nutrition-assistance
-program)
Older adults with limited income may
qualify for SNAP, a federal program that
provides temporary benefits to help individuals purchase foods and beverages to
support a healthy dietary pattern when
resources are constrained.

For more information on available services,
contact your state's Division or Department
of Aging.

BIBLIOGRAPHY

Dahl, W. J., and M. L. Stewart. "Position of
the Academy of Nutrition and Dietetics:
Health Implications of Dietary Fiber." *Journal of the Academy of Nutrition and Dietetics* 115, no. 11 (2015): 1861–70.

Deutz, N. E. P., J. M Bauer, R. Barazzoni,
et al. "Protein Intake and Exercise for
Optimal Muscle Function with Aging:
Recommendations from the ESPEN Expert
Group." *Clinical Nutrition* 33, no. 6 (2014):
929–36.

Domecq, J. P., G. Prutsky, and A. Leppin.
"Clinical Review: Drugs Commonly Asso-
ciated with Weight Change: A Systematic
Review and Meta-Analysis." *Journal of
Clinical Endocrinology and Metabolism* 100,
no. 2 (2015): 363–70.

Doty, R. L. "Treatments for Smell and Taste
Disorders: A Critical Review." *Handbook of
Clinical Neurology* 164 (2019): 470–71.

Gill, H., B. Gill, and S. El-Halabi. "Antidepressant Medications and Weight
Change: A Narrative Review." *Obesity* 28,
no. 11 (2020): 2064–72.

Lichtenstein, A. H., H. Rasmussen, W. W.
Yu, et al. "Modified MyPyramid for Older
Adults." *Journal of Nutrition* 138 (2008):
5–11.

ter Borg, S., S. Verlaan, D. M. Mijnarends,
et al. "Macronutrient Intake and Inadequa-
cies of Community-Dwelling Older Adults:
A Systematic Review." *Annals of Nutrition
and Metabolism* 66, no. 4 (2015): 242–55.

Tsai, A. G., and D. H. Bessesen. "Obesity."
Annals of Internal Medicine 170, no. 5
(2019): ITC33–ITC48.

US Department of Agriculture, Agricultural
Research Service. "Usual Nutrient Intake
from Food and Beverages, by Gender and
Age, What We Eat in America, NHANES
2015–2018." January 2021. https://www
.ars.usda.gov/ARSUserFiles/80400530/pdf
/usual/Usual_Intake_gender_WWEIA_2015
_2018.pdf.

Wilson, M. G., D. R. Thomas, L. Z. Rubenstein, et al. "Appetite Assessment: Simple
Appetite Questionnaire Predicts Weight
Loss in Community-Dwelling Adults and
Nursing Home Residents." *American Journal of Clinical Nutrition* 82, no. 5 (2005):
1074–81.

CHAPTER 16

Sex Talk

As we age, our openness and desire to have sex and be intimate may change. Our bodies look and function differently, we may feel uncertain about our attractiveness, or we may just feel done with sex. Arousal and orgasm, which may have occurred quickly when younger, now may take more time. Adaptations may be needed based on health conditions or physical limitations. Medications may make sex difficult, or, conversely, we may need medications to make sex better. Some of us find ourselves without a partner, or having sex with a new partner for the first time in many years. The times we live in are changing as well, and the rules about sex and relationships are not the same as when we last dated.

This chapter explores how sexual responses change with normal aging, how to adapt to these physical and emotional changes, what you can do to overcome some of the barriers that arise to having sex alone or with a partner as you age, what's different from when you last dated, and how to discuss sex and relationships with new partners, your family, and your health care providers.

For an overview of the stages and physiology of the sexual response, see box 16.1.

What's Normal with Aging?

For a deeper dive into age-related changes in the stages of the sexual response and sex hormone levels, see box 16.2.

We've been married for many years, and over the past few years we've been having sex less often. Does interest in sex decrease in long-term relationships?

The numbers of partnered older adults who are sexually active does decrease with age and health status. For those 76–80 years old and in good to excellent health, 50 to 60 percent are sexually active, whereas for those ages 81–85, 45 to 55 percent of men and 20 to 45 percent of women are. Being in fair or poor health markedly reduces these numbers. For some people, being with the same partner for many, many years can cause some loss of interest or other concerns that can decrease sexual activity (see the book *Mating in Captivity* in the Resources section at the end of this chapter).

BOX 16.1

The Sexual Response 101

THE SEXUAL RESPONSE CYCLE

Emotions and physical feelings cause sexual arousal and activity, and vice versa. The sexual response cycle for both men and women is similar and has four stages: desire, arousal, orgasm, and resolution. These stages occur whether the activity is intercourse, self-stimulation, or stimulation by another. Each stage is unique, although their order and duration may differ by individual and situation.

Stage 1: Desire

Desire is the urge to engage in sexual activity. It is also called *libido*. Learned responses, motivation, including a desire for intimacy, and hormonal status play a role in feeling desire.

Stage 2: Arousal

Arousal is the state where thoughts and fantasies, nongenital physiologic changes like salivation, sweating, flushing, nipple erection, and genital engorgement bring one to the brink of orgasm. For women, arousal tends to require foreplay, or tactile stimulation. Achieving orgasm often requires direct stimulation of the clitoris or its surrounding tissues.

Stage 3: Orgasm

Orgasm is the altered state of consciousness that occurs when genital stimulation, by causing neurotransmitters to discharge, results in the release of sexual tension and the feeling of sensory pleasure. This stage is the climax of the sexual response cycle and generally lasts only a few seconds. In men, orgasms tend to be sudden, forceful, and occur once during a sexual encounter. They are followed by a *refractory period*, during which time another orgasm cannot occur. Women's orgasms are more variable. They can be sudden and forceful or more gradual, rising and falling, occurring once or several times during the encounter. Women do not have a refractory period, and with further stimulation, they may have another or several orgasms.

Stage 4: Resolution

During this phase, the body slowly returns to its unaroused state, and swollen and erect body parts return to their previous size and color. This phase is marked by a general sense of well-being and, often, fatigue.

PHYSIOLOGY OF THE SEXUAL RESPONSE

Although the external genitalia of women and men look different, our bodies' response to sexual feelings and activity is similar. During the first three stages of the sexual response, muscle tension, heart rate, breathing, blood pressure, and skin flushing increase, reaching their maximum at orgasm. With arousal, nerve impulses cause lubrication to begin and blood to flow to the erectile tissues of the genitals, enlarging the clitoris or the penis.

(continued)

BOX 16.1 *(continued)*

In women, a number of neurotransmitters, including nitrous oxide and vaso-active intestinal peptide, are critical to arousal and orgasm. These neurotransmitters cause blood vessels to dilate, increasing flow and causing the clitoris, labia, and vagina to swell. The vagina lengthens, dilates, and lubricates, the clitoral hood retracts, and the clitoris enlarges and hardens. With orgasm, the muscles of the pelvic floor, uterus, and vagina contract, producing a sensation that begins at the clitoris and spreads throughout the pelvis.

In men, the same process results in an *erection*. The penis is composed of spongelike erectile tissue. When its blood vessels relax, often in response to nitrous oxide, the penis fills with blood. The expanding tissue presses up against a dense membrane that surrounds these vessels, trapping the blood and causing the penis to enlarge and become rigid. With orgasm, rhythmic contractions of the muscles at the base of the penis result in the ejaculation of semen and opening up of the veins that allow blood to drain out, causing a return of the penis to its non-erectile state.

My mother is in her seventies and recently divorced. She's now starting to date. Do you think she'll be having sex at this age?

Our need for sexual intimacy does not stop simply because we get older. In fact, the best predictor of sexual interest and activity in our later years is our frequency of and interest in sexual activity when we were younger. If sex was important to you when you were 30, it is likely to still be important when you're 65 and older. According to a recent University of Michigan and AARP poll, nearly two-thirds of older adults say they are interested in sex, although men seem to have a stronger drive and interest than women, a gap that widens with age.

I'm on my own and not interested in having sex or a relationship. Is this normal?

It's certainly not abnormal. Women are more likely than men to report lack of interest as a reason for sexual inactivity; this was especially true among those who are not currently in a relationship (51 percent of women versus 24 percent of men). Some people have never been very interested in sex. Many people like being and living alone, and don't want to complicate things with the needs and desires of another person. Don't feel pressured; many of my patients find life incredibly fulfilling on their own.

Sex doesn't seem to be as spontaneous as when I was younger. This makes me frustrated and less interested. Is there something wrong with me?

No. It's not unusual for older adults to have concerns about sex. A 2007 study (the most recent that was published) found that almost half of all sexually active older people reported at least one "bothersome" sexual problem. For women, these were most often lack of interest in sex (43 percent), difficulty with vaginal lubrication (39 percent), and inability to orgasm (34 percent). For men, the concerns were difficulty achieving or maintaining an erection (also known as erectile dysfunction, or ED) (37 percent), lack of interest in sex (28 percent), climaxing too quickly (28 percent), performance anxiety (27 percent), and inability to orgasm (20 percent).

Many of these problems are *normal aging*. As we age, it takes longer to become sexually aroused. Woman need longer and more direct clitoral stimulation to reach orgasm. Lubrication declines, and the vaginal tissues become thinner, less elastic, and dry. Older men also need a longer amount of time and more direct stimulation to have an erection. The erection may be less firm, and occasionally it's difficult to maintain. It can take longer for men to reach orgasm, the orgasm may be shorter or less intense, and they may produce a lower volume of ejaculate than when younger. There are also physical and psychological conditions that can interfere with sex that will be discussed later in this chapter. See the next section for some suggestions on how to adapt to these changes.

What about hormone replacement? Will that help my sex life?

For some people, hormone replacement can increase desire. Many women experience a decrease in sexual interest and response with menopause. Oral estrogen or estrogen-progesterone therapy can produce a small increase in arousal and fantasy in woman during the first five years or so after menopause, but after this period the risks may outweigh the benefits, especially for those over 60 or with a cardiac condition. Women who have had a hysterectomy are prescribed oral estrogen, which can increase the risk for stroke and blood clots, while women who still have a uterus are prescribed estrogen-progestin combinations, which can increase the risk for cardiovascular disease and invasive breast cancer. Vaginal estrogen therapy can improve symptoms of vaginal atrophy, but it has little effect on libido or sexual satisfaction. Testosterone increases sexual desire in women; however, the appropriate dose and long-term safety, particularly the risk of breast cancer, are not known. At this time, the US Food and Drug Administration has not approved any testosterone preparations for women.

In men, testosterone levels may decrease as part of normal aging, and low levels may be the reason for decreased libido. Testosterone does not improve sexual performance if you have normal testosterone levels, and it puts you at risk of numerous serious adverse effects, so your hormone levels must be measured accurately. Testosterone levels vary by time of day, so your testosterone should be measured in the early morning, and if low, the measurements should be repeated once or twice for confirmation. If testosterone is persistently low, your medical provider needs to determine whether the problem is in the testes or the pituitary gland (see box 16.2) by measuring pituitary hormones.

If your testosterone levels and your sexual desire are low, a three-month trial of testosterone will determine whether you will benefit from testosterone replacement. Adverse effects of testosterone include acne and skin changes, water retention, gynecomastia (enlarged breast tissue), an increased risk of male breast and prostate cancer, exacerbation of benign prostatic hypertrophy and sleep apnea, aggressive behavior, and overproduction of red blood cells, a condition called polycythemia, which is associated with an increase in heart attacks and strokes.

I would really like to be sexually active, but I'm afraid I won't be successful. What can interfere with having sex as you get older?

These are really two different questions. Success is in the eye of the beholder. For some, intimacy and touching are as sat-

isfying as having an orgasm. Others find that attaining orgasm through manual or oral stimulation can be as pleasurable, or at times more pleasurable, than intercourse. Make sure you're aware of the changes that occur with normal aging discussed above, as "right-sizing your expectations" can prevent you from obsessing if your experience isn't the same as when you were younger.

I look in the mirror and am not crazy about what I see. I certainly don't look like I did the last time I dated or when I got married. Why would anyone want to have sex with someone who looks like me?

Everyone's body changes with aging, whether it's through normal aging, lifestyle, or disease. Skin is looser, muscle

BOX 16.2

What Happens with Aging: A Deeper Dive

Foreplay is more important for both men and women, and orgasms may be less intense.
Desire often decreases for women after menopause. Men may be used to achieving a full erection from a thought or an image, but with aging, both men and women need foreplay that includes longer and stronger genital stimulation to get aroused and have erections and orgasms. Orgasms may be shorter or less intense in older adults. For men, the erection may be less firm, the volume of ejaculate less, and the refractory period, the time between orgasms, longer. The decrease in the fullness and rigidity of the erection can increase the importance of direct clitoral stimulation during intercourse for the woman to achieve orgasm.

Estrogen levels decline.
After menopause, women's estrogen levels decline, causing vaginal and bladder symptoms in almost half of postmenopausal women. Estrogen is important for maintaining vaginal, bladder, and rectal mucosal and musculoskeletal integrity, vaginal pH, genital blood flow, and sensation. As a result, the tissues of the vagina and vulva become thinner, less elastic, and dry, and the vagina itself becomes shorter and stiffer, with a smaller opening. This vaginal atrophy can cause pain with intercourse. The increase in vaginal pH increases the risk of bacterial vaginitis and urinary tract infections.

BOX 16.2 (*continued*)

Testosterone levels decline.
Testosterone levels decrease with aging in both women and men. Androgens are the "male" sex hormones, the majority of which are testosterone. In women, androgens are produced in the ovaries and adrenals. Libido decreases in the absence of these organs, such as after surgical removal. Studies have shown that testosterone increases sexual desire in postmenopausal women with low libido; however, the appropriate dose and long-term safety, particularly the risk of breast cancer, is unclear.

For some men, decreased libido may be due to low testosterone. Testosterone levels peak when a man is a teenager or young adult, and then decline as a natural part of aging. Testosterone is produced in the testes, and its level is regulated by two pituitary gland sex hormones, luteinizing hormone (LH) and follicle stimulating hormone (FSH). *Hypogonadism* is the term for low production of sex hormones. In *primary hypogonadism*, the testes don't produce enough testosterone, while in *secondary hypogonadism*, the pituitary gland doesn't produce enough LH and FSH to signal the testes to release testosterone. See the Yellow Alerts section for more information on testosterone replacement.

tone decreases. Our altered appearance can affect how we see ourselves and how we feel about our sexual attractiveness. Our physical changes with aging do not have to translate to unsatisfying or nonexistent sex or love. It's critical that we become comfortable with our bodies as we age if we expect others to be comfortable with our bodies.

Remember, people your age look like you. One of my patients had been widowed twice, and at 87 fell in love with an 89-year-old man, who also had been twice widowed. They were madly in love and swore that they were having the best sex they had ever had in their lives. And I believed them!

My adult children are giving me a hard time about my wanting to date at this stage of my life. I don't know if they're afraid I'll get duped or afraid they'll lose their inheritance. Can you give me any insight into what might be going through their minds, and how I can reassure them?

Your children's reactions are unfortunately common, especially if the only person they've ever seen or imagined you with was their other parent. Additionally, our society can be ageist about romance and sex in older adults. How many times did you imagine your parents had sex? For many of us, the answer is the number of children or pregnancies they had. I bet you never thought they'd be having sex in old age!

Our children are also concerned about our safety and our financial stability during the rest of our lives. It is important to talk openly and honestly with them about the issues that surround new relationships. Make sure they understand why the relationship is important to you, and be open to hearing and discussing their concerns. Most of these concerns can be addressed without endangering either your relationship with your family or with your new love interest.

I had a traditional marriage for many years, and my husband recently died. Now I'm finding that I'm having strong romantic feelings toward one of my female friends, and I think she's flirting with me. Is it ridiculous to "come out" at 75?

Coming out is ageless. Sometimes it coincides with life changes, like the death of a spouse, or grown children moving out of the home. More than 1.1 million people over the age of 65 identify as lesbian, gay, bisexual, transexual, or queer (LGBTQ), and this number is expected to at least double over the next 40 years. Baby boomers grew up in a time when homosexuality was a crime, classified as a psychiatric disorder, and could cost them their job or family ties. Many people had romantic feelings toward people of the same sex but never allowed themselves to consider this option. Much has changed over the past 50 years.

Some people are reluctant to disclose their sexual orientation or gender identity to their families, friends, and health care providers. If you are thinking of coming out, educate yourself on ways to find community and support (see the Resources section at the end of this chapter). Although medical providers should routinely ask questions about sexual orientation, the majority do not. It is important to have this discussion, as it can open the door to important conversations about what matters to you in your life and health care.

Adapting to Your New Normal

Both physical and emotional issues play a role in one's sex life. Forms of sexual expression differ among people and may include intercourse, self-stimulation, stimulation by others, oral sex, sexual aids like vibrators or dildos, hugging, or caressing. Desire or arousal may be spontaneous or evoked by a variety of stimuli, including touch, fantasy, dressing up, erotic stories, or videos. With aging, aspects of your sexual response will differ from when you were younger (box 16.2). This section answers questions about what you can do to make your sex life more comfortable, enjoyable, and fulfilling as you age.

My wife and I used to have a good sex life, but lately it's just not working. I have no idea what the problem is, or even how to bring it up in conversation. Any thoughts on how to start?

Communicating about sex can be difficult for couples of any age, but the changes that occur with aging (needing more time and genital stimulation, having less desire, problems with body image, medical conditions, or pain or discomfort during sex) may cause you to shy away from making love. If you and your wife aren't familiar with the normal changes that come with aging, your encounters may leave you feeling disappointed, frustrated, or thinking that your partner no longer finds you attractive. Frank, open, and loving discussions about these problems, and learning how the sexual response changes with age, are the first steps to developing creative solutions that work for both of you. Other conditions like depression or medical concerns could also be interfering.

Many of the "forms of expression" you mention are things I've never done and am uncomfortable even thinking about. Why should I consider them?

What we are discussing is *opening yourself up to new ways of achieving sexual arousal and release.* When I was growing up, speaking about sexual fantasies and masturbation was taboo, sex was defined as vaginal penetration by a man's penis in the missionary position, and vibrators were only sold in pornography shops. These are no longer commonly held beliefs, and many previously taboo practices can help older adults have more satisfying and pleasurable sex. About 50 percent of older men and 25 percent of older women masturbate, whether or not they have a partner. Both hands and vibrators are used for self-pleasuring (see the book *Sex for One* in the Resources section at the end of this chapter for suggestions). Vibrators can be particularly helpful because genital stimulation needs to be stronger and more time is needed to achieve

arousal and climax with aging. Fantasies, stories, and movies help some people increase desire and arousal.

What else can be done to enhance my sexual experiences? I'm especially concerned about the lack of spontaneity.

In a few words, *plan for sex and increase foreplay.* We'd all love sex to be like in the movies, spontaneous and easy, but we also want it to have a high likelihood of providing the pleasure we're seeking. Lack of "success" can lead to upset, anxiety, questions about ourselves and our partners, and a reticence to try again. Physical discomfort and pain as well as erections and orgasms that aren't as reliable as when we were younger are often part of aging. By denying this and going on with "business as usual," you'll be sabotaging your chances of having enjoyable sex as part of your life.

The term *foreplay* sounds like something you do while waiting to get to the main event. Yet as many of us, particularly women, know, it's anything but. *Touch can often lead to desire.* Younger men may only need to think about having sex or picture a certain person or scene to achieve a full erection, but this is rarely the case as you get older. Older men *and* women need longer and stronger physical stimulation to the penis and clitoris to get aroused and have erections and orgasms.

I have pain in my genital area during sex. Is there anything I can do to decrease this discomfort?

In women, pain during sex, particularly during penetration, is most often due to vaginal dryness. This may be due to lack of arousal, menopause, medications, or certain medical conditions. For some women, use of over-the-counter lubricants or longer periods of foreplay may help. Vaginal atrophy occurs with the decline in estrogen after menopause, causing dryness that can result in pain, irritation, friction, and even bleeding during sex. Estrogen applied locally to the vagina as a cream, tablet, or internal ring can improve vaginal atrophy, dryness, and itching without the estrogen being absorbed into the body and causing harmful side effects. Using different positions, pillows, lubrication, or sexual aids may also help improve comfort during sex. Pain that doesn't respond to lubrication or vaginal estrogen should be discussed with a gynecologist.

In men, pain or discomfort during sex should be discussed with a urologist or primary care provider, as this could be due to an infection of the prostate, urethra, or testes, or by sexually transmitted diseases like chlamydia and genital herpes. It may also be due to an allergic reaction to spermicide or condoms.

My partner has conditions that cause body discomfort, pain, and occasionally embarrassment during intercourse. As a result, we've essentially stopped having sex. Do you have any suggestions for what might be able to help?

Necessity if the mother of invention, they say. Discomfort can motivate us to consider new ways of being intimate. Using alternative positions, including standing or lying side to side and making creative use of pillows or cushions may help if there's back, hip, or knee pain. If

one of you has occasional urinary incontinence, you'll want to avoid positions that put pressure on the lower abdomen. Hand or jaw arthritis may worsen with manual stimulation or oral sex. Vibrators and other sex aids can often help. When you're going to have sex, make sure the vaginal lubricant, special pillows or cushions, and other sexual aids are nearby or easily available.

Expanding your view of sex beyond penetration and orgasm can also be beneficial. Many older couples work around these changes to a find new satisfying ways to make love. There may be more of an emphasis on extended foreplay and less of a focus on intercourse and orgasm. Intimate touch in a comfortable setting and position can bring lots of pleasure.

Are there things I can do about my health that will improve my sex life?

Absolutely. Remember, *heart health is sexual health* (as well as brain health). Smoking, increased cholesterol, high blood pressure, and diabetes can compromise sensation and decrease blood flow to the genitals, impeding arousal and orgasm. These may improve if you stop smoking and control your blood pressure, weight, sugar, and cholesterol. Watch your drinking, as too much alcohol can interfere with having erections and orgasms. Some studies suggest that exercise can help improve erectile function, probably by improving blood flow to the penis.

I'm meeting and "seeing" several new love interests. The last time I dated, the only thing I had to worry about was unwanted pregnancy. That's no longer a problem, but at my age am I still at risk for other sexually transmitted diseases?

Unfortunately, age doesn't protect you from sexually transmitted diseases (STDs), but being smart and taking precautions does. STDs like syphilis, gonorrhea, chlamydia, genital herpes, hepatitis B, genital warts, and trichomoniasis are increasing in older adults. Adults over the age of 50 make up half of the total population of people with HIV infection. Why? Simply put, people are having more sex with new and different partners, increasing their exposure to STDs. Drugs that treat erectile dysfunction, more people divorcing in midlife, and the rise of the Internet increase the ability to find a partner and have sex.

When you were younger, condoms were mainly used to prevent pregnancy. Nowadays, they are critical to preventing transmission of STDs. It doesn't matter how old you are—talk openly and honestly with your partner about sexually transmitted diseases. Always use a condom if you're a male having sex with a new or different partner.

I haven't dated in 45 years, and it's a whole new world out there. How do I start?

There are plenty of places to meet new people. Some ideas: a church or synagogue group, a local book club, a fitness or wellness program in your community, a senior center, or a senior travel program. Meeting someone while doing something you enjoy essentially guarantees that the two of you will have at least one thing in common. That's a good place to start.

You are never too old to fall in love. Think about what you are looking for. Is it companionship, casual sex, possibly marriage? It is important at the outset to think through your relationship goals, and to be open in your communication about them.

I've heard good and bad stories about online dating. Should I try it?

Several of my patients have found wonderful partners through Internet dating. Online dating apps or websites are an easy way to meet new people, but you must be cautious. You want to be sure the people you meet are like you, interested in a relationship, and not trying to scam you. It's a good idea to use an established website or app that is tailored to older adults (like eharmony, match.com, Our Time, or Silver Singles). Be honest and realistic about your expectations, and trust your instincts when talking or texting with potential partners.

Make sure you take precautions. Try to verify what someone tells you about themselves by doing an online search to be sure the details are accurate and match up. Your first meetings should be in a safe and neutral place like a coffee shop, not your home. You should also tell a friend or family member where and when the meeting will happen. Never send intimate photos or give out personal financial details to anyone you have just met or have only met on the Internet.

Unfortunately, online love scams are common. In 2019, the Federal Trade Commission (FTC) reported that more money was lost online in romance scams than any other type of fraud.

One sign that you are being scammed is that the person you are communicating with will quickly want to leave the dating website and communicate via email or instant messaging. There may be constant planning for in-person meetings, but somehow they never happen. Eventually, you may receive a sudden request for money to enable them to visit you or in response to an emergency, like a medical problem. If you suspect you're being scammed, stop communicating with the person immediately, and talk to someone you trust about what has been happening. You can also report it to the FTC at ftc.gov /complaint to be sure others aren't also victimized.

What Isn't Normal Aging?

 Red Flags: Symptoms Needing Prompt Medical Attention

For women:
- Pain during intercourse that doesn't respond to lubrication.
- Postmenopausal vaginal bleeding.

For men:
- Pain during intercourse.
- Painful or persistent erection that lasts more than four hours.

For women and men:
- Hypersexuality. This may be due to primary or secondary mania (see chapter 8), disinhibition in people living with dementia, or the use of dopamine-increasing medications like those used to treat Parkinson's disease.

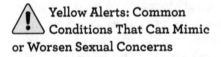 **Yellow Alerts: Common Conditions That Can Mimic or Worsen Sexual Concerns**

Medications

Many medications can inhibit your libido or interfere with sexual function. For a list, see table 16.1.

Depression, Antidepressants, and Sex

Depression can cause sexual dysfunction, and so can many antidepressants. All parts of the sexual response cycle can be affected by antidepressant medication: desire, arousal, orgasm, satisfaction. Sometimes the sexual dysfunction improves with time or a lower dose; however, for some, the medication continues to interfere with satisfactory sexual activity. The drugs most likely to cause a problem are selective serotonin reuptake inhibitors (SSRIs), serotonin-norepinephrine reuptake inhibitors (SNRIs), and tricyclic antidepressants (TCAs) because they increase serotonin levels. Increasing the level of serotonin improves depression and anxiety, but it also can result in decreased libido and orgasm in women and men, decreased lubrication in women, and ED in men. The lowest rate of sexual side effects occurs with bupropion (Wellbutrin), mirtazapine (Remeron), vilazodone (Viibryd), and vortioxetine (Trintellix).

TABLE 16.1
Medications That Can Cause Sexual Impairment

Drug Classes and Examples	Loss of Libido	Erectile Dysfunction	Anorgasmia
Blood pressure, cardiac, and diuretic medications			
Diuretics: chlorthalidone; metolazone (Zaroxolyn); triamterene-hydrochlorothiazide (Dyazide); furosemide (Lasix)		X	
Beta-blockers: carvedilol (Coreg); metoprolol (Lopressor); propranolol (Inderal)	X	X*	
Statins: pravastatin (Pravachol); simvastatin (Zocor); atorvastatin (Lipitor)		?	
Pain relief			
GABA-ergic neurogenic pain medications: gabapentin (Neurontin); pregabalin (Lyrica)	X	X	X
Neurological, psychological, and sleep medications			
Antianxiety: diazepam (Valium); alprazolam (Xanax); lorazepam (Ativan); clonazepam (Klonopin)	?	?	?
Antidepressants			
Tricyclic antidepressants: amitriptyline (Elavil); imipramine (Tofranil); desipramine (Norpramin)	X	?	X
SSRIs: citalopram (Celexa); paroxetine (Paxil); sertraline (Zoloft)	X	X	X
SNRIs: venlafaxine (Effexor); duloxetine (Cymbalta)	?		X
Antipsychotics: haloperidol (Haldol); thioridazine (Mellaril); olanzapine (Zyprexa); quetiapine (Seroquel)	X	X	X
Anticonvulsants: phenytoin (Dilantin); primidone (Mysoline); carbamazepine (Tegretol); topiramate (Topamax)	X	X	
Valproic acid (Depakote)	X		X

(continued)

TABLE 16.1 *(continued)*

Drug Classes and Examples	Loss of Libido	Erectile Dysfunction	Anorgasmia
Urinary medications			
BPH alpha-blockers: doxazosin (Cardura); terazosin (Hytrin); alfuzosin (Uroxatral); tamsulosin (Flomax)	?	?	
Prostate shrinkers: finasteride (Proscar); dutasteride (Avodart)	X	X	

Note: X, may cause this condition; ?, studies conflict as to whether these drugs cause this symptom. Abbreviations are as follows: BPH, benign prostatic hyperplasia; GABA, gamma amino butyric acid; SNRI, serotonin-norepinephrine reuptake inhibitor; SSRI, selective serotonin reuptake inhibitor.

*Nebivolol (Bystolic) does not cause erectile dysfunction.

Relationship Issues and Overall Outlook on Life

Your relationships and perspective on life can interfere with all parts of the sexual response cycle. If you're depressed or anxious, or if your relationship is strained, sex may be the last thing on your mind. Depression and anxiety are *not* normal aging, and you may benefit from some help (see chapter 8). If you're having relationship troubles, consider individual or couples counseling. It is unusual for relationships to improve without some outside help, whether it be with a therapist, clergyperson, or another person or group where you can both be open and honest about what's going on. Communication with your partner is key. Talk honestly about both physical and emotional issues that may be interfering with your relationship and sex life. Consider a referral to a professional who specializes in treatment of sexual disorders.

Loss of Interest in or Desire for Sex

As discussed above, there are many reasons for loss of interest in sex among older adults, including medications, medical conditions, degree of life-long interest in sex, and psychological and relationship concerns. Depending on the circumstances, psychotherapy or cognitive behavioral therapy may helpful.

Widower's or widow's syndrome occurs when the person involved in a new relationship has difficulty with sex because they feel as if they are being unfaithful to their deceased spouse. This is something that may improve with the passage of time, or through discussions with your partner or a therapist.

Inability to Orgasm

Anorgasmia, or the inability to achieve orgasm, can affect both men and women. As discussed above, desire and relationship concerns often play a role, as do medications (see table 16.1), medical conditions, and pain. If you are able to have an orgasm when alone, through manual self-stimulation or by using a vibrator, or if you are a man and you have morning erections, your inability to have an orgasm during sex is most likely not due to a medical condition or a medication. Individual counseling to help with stress or depression, couples counseling, or referral to a mental health professional specializing in treatment of sexual disorders may provide insight and interventions that may help.

Erectile Dysfunction

Erectile dysfunction, or ED, is the inability to get and keep an erection firm enough for sex. It's important to recognize that even with ED, a man may still have desire and be able to orgasm and to ejaculate.

Having an erection depends on your brain and emotions as well as hormones, blood vessels, nerves, and muscles, so, not surprisingly, there are many causes and possible treatments. Any condition that affects the blood vessels or nerves going to the penis—including diabetes, heart disease, hypertension, prostate surgery, neurological disorders like spinal cord disease, Parkinson's disease, or multiple sclerosis—can cause ED. Medications are often involved (see table 16.1), as are psychological concerns like depression, anxiety, stress, and relationship issues. Hormones like thyroid, testosterone, and the pituitary hormone prolactin may rarely play a role.

Treatment for ED begins with identifying and optimizing the underlying conditions. As discussed earlier in this book, better management of diabetes

and heart disease, including exercising, losing weight (if needed) and decreasing smoking and drinking may significantly improve the ability to have an erection.

Testosterone deficiency alone isn't a cause of ED. Men with lower levels of testosterone can attain erections in response to direct penile stimulation; however, in response to fantasy, their erection is smaller and develops more slowly. This condition can improve with testosterone replacement.

The most common first-line therapy for ED are *phosphodiesterase inhibitors* (medications like sildenafil [Viagra], tadalafil [Cialis], verdenefil [Levitra], and avanafil [Spedra]). These easy-to-use medications are effective in 45 to 90 percent of men and generally have minimal side effects. They are not as effective if the underlying problem is related to previous prostate surgery or uncontrolled diabetes. Men who don't respond to these drugs should be tested for testosterone deficiency. They may respond once testosterone is replaced.

Phosphodiesterase inhibitors work by enhancing the effects of nitric oxide, which increases blood flow to the penis. Be aware that the response is not automatic; sexual arousal and manual stroking are needed for an erection to occur. They should not be used if you are taking any medication that contains nitrates, which are commonly used for treatment of ischemic heart disease. Speak with your medical provider to see if these medications may help treat your ED.

If Viagra-like drugs don't work for you, consult with a urologist to discuss other options, including vacuum-assisted erection devices, self-injections, penile suppositories, pumps, implants, or surgery, depending on the cause of the problem. If there are psychological concerns, consider seeing a mental health or other professional specializing in treatment of sexual disorders for further evaluation and treatment.

Getting Evaluated for Sexual Concerns

Although most people experience some concerns about their sexual functioning as they age, it's unusual for them to discuss these with medical providers. In one study in the United States, only 38 percent of men and 22 percent of women reported that they had discussed sex with a physician after they turned 50. Many are uncomfortable discussing sex at all, let alone with their doctors. Yet for those who'd like a more satisfying sex life, we've discussed many physical, medical, and psychological conditions that, if attended to, could improve one's experiences.

Should I See a Specialist?

Primary care providers can initially evaluate and treat your concerns. They may then refer you to a urologist, gynecologist, endocrinologist, therapist, or psychiatrist. A urologist can evaluate the reasons a man may be having pain during sex and help determine the right treatments for ED. A gynecologist can determine reasons a woman may be having pain during sex; suggest pelvic physical therapy if there is a pelvic, abdominal, or low-back component to the pain; and prescribe vaginal estrogens to assist with lubrication. If low testosterone is a consideration, see an endocrinologist to make sure the diagnostic tests, replacement dose, and monitoring are right for you.

Preparing for Your Visit

Discussing your sexual concerns with your medical provider may be uncomfortable or embarrassing for you, and you may worry that your medical provider feels the same way. But your sexual life is an important part of your well-being, and believe me, you're not telling your provider anything they've never heard before. Filling out the chapter 16 pre-visit checklist on page 390 in Appendix 3 can be a good way to organize your thoughts before your appointment, and make it easier to find comfortable language for discussing your concerns. Bring it to the visit and review it with your provider.

Advice for Loved Ones

Whether your loved one is in a relationship or rediscovering dating, their desire and yours should be that they find companionship and happiness. Be open about your concerns and feelings, but also understand that love and intimacy are important parts of life, regardless of age. Although these discussions can be difficult, in the end they are worth having, as they will enrich your connection.

Bottom Line

Your interest in and ability to have sex may change with aging, but knowing what to expect and how to adapt can help a lot. If you have a partner, it's important that you be able to discuss your experiences and feelings together without discomfort. Sometimes this will require the help of a behavioral health or medical provider. If you enjoyed sex when you were younger, you're likely to want to have sexual relationships as you age; if not, there are other forms of intimacy that may work for you. Above all, allow yourself the freedom to try new things. You may find it's well worth it.

RESOURCES

Dodson, B. *Sex for One: The Joy of Selfloving.* New York: Harmony, 1996.

Perel, E. *Mating in Captivity: Unlocking Erotic Intelligence.* New York: Harper, 2017.

SAGE
(https://www.sageusa.org)
This organization provides advocacy and services for LGBT elders.

BIBLIOGRAPHY

Imprialos, K. P., K. Stavropoulos, M. Doumas, et al. "Sexual Dysfunction, Cardiovascular Risk and Effects of Pharmacotherapy." *Current Vascular Pharmacology* 16, no. 2 (2018): 130–42.

La Torre, A. G., A. Conca, D. Duffy, et al. "Sexual Dysfunction Related to Psychotropic Drugs: A Critical Review. Part II, Antipsychotics." *Pharmacopsychiatry* 46 (2013): 201–8.

La Torre, A. G., G. Giupponi, D. Duffy, et al. "Sexual Dysfunction Related to Psychotropic Drugs: A Critical Review. Part I, Antidepressants." *Pharmacopsychiatry* 46 (2013): 191–99.

La Torre, A., G. Giupponi, D. Duffy, et al. "Sexual Dysfunction Related to Psychotropic Drugs: A Critical Review. Part III, Mood Stabilizers and Anxiolytic Drugs." *Pharmacopsychiatry* 47 (2014): 1–6.

La Torre, A. G., G. Giupponi, D. Duffy, et al. "Sexual Dysfunction Related to Drugs: A Critical Review. Part V, α-Blocker and 5-ARI Drugs." *Pharmacopsychiatry* 49 (2016): 3–13.

Lindau, S. T., L. P. Schumm, E. O. Laumann, et al. "A Study of Sexuality and Health among Older Adults in the United States." *New England Journal of Medicine* 357, no. 8 (2007): 762–74.

Yang, Y., and X. Wang. "Sexual Dysfunction Related to Antiepileptic Drugs in Patients with Epilepsy." *Expert Opinion on Drug Safety* 15, no. 1 (2016): 31–42.

Difficult Decisions

Difficult Decisions

CHAPTER 17

Making Difficult Decisions

We spend our lives making decisions. Some decisions can be relatively easy, like where to eat, who to be friends with, or how to spend our time, while others are more complex. The three decisions we'll be discussing in Part III are those my patients tell me are the *most difficult* decisions they are faced with.

Chapter 18. *Everyone's telling me to move out of the house I've lived in for 30 years . . . to be near my children, to go to an independent or assisted living facility, to downsize, to live in a "better" neighborhood. I'm reluctant to leave what I know. What should I do?*

Chapter 19. *I don't want to stop driving . . . my daughter thinks I should, but my wife and I disagree.*

Chapter 20. *Who will decide what happens to me if I get sick and can't speak for myself, and will they do what I would want?*

These dilemmas are not just faced by older adults, but also by their spouses, families, and friends. People differ greatly in how they deal with these types of issues. Their decisions are often based on their understanding of the issues, cultural and religious beliefs, family dynamics, social and physical support structures, and personal beliefs and values.

This chapter will help you develop a framework for how to think about these dilemmas, make decisions, and discuss them with others. The Advice for Loved Ones applies to all Part III chapters, since these tips are applicable regardless of the decision you are making.

These types of decisions overwhelm me. I don't know where to begin. I figure I'll make them if I need to. Maybe I'll never have to deal with them.

The following six pieces of advice will help you confront the uncertainty of making difficult decisions.

Don't Be an Ostrich

These dilemmas are part of aging for many older adults, even if we'd rather not think about them. Remember the ostrich, the worry wort, and the wise old owl we talked about in chapter 1? Be a wise old owl and follow the Boy Scout motto: Be Prepared.

Think about These Concerns Early and Often

I'm not saying that you should dwell on them, but don't wait for an emergency to occur before you start considering what you would do in these circumstances. Beginning a conversation opens the door to further discussion. Talking with friends, family, and your medical provider in a calm, no-pressure environment gives you time to iron out the details and make a plan that can work for all involved. Most of the time there's no absolutely right answer, and the situation you're in may change, so these discussions and decisions may have to be reconsidered.

Involve Family and Friends

As independent as you are, and want to remain, the truth is that your decisions will affect others besides yourself. It helps to let these others know what your concerns are and to have them participate in the fact-finding and problem-solving we discuss in these chapters. Making some of these decisions can be emotional, and identifying differences in opinions early on allows time to try to work things out before an emergency requires an immediate decision to be made, often by someone other than you.

Exercise Patience and Practice Your Listening Skills

This may be harder than it seems. Be honest about your feelings and thoughts, and allow others to do the same. People often have strong opinions about what should be done in these situations. Allowing everyone to speak lets everyone feel heard, even if in the end some don't agree with the decision. Some concerns may be premature and never materialize, while others may become more pertinent with time.

Reach Out for Help

Don't try to make these decisions without taking advantage of the resources that can help support you. These include community organizations and professionals who can help provide context and advice (see the Resources section at the end of each chapter). Making decisions is a process, and it may involve some homework, such as visiting assisted living centers, sitting down with a social worker to discuss local services that may be helpful to you, or even having your driving skills reevaluated.

Once Again, Never Say Never

We may refuse to try new things that may improve our lives out of fear or misconceptions. Hearing aids, assisted living, and joining a senior center are just some of these. Check your beliefs against reality, and consider giving things that may benefit you a trial.

There are so many things to consider in making these decisions—what I want, what others want, the pros, the cons— where do I start?

For any decision as personal as these, the first question is not "What do I want?" but "What really matters to me?" The answers to these two questions are often not the same. *What matters* should be the first thing you explore, because it will allow you to evaluate your options in a different light. What matters may differ depending on what decision you're making, but generally there are some core things that are most meaningful to you.

What matters to you? What makes life meaningful? As discussed in more detail in chapter 4, the patient-centered practices (see the Resources section at the end of chapter 4) can help you conceptualize your core values by completing the following:

I want to be able to _____ (live, drive, get health care, whatever decision you need to make) so that I can:

- Connect and relate to others—family, friends, significant others, religious or spiritual community
- Enjoy life—play tennis or bridge, travel, do work that is meaningful to me, learn or create new things
- Function independently—take care of myself, maintain my dignity, not be a burden to others
- Manage my health to meet my goals, whether this be living as long as possible or living for less time but enjoying a better quality of life.

Be specific and dig deep, unpeel the onion, and try to understand why these things are so important to you and how you might still get what you need even if you can't keep doing what you used to.

Let's say that being able to play tennis is what really matters to you.

Why? Is it the exhilaration that you feel when you play, is it spending time outdoors or with your tennis buddies, the thrill of competition, that you take pride in being able to say you're a tennis player, or something else? Keep digging.

Does not being able to play tennis as you did make you feel "old"? What does that mean to you? That you aren't as strong or vigorous as you once were? That you have to give up things that you love? That life is not limitless? That this is the beginning of the end, you will continue to lose your abilities? Don't make these changes into more than they are. Sometimes a cigar is just a cigar.

It's possible that even though you can't play as you did, you can get what you're looking for in another way. I have patients who have used their desire to get back on the court as motivation to exercise and participate more in physical therapy, others who have become avid spectators of televised and in-person tournaments, some who just love hitting the ball on the court, and others who have switched to something that's easier for them to do, but just as much fun, like pickleball. The point is that once you identify what really mattered to you about an activity, you can start to look for something else that gives you a similar feeling. Try to look at the glass as half full rather than half empty.

Advice for Loved Ones

Loved ones often question whether an older adult has the mental ability to make a particular decision, particularly if the decision is something they may not agree with—like opting not to pursue chemotherapy for a newly diagnosed cancer. What they're asking is whether the person has *capacity*, which can be determined by a physician. Older people are adults, and adults are assumed to have the capacity to make decisions for themselves. Capacity can be affected by certain diseases and disorders, however. Also, one can have capacity to make some decisions, like whether to go to a wedding, but not others, like having surgery or living alone. Someone has capacity to make a specific decision if they're able to describe all their options, the option they chose and why, and its consequences (risks and benefits), and then provide rational reasons for their decision. Their reasoning has to be clear and consistent. You may not agree with their choice, but you have to decide if this is a battle you want to fight. Remember, most of these decisions can be revisited, particularly as circumstances change.

Capacity is often confused with *competency*, a legal term that refers to someone's ability to make a specific decision and then to carry out the actions needed to make that decision happen, like managing their finances, caring for themselves, signing a contract. Only a judge can determine competency. People who are judged to be incompetent must have a guardian or a conservator appointed. Laws for appointing a conservatorship differ by state.

Discussions about health care decisions can be challenging. Give your loved one the space to be the expert in what matters most to them. See if they might be comfortable having you present when they utilize the Patient Priorities Care website described in chapter 4. This can be an ideal time to understand their thinking and reasoning about their health care and health goals, even if you disagree with them. These times offer opportunities for deeper conversation, helping you connect even more. You may be surprised by what you discover. What you learn will help you if you ever need to make decisions for them when they can't (see chapters 4 and 20).

RESOURCES

Patient Priorities Care
(https://myhealthpriorities.org/)
This website helps patients, caregivers, and families navigate health care decisions.

CHAPTER 18

To Move or Not to Move

One of the most difficult decisions for my patients and those who care about them is whether to "age in place," that is, to keep living in the same home where they've lived for many years. For most, a home is much more than its rooms and furniture. It's filled with memories of good times and bad, of celebrations and other important occasions, and of people we have known and loved, some of whom may no longer be in our lives. To many, staying in one's home means staying within a community filled with familiar people and places, where you make your own decisions about what you're going to do, when, and with whom. Moving late in life can be an exciting adventure, but too often it happens due to necessity, not desire. This is another one of those times where it really makes sense to think through your options ahead of time.

In this chapter we'll discuss reasons to consider moving; what you might need to age in place, including in-home help; and different living options, should you decide a move is what's right for you.

I've been living in my home for 50 years, 20 of them by myself. Why would I even think of moving?

There are some major issues that raise questions about our ability to age in place, especially with regard to safety,

doing everyday activities, having local support, and the possibility of becoming socially isolated.

Home Safety

The home that worked for you when you were 60 may not work when you're 80. Going up and down flights of stairs and traversing narrow passageways can be hard, especially if your mobility is limited. Bathrooms and showers can be especially difficult to negotiate. If you injure yourself while living alone, it could be days before someone finds you. If your memory is slipping, you could accidentally leave the oven on or the door to your home open.

Everyday Needs

Even if your home is perfectly designed for aging, you need to have food to eat; be able to pay bills, manage medications and finances, connect with the outside world by using the phone (or computer); and access transportation. At some point you might need help with getting to the bathroom, bathing or showering, dressing, or walking safely.

Local Support

Local support doesn't always mean having a family member close by, but there needs to be someone who is willing and able to be there if you need help. Sometimes you may not be able to make a call, like when illness presents subtly as confusion or falls, or if an accident happens. You need a plan for these occasions. Not having one can result in serious illness or injury.

Social Isolation

Sometimes your home may be fine for aging in place, but the day-to-day experience of living there may be quite different than it was in years past. The neighborhood may have changed, with neighbors, friends, and community connections no longer there. Public transportation may be limited. If it exists, it may be hard to access, requiring the use of stairs or a working elevator. Even if none of these are the case, when you're living alone, you may find it harder to get motivated to go out and take advantage of your neighborhood. This can lead to isolation, depression, and feeling like there's no reason to get up in the morning. Having others nearby can help you avoid becoming isolated.

Adapting to Your New Normal

I really want to stay where I am and age in place. Do you have any tips for what I can do now to make this more likely to happen?

The question you're asking is whether there are realistic changes that you could make to alleviate the concerns noted above. Some can be easily addressed, others not so much. This section covers ways you can prepare for aging in place.

Home Safety

Perhaps the most important thing you can do when planning to age in place is to retrofit your home to prevent falls and injury (see chapter 9). Below is a list of home safety modifications you might want to consider (see also the Resources section at the end of this chapter).

- Improve lighting and your vision (chapter 12).

- Remove throw rugs and clutter from the floor and stairs, make sure there are no power cords in places that you might trip over. Also, ensure that hand railings are secure.

- Install grab bars in the shower and around the toilet seat. Consider installing a raised toilet seat.

- Use nonslip bathmats with rubber backings in the bathroom. Use nonskid rubber mats or strips in the tub.

- Consider changing round doorknobs or sink dials to single-lever handles.

- Reorganize the kitchen and closet by moving objects from high shelves and bringing them to a more reachable location.

- Be sure smoke and carbon monoxide detectors have working batteries.

- Set the bathroom water thermostat at less than 120°F.

More expensive home modifications include the following.

- Home stair lift for ascending and descending stairs
- Bathroom that meets ADA (Americans for Disability Act) guidelines
- Walk-in tub or shower
- Ramps at entryways
- In a multi-floor dwelling, moving all activities (cooking, eating, sleeping, bathing and toileting, living area) to the first floor

Everyday Needs

- Use pill organizers or blister packs to help manage medications (chapter 3).
- Set up an automatic bill-paying service through your bank or another online system.
- See what transportation options are available in your area (chapter 19).
- If you have difficulty using your hands or dressing, work with an occupational therapist who can identify specific tools that may help you do the things you're having difficulty with.
- Utilize adaptive devices like grabbers or telescoping reachers to help reach high or low objects.
- Purchase a nonskid shower chair and a hand-held shower head to make bathing easier.
- Identify your local Meals on Wheels program for access to nutritious and hot meals (see the Resources

section at the end of chapter 15). There are also mobile apps you can use to shop for food and ready-to-eat meals that will then deliver your items to your home. Most big supermarkets offer this service.

Local Support

- Work out a system so that a friend, family member, or local community agency calls you daily to check in. You could make this a buddy system with a friend. Give them a key, or make sure they know whom to contact to enter the home if you don't answer the phone.
- Get a personal emergency response system (see Appendix 1).

Social Isolation

- Check out local senior centers and community resources for activities and clubs. Many provide transportation.
- Friendly visitor programs are available in some areas through senior centers, community programs, or religious organizations.
- Learn to use the Internet. Community agencies and senior centers often have free classes on how to use the computer and access the Web. Once you've learned this technology, you can use video to connect with loved ones, take classes online, and participate in book groups, current event discussions, or other activities offered by community agencies.

I need help with some of my daily activities, but I'm not sure I want a stranger in my home. What are my options?

As we discuss above, many of the tasks that older adults need help with can now be done "virtually," like getting nutritious, ready-to-eat food delivered or bills paid. Many people rely on family and friends for informal practical support, like helping with shopping and household chores.

If you need a person to assist you, look into a paid caregiver. There are several types of paid caregivers, including the following.

Companions who can assist with housework, shopping, meal preparation, and transportation to medical appointments. This option is suitable for people who are otherwise independent in personal care but don't have the endurance to do household chores.

Home attendants and personal care aides assist with household chores and meal preparation as well as with basic personal care needs such as bathing, dressing, and grooming. People with some mobility issues but who are able to follow directions and assist the caregiver in managing some aspects of their own care may benefit from this type of caregiver.

Home health aides are trained to assist those with significant cognitive and/or functional issues. They are skilled at helping people move from a bed to a chair and assisting in the personal care of those who may be wheelchair-dependent or bed-bound. Under the supervision of a registered nurse, they can give oxygen, perform basic range-of-motion exercises, and help with other tasks, depending on your state's regulations.

How much will a paid caregiver cost me?

When a paid caregiver is hired through an agency, the hourly charge is often more than if you are hiring privately, but there are advantages, such as supervision and back-up (see box 18.1). Costs also vary by geographic area. Average hourly rates can vary from $25 to $35. Medicare does not cover long-term home health aide services.

Long-term care (LTC) insurance policies can be activated when a person needs the assistance of someone else for at least two activities of daily living (personal hygiene and grooming, dressing and undressing, movement and mobility, toileting, preparing food and feeding) or if diagnosed with dementia.

For seniors with lower incomes who do not have LTC insurance, Medicaid-funded home health services can be an option. Elder law attorneys may be of assistance in qualifying a low- or middle-income senior for Medicaid-funded home care benefits. For information about Medicaid financial criteria and how to access Medicaid benefits, call your state's Department of Aging or aging ombudsman (see the Eldercare Locator in the Resources section at the end of this chapter).

Medicaid and the US Department of Veterans Affairs have programs that allow family members or friends to be paid as a caregiver for a loved one (see the Resources section at the end of this chapter).

BOX 18.1

How to Find a Paid Caregiver

Take some time to think about your care needs before you begin looking for a caregiver. Are you looking for a *companion, home attendant or personal care aide*, or a *home health aide* (see page 338)? Generally, aides will not commit to a job unless they are hired for a minimum of four hours a day, two to three days a week.

Ask the right questions.
Jot down questions you need to ask a prospective caregiver. You might want to ask about how they interacted with previous clients, and what duties they are accustomed to carrying out. Be sure to clarify any additional tasks you would require them to do, such as cooking, grocery shopping, and transporting you to medical appointments or to the store. Also ask how they handle emergency situations (for example, are they certified in CPR?). If you need the caregiver for a partner or family member with a physical disability or dementia, ask about the caregiver's experience with these issues and how they navigate caring for somebody who might not be fully cooperative.

Personal recommendations are preferable.
If you prefer to hire a caregiver privately, try to get a personal recommendation if at all possible, since this does provide some assurance that the caregiver is reliable and trustworthy. But even if you do manage to find a suitable caregiver based on word of mouth, you should take some security precautions. Ask to see photo identification (driver's license, passport) for anybody you interview. Also ask for references (ideally three, two of which should be former employers), and contact them. A background check is also advisable, as it can tell you if a potential caregiver has been convicted of elder abuse or other crimes in a different state. You can use an online "people search" to confirm that the information a prospective caregiver has provided to you is correct. The cost ranges from about $10 upward, but keep in mind that all records may not be available depending on individual state penal codes. Be sure to get your prospective caregiver to sign a background check disclosure or authorization form (find one at http://bit.ly/1Fa9FrA)—if they are unwilling to do so, they may not be a suitable candidate.

Using an agency.
When a paid caregiver is hired through an agency, the hourly charge is often more expensive than if you are hiring privately. There are advantages that come with the additional expense. Home health aides who are hired through an agency must have training—this typically involves a 75-hour course offered by the agency itself or by a paraprofessional training school. Agencies also offer a level of supervision that you won't get with a private hire: a registered nurse will screen you and develop a care plan that the caregiver must follow. If an agency caregiver calls in sick, the agency must supply a substitute caregiver. If you are going through an

(continued)

BOX 18.1 (*continued*)

agency, verify that it carries out criminal background checks and drug screening on its employees—some research suggests that nearly half of caregiver agencies fail to perform these vital security precautions. Also check whether the agency regularly evaluates the quality of care provided by its employees, and how that supervision is carried out (for example, will a supervisor visit you at home to ask you about the care you're receiving?).

I really don't want to pay someone for time that they're not helping me. My friends tell me about aides who watch TV, read, and talk or play games on the phone when they're supposed to be working. What can I do to prevent this?

Most aides work a minimum number of hours a day, at least two to three days a week. Remember, it needs to be worth it to them to come to your home. They also need time for breaks and meals. What they are allowed to do depends on the person's care needs, whether the caregiver is working privately or hired through an agency or by Medicaid, and state regulations.

Aides hired privately work directly through the patient and family. They are not restricted in their job description and can also give medications. When they are hired, you can decide with them how they will spend their time. Privately hired aides can work for a few hours at home and then accompany you on a walk, shopping, to a movie or museum, or they can help with projects like organizing papers or photographs. Aides hired through an agency typically work from a structured care plan that is developed by a nurse from the agency who has been in contact with the person and/or

their family. Medicaid-funded aides work from a "task-oriented care plan," where each task is assigned a time frame for completion. These care plans include assistance with personal care, light housework, meal preparation, and possibly some outside activities. Discuss what you'd like your aides to be doing with the nurses who develop these care plans.

If you're not sure how much help you need, you can hire aides for fewer hours and increase them as needed or as you get more comfortable with having someone in your home.

My family doesn't think it's safe for me to live alone; they also think my home is too big for me to keep up with the cleaning and repairs. They'd like me to either move in with them, enter a senior housing community, or just move to a smaller place, preferably with a doorman. I want to stay where I am. The only thing we agree on is that we're getting more and more upset with each other. What can we do?

The concerns mentioned above and others can force the question of whether you need help in your home or even if you should move out of your current home. If you and your loved ones have different opinions, it's important to understand everyone's concerns. If you're really against the idea, unpeel the onion to determine what really matters to you. Can you still have the life you want where you currently live, or might there be a silver lining if you were to move? These are tough decisions, and it will take time to identify the issues and discover what options exist.

The worksheet in table 18.1 will help clarify your thinking and options. Remember, we never know what the future will bring. These are some of the major activities that you will need to do, or have done for you, if you want to age in place. Fill out what your options are for each of these activities. Be as specific as possible, and remember that cost needs to be considered.

If I need to move, what are my options?

Your options depend on where you currently live, your finances, if you qualify for senior housing or nursing home residence, and whether you can afford housing in a different neighborhood or an independent or assisted living community. If you're considering moving to be near your children, have an open and honest discussion about how each of you envisions what living nearby or together would look like. Would you be able to have your own place or room? Do you have similar expectations in terms of housekeeping, babysitting, and financial contributions? Discuss these issues (and any others you think apply) to help you make your decision.

What is senior housing, and should I consider it?

For the most part, only older adults live in senior housing communities. Options vary depending on functional needs and financial abilities. Generally, senior housing is offered by private organizations and can be a significant financial investment. For lower-income people, there are independent senior housing options offered through federally funded programs (known as Section 202) and nonprofit organizations. Costs vary according to geographic area and amenities that are offered. There are organizations and professionals that can assist in selection of senior housing, the majority of whom are paid by the senior housing management when the senior commits to moving into their housing.

Options for senior housing include the following.

Independent living. These are regular apartments in a building with social services, home care, and other supports. Some independent living communities serve meals in a communal dining room. If you like, you can participate in organized activities and trips. If help with personal care is needed, you can hire an aide from an on-site agency. Some independent living buildings allow their residents to use outside home care providers. Many seniors move into independent living buildings to be closer to their children or because their current home is inaccessible. Independent living is for people who are independent but want meals and housekeeping services provided.

TABLE 18.1

Aging in Place

We never know what the future will bring. These are some of the major activities that you will need to do, or have done for you, if you want to age in place. Fill out what your options are for each of these activities. Be as specific as possible, and remember that cost needs to be considered.

Activity	Who Does This Now?	If You/They Couldn't, How Could You Get This Done?	Who Would Do/Arrange/Pay for This?
Housework			
Laundry			
Food shopping			
Cooking			
Local transportation			
Medication management			
Bills and finances			
Home repairs			

TABLE 18.1 *(continued)*

Activity	Who Does This Now?	If You/They Couldn't, How Could You Get This Done?	Who Would Do/Arrange/Pay for This?
Computer use			
Stair climbing			
Walking			
Bathing			
Dressing			
Grooming			
Toileting			
Getting out of bed/chair			
Eating			

Assisted living. To qualify for assisted living, you must need some help with personal care. In addition to the amenities listed under independent living, varying amounts of help tailored to your individual needs are available. Care is provided by a staff of home health aides who move in and out of the apartments and help with dressing, bathing, and toileting. Most assisted living programs are financed privately.

Nursing home care. These facilities offer care for the totally dependent person who has skilled nursing needs and who can no longer have their care needs met at home. Nursing homes are expensive, and Medicare only covers a limited period of skilled services after a hospitalization. If nursing home services are still required after this time, one may pay privately or use long-term care insurance, if they have it. Most nursing home residents eventually apply for Nursing Home Medicaid when their financial assets are depleted and they become eligible for Medicaid. This process is complicated, which is why planning is essential. Elder law attorneys specialize in this kind of planning. (See the Resources section at the end of this chapter.)

Continuing care facilities. These facilities provide all levels of care, from independent to assisted living to nursing home. There are usually separate buildings or areas on the same campus for each level of service. Continuing care facilities are financed privately and allow an individual to stay on within the same facility as their care needs progress.

Advice for Loved Ones

After two hospitalizations for confusion and heart failure, Mary's family wanted her to have a live-in aide. Even though Mary was no longer confused, her family members lived out of state and were afraid that she would end up back in the hospital with heart failure, confusion, or a fall. Mary disagreed—she wanted her privacy and didn't want someone telling her what to do. To her, the heart failure had been treated and she was no longer short of breath, so why couldn't she go back to living alone as she had for years?

The disagreement between Mary and her family is no surprise. Neither is her family asking me what they can do to get her to accept a live-in aide. The real question is whether she actually needs one. As an intermediate step, her care provider can order *Medicare short-term home care* for a few months. Medicare provides skilled services such as a visiting nurse to teach Mary how to manage her heart failure medications, diet, and fluid intake, and to regularly weigh herself and take her blood pressure. Depending on her care needs, she can also get a home physical or occupational therapist as well as home health aides for a maximum of 20 hours a week. If she improves and can take care of herself, she may not need a live-in aide. If she doesn't, she will have experience in how additional care may be able to help her.

It's unlikely that someone like Mary would accept additional help if she doesn't feel part of the process. "Nothing about me without me," as Valerie Billingham put it in a 1998 session entitled "Through the Patient's Eyes."

The older adult needs to be involved in identifying the aide's activities. If possible, have them participate in the interview process. This is routine when hiring privately, but it may require your advocacy in negotiating with the agency or Medicaid supervisor.

If you can't reach an agreement about an aide, it's important to identify what really matters to the older adult and what the family can live with. I have found that many times an older adult will say no to an aide, only to be open to one 6 to 12 months later. Timed trials of part time help may be a start.

And sometimes, like my patient Rose, help in the home is just not an option.

Rose was adamant that she be able to keep living live alone in her home despite having had multiple falls. Her children wanted her to move in with them or have someone live with her. She refused. She knew that she could fall, break a hip, or even die, and said she could live with these possibilities as long as she could live by herself in her own home. She had the capacity to make the decision (see chapter 17 for more on capacity versus competency).

In speaking with her children, it was clear that this was Rose being Rose, and it was unlikely she was going to change now. She never enjoyed spending more than a few days at their homes and valued her privacy. They worked to get comfortable with the idea that she might not be safe, but she would be content. They did some home modifications, engaged home physical therapy to try to decrease her risk of falling, purchased a personal emergency response system (see Appendix 1) so that if she fell she could get help, and accepted her choice. Eventually, Rose died from a fall. Her children did not regret their decision; they were actually at peace knowing that they had honored her wishes.

Remember, the relationship is the most important thing. Keep an eye on what's important and acceptable to the older person you love, not what will make you feel better but possibly make them miserable. Also, remember that these are dynamic, not static, situations—things change, as do people.

RESOURCES

Local Services

Eldercare Locator
(www.eldercare.acl.gov)
This service of the US Administration on Aging assists in finding older adult resources in any community in the United States.

National Association of Area Agencies on Aging
(n4a.org)
This website gives information on local resources for seniors.

National Council on Aging
(www.ncoa.org; 571-527-3900)
Provides information on resources, benefits, senior centers, and state Departments of Aging.

For information on access to food and meals, see the Resources section at the end of chapter 16.

Home Modification

National Resource Center on Supportive Housing and Home Modification of the University of Southern California
(www.homemods.org)
Provides an information clearinghouse on home modification to equip professionals and consumers with a comprehensive inventory of resources, such as a National Directory of Home Modification and Repair Resources.

Safety Checklists

Falls and Fire Prevention
(https://www.nfpa.org/-/media/Files /Public-Education/Resources /Education-programs/remembering -when/RWHomeSafetyChecklist.ashx)
The National Fire Protection Association offers a fire and fall prevention program for older adults.

Home Safety

The US Centers for Disease Control and Prevention offers checklists to help you ensure your home is safe as you age:

https://www.cdc.gov/steadi/pdf/check_for _safety_brochure-a.pdf

https://www.cdc.gov/steadi/pdf/STEADI -Brochure-CheckForSafety-508.pdf

Programs That Pay Family or Friends to Be Caregivers

Medicaid
(https://www.medicaidplanningassistance .org/getting-paid-as-caregiver/)
This information from the American Council on Aging describes how individuals may receive financial compensation in helping to care for a loved one on Medicaid.

US Department of Veterans Affairs
(https://www.va.gov)
Contact your local VA or regional benefits center for eligibility requirements and a referral.

Medicaid Eligibility

Elder Law Attorneys
(https://nelf.org/)
The National Elder Law Foundation provides this directory of certified elder law attorneys.

Rules for Spending Down to Become Eligible for Medicaid
(https://www.medicareinteractive.org /get-answers/cost-saving-programs-for -people-with-medicare/medicare-and -medicaid/spend-down-program-for -beneficiaries-with-incomes-over-the -medicaid-limit)
To qualify for Medicaid, one's income and assets must be below a certain amount. If you exceed that amount, you may still be able to qualify by spending down with monthly medical expenses. Medicaid financial requirements differ by state, and not all states have a spend-down program. Use the information in the link above to learn more about this option.

BIBLIOGRAPHY

Billingham, Valerie. "Through the Patient's Eyes." Session 356, presented at the Salzburg Global Seminar. Salzburg, Austria, 1998.

CHAPTER 19

Do I Need to Stop Driving?

For most older adults in the United States, driving is as much a part of life as breathing, and public transportation doesn't come close to providing the convenience of getting in a car and driving yourself wherever you want to go. Questions surrounding an older person's ability to drive can be a major area of conflict among older adults and their loved ones, and it's one I'm often asked to weigh in on. Just as thinking about your options in advance is important when considering whether to move, you need to consider your options for getting around if your ability to drive becomes impaired. Your vehicle, your driving patterns, and even you can be modified (by cataract removal, for example) to make you a safer driver.

This chapter discusses age-related changes in driving abilities, provides ways to remediate some of them, and helps you identify transportation options if you temporarily or permanently lose the ability to drive.

I've been driving since I was 16, and I have a stellar record. Why are people concerned about my ability to drive now that I'm 85? Is this just another form of ageism?

Actually, it isn't. Motor vehicle crash and fatality rates per mile driven begin to increase significantly at age 70. Drivers 85 and older have the highest rates of fatal accidents per mile driven. The rate for drivers 80–84 years old is similar to that for teenagers. In 2018, 58 percent of those killed in accidents involving drivers aged 70 and older were the older drivers themselves, 13 percent were their passengers, and 28 percent were occupants of other vehicles, motorcyclists, and pedestrians. Drivers 70 and older are three times more likely to die and 50 percent more likely to sustain a serious injury than drivers aged 35–54. This is likely because of their increased vulnerability, especially to head and chest injuries, and to the use of older cars with fewer safety features.

What is it about aging that makes our driving less safe?

The most common causes of car crashes for older adults are not being able to stay in one's lane (when turning, driving on a straight away, or changing lanes), yielding improperly, and choosing to cross in front of oncoming traffic without having enough time or being far enough away from oncoming traffic. In fact, the most frequent traffic citations for older drivers are for failure to yield, improper use of lanes, and improper left turns.

These errors are related in part to physical, visual, and/or cognitive changes associated with aging, medications, and disease, which can cause difficulty reading road signs, responding to traffic signals or GPS directions, following lane markings, or being able to find the beginning of a left turn lane. Examples include:

- Vision and hearing impairment (chapter 12).

- Cognitive changes, including decreased ability to switch tasks and attention quickly enough to respond to unexpected situations like a change in road sign information, vehicle movements, pedestrian movements, or potential hazards.

- Slower reaction times, especially in response to unexpected situations where you need to immediately brake, steer around an obstacle, or accelerate.

- Less flexibility when turning one's head and neck to see into blind spots, when backing up, or when merging lanes.

Older adults are less likely to speed, tailgate, consume alcohol before driving, or engage in other risky behaviors, but a third of all their fatal accidents, and more than half that involve drivers 80 or older, happen at intersections.

Why are intersections such a problem?

Driving through an intersection requires the ability to multitask, especially if you're turning. You must anticipate the movements of other drivers and pedestrians; be in the correct lane and turn into the correct lane; yield if it is either a two- or four-way stop, a right turn on red, or a lane merge; and judge the speed of other vehicles and the space available to safely go through the intersection. Making a left-hand turn is particularly challenging.

Are there specific medical conditions or medications that may interfere with safe driving?

Absolutely. This is why it makes a lot of sense to involve your medical provider in optimizing your ability to drive safely. Medical conditions such as cataracts, diabetes, glaucoma, macular degeneration, Parkinson's disease, stroke, and sleep apnea can affect your ability to drive, so they need to be identified and managed.

Having a seizure, or epilepsy, is a particular risk for crashes, and many states require that you be seizure-free for a certain amount of time before allowing you to resume driving. You should stop driving until you are evaluated by a doctor if you develop a new condition where you lose consciousness or have dizziness or angina.

Sedation, blurred vision, impaired cognition, tremor, poor concentration, light-headedness, sleep attacks, and hypoglycemia can increase the risk of a crash. Do not drive if you are having any of these symptoms, and have your doctor review your medications to determine whether one or more could be causing them.

I'm in a quandary. My wife has early dementia, and since I don't drive, she's the one responsible for getting us places. At times I act as her co-pilot. Is this safe?

In some circumstances, the answer is yes. Studies show that more than 75 percent of drivers with dementia can pass a road test, but as you know, this is only one part of what needs to be considered in determining whether someone is a safe driver. As dementia progresses, many people lose the insight and judgment needed to drive. Your medical provider can be helpful with determining whether dementia has progressed to a point where it is no longer safe to be behind the wheel.

Another good way to tell is to *honestly* answer the question, "Do you feel safe in the passenger seat?" By honestly, I mean that you need to put aside any possible conflict of interest if you're dependent on the person with dementia for transportation. Answering yes to this question correlates with accidents caused by drivers with dementia. So does a history of accidents or citations, impulsive or aggressive behavior, and inability to follow basic commands or to repeat simple movements.

Adapting to Your New Normal

How do I know if I'm becoming an unsafe driver?

Review the questions in table 19.1 (on page 351). If you answer "yes" to any of these, it may be time to talk with your doctor about driving or have a driving assessment. *This doesn't necessarily mean it's time to take away your keys.* The purpose is to identify ways to help you maintain the ability to drive on your own.

What can I do to make my driving safer?

Optimize Your Medical Treatment and Function

Interventions for certain conditions (such as treating obstructive sleep apnea, cataract removal, and medication management) and improving functional deficits (such as endurance or range of motion) may lower your crash risk or enhance or maintain your current driving performance. Physical, occupational, and vision rehabilitation specialists may be able to help. The latter can provide training for neurologic conditions that cause visual impairments that affect driving.

Reconsider Some of Your Driving Habits

Many older adults adapt by driving less, especially at night, during rush hour, or on major highways. Instead of taking a left turn at an intersection, they may opt to take a series of right turns to go around the block so that they can drive straight through the intersection. Not using your cell phone while driving helps keep your attention focused so that you can react more quickly to unexpected situations. Does making these changes actually decrease crashes? It's not clear, because the reasons for declines in driving ability are different for each person, and the changes made would need to match these. But they certainly can't hurt, and they may make you more mindful when you're driving.

Drive a Safer Vehicle

Newer cars have several effective crash avoidance technologies that may be standard or optional features. In one study, police-reported crashes decreased 56 percent when vehicles had forward collision warning systems with autobrakes, 27 percent with the warning system alone, 21 percent with lane departure warnings, and 23 percent with blind spot detection. Rear-end accidents decreased 62 percent with rear automatic braking, 17 percent with rearview cameras, and 22 percent with rear cross-traffic alerts. Electronic stability control, which improves your control on curves and slippery roads, has been standard on all cars sold since 2012. The National Highway Traffic Safety Administration estimates electronic stability control has reduced fatal single-vehicle crashes by 38 percent and sport utility vehicle crashes and rollovers by 56 percent, so if your vehicle was manufactured in 2011 or earlier, you should strongly consider trading up to a newer model.

Modify Your Vehicle to Improve Your Ability to Drive

Advancement in vehicle technology allows compensation for a wide range of physical and some visual impairment. There are foot pedal extenders and seat raisers if you've lost height and can't see over the steering wheel or reach the pedals, padded steering wheel covers for pain or weakened grip, and extra and larger mirrors for those with restricted range of motion or flexibility, such as happens with arthritis.

My son doesn't think I should be driving anymore, but I think I'm a safe driver. I don't go on highways, just locally to the grocery store and the mall. He's now refusing to let his kids be in the car with me. Is there anything I can do to convince him that I'm okay to drive?

What should make a difference is to get a *driving evaluation*. Driving evaluations are done by driving rehabilitation specialists who can provide driving simulation and actual on-road evaluation. Based on the results of the evaluation, they determine any areas of concern as well as whether you would be a candidate for adaptive driving instruction or driver retraining, would benefit from vehicle modifications, or should stop driving.

There are several different types of driving improvement and driver rehabilitation programs. The American Occupational Therapist Association has a handout comparing the various programs that are available (see the Resources section at the end of this chapter).

The cost of a driving evaluation program is generally not covered by insurance, including Medicare. If you are a veteran, a US Department of Veterans Affairs facility in your area may provide this service. Suggestions for how to find local providers can be found in the Resources section at the end of this chapter. When you call, make sure to ask about costs for the program, adaptive

TABLE 19.1
Indications That One Might Be Having a Problem Driving

The National Institutes of Health and AARP suggest that you ask yourself the following questions (check any that apply):

- ☐ Do other drivers often honk at me?
- ☐ Have I had some accidents, even if they were only "fender benders"?
- ☐ Do I get lost, even on roads I know?
- ☐ Do cars or pedestrians seem to appear out of nowhere?
- ☐ Do I get distracted while driving?
- ☐ Have family, friends, or my doctor said they're worried about my driving?
- ☐ Am I driving less these days because I'm not as sure about my driving as I used to be?
- ☐ Do I have trouble staying in my lane or navigating turns?
- ☐ Do I have trouble moving my foot between the gas and the brake pedals, or do I sometimes confuse the two?
- ☐ Have I been pulled over by a police officer about my driving?
- ☐ Do I have difficulty turning my head to see when backing up?
- ☐ Am I hitting curbs, or have I scraped or dented the car, mailbox, or garage?
- ☐ Am I getting more agitated or irritated when driving? Why?
- ☐ Have I failed to notice traffic signs or important activity on the side of the road?

equipment, and whether they will help you explore funding options for vehicle modifications.

I'm not keen on a driving evaluation. What if they tell me I have to stop driving?

The driving rehabilitation specialist will review the results of the evaluation with you, explaining what the findings indicate about your function and its relationship to driving. Your needs will also be taken into account, ideally resulting in adaptive driving instruction, retraining, or modifying your vehicle.

If the recommendation is that you stop driving, however, you need to seriously consider what this means. How would you feel if you kept driving and caused an accident? Remember, older drivers have the highest rate of fatal crashes, and the fatalities are the drivers themselves, their passengers, and bystanders—those in other vehicles, pedestrians, bicyclists, or motorcyclists.

If I have to stop driving, how will I get around?

There are other ways to get around, but some are more realistic for certain individuals than others:

- Walking
- Train or subway
- Bus
- Taxi or ride-hailing services
- Family and friends
- Community transportation services
- Hospital shuttles

- Medi-car
- Volunteer drivers (such as from a church, synagogue, mosque, or community center)
- Private for-profit senior care services

This chapter's Resources section has links to organizations that can provide information on local transportation. You may also be able to get certain things that you need—like prescriptions, newspapers, and groceries—delivered.

Oftentimes, older adults are loath to ask family and friends for help with transportation. But I would guess that you have been giving rides to people throughout your years of driving. Now you can let others return the favor. It helps to schedule a specific time to have someone stop by with their vehicle and be available to help with your transportation needs. Having a regular schedule frees you from feeling like you're always having to ask for a favor and lets you plan ahead.

Advice for Loved Ones

Some people can't imagine not driving and refuse to consider a driving evaluation or alternatives to driving. In having these discussions, it's important to emphasize that both of you are wishing for the same thing, that they be an independent and safe driver.

It's okay to get medical providers involved if these discussions get sticky. Ask if you could be at their next visit, in person or on the phone, to discuss your concerns. I've also had patients' families call with a concern about driving when I was unaware of the issue. I listen but don't provide any medical information unless I have the patients' prior consent. This alerts me to raise the issue at our next visit, and to suggest a driving evaluation if it seems warranted.

If someone needs to stop driving for their own or others safety, it's important that they know you recognize this is yet another loss, but that you can work together to help identify realistic alternatives like those mentioned above. It still

won't be the same as being able to jump in the car and go whenever the impulse strikes, though.

Many of my patients are concerned about the cost of alternative forms of transportation. Remember, having a car isn't cheap. Calculate how much it is currently costing to have a car, adding up the cost of insurance, license, registration, gas, maintenance (oil changes, tires, and tune-ups), repairs, car payments, parking, and so on. Without a car, this money can be used on cabs, car services, or even paying a neighbor. Find out about local transportation options. The daughter of one of my patients created a Lyft account for her mother and deposited some money in it as a holiday present. My patient initially refused the whole idea, but eventually she tried it out. By the time the money needed to be replenished, my patient was happy to use her own money to keep it going.

If someone is still unwilling to stop driving, there may be an opportunity when it's time for them to renew their driver's license. Most US states have one or more renewal provisions specific to older drivers, such as shorter renewal cycles, required vision or road testing, and in-person rather than mail or electronic renewal. Surveys find that the majority of older adults think this is appropriate. The ages at which special regulations are required vary by state (see the Resources section at the end of this chapter).

If your loved one continues to drive, inform their medical provider that in your opinion (or that of the driving specialist), she shouldn't be. Each state has its own rules about medical providers reporting that someone is at risk as a driver, but even when it's not mandated, most take the risk to public safety seriously. I speak with my patients about their driving, tell them that there is concern (often the concerned person is in the room during this discussion), and that we're worried they may be respon-

sible for significant injury to someone if they continue to drive. We discuss why continuing to drive is so important to them, and explore each of these reasons. For many older adults, it's the sense that asking for help getting places makes them dependent or a burden to others. Reiterating what we discussed above about alternative ways to get around can help.

There are always some people who insist that they can continue to drive despite others' concerns. I let these patients know that I am contacting the Department of Motor Vehicles because I have concerns about their driving and think that they need to be evaluated. Obviously, this can cause strain in the patient's relationship with both me and their loved one, but I make it clear that this is not personal, and it has to do with avoiding injury to them and others. Have I lost patients because of this? Yes, but very rarely. Most people understand the stakes.

RESOURCES

Assessment of and Information on Older Adult Driving

American Automobile Association
AAA offers numerous tools to help older drivers assess their fitness to drive an automobile:

- Drivers 65 Plus Assessment Tool (https://exchange.aaa.com/wp-content /uploads/2021/03/Driver-65-Plus.pdf) This self-guided publication helps drivers 65 and old assess their driving performance and offers suggestions for safe driving.
- Foundation for Traffic Safety Resources (https://aaafoundation.org/resources/) Contains online free resources to help

older adults assess personal driving readiness and make informed choices about their driving.
- Senior Driving Safety and Mobility (https://seniordriving.aaa.com/) Provides users with general information to help them better understand the traffic safety implications of certain health conditions and human behaviors as we get older.

Centers for Disease Control and Prevention (https://www.cdc.gov/motorvehiclesafety /older_adult_drivers/mymobility/index .html)
The CDC's *MyMobility Plan* provides general guidance for older adults seeking to

maintain both individual and community mobility.

National Highway Traffic Safety Administration
(https://www.nhtsa.gov/road-safety /older-drivers)
NHTSA's Older Drivers site has download-able materials and short video clips that show how aging can affect driving and what drivers can do to continue driving safely as they age, such as adapting a vehi-cle to meet specific needs.

National Institute on Aging
The NIA provides safety information to older adults who may be worried about their driving, including:
- Driving and Transportation (https:// www.nia.nih.gov/health/topics/driving -and-transportation)
  Read and share this infographic about ways to help keep older drivers safe, especially if you have concerns about a loved one's driving ability.
- Older Drivers Website (https://www.nia .nih.gov/health/older-drivers)
  Some older drivers may have problems when yielding the right of way, turning (especially making left turns), changing lanes, passing, and using expressway ramps. Among the NIA's safe driving tips is to have your driving skills checked by a driving rehabilitation specialist, occupational therapist, or other trained professional.
- "Research Helps Older Drivers Stay Safe and Independent." November 6, 2011. https://www.nia.nih.gov/news/research -helps-older-drivers-stay-safe-and -independent
  This article presents research on train-ing that may improve driving skills and reduce accidents. It also discusses the usual field of view (UFOW), the window of attention within which an individual can rapidly be alerted to visual stimuli. The UFOW can be measured and often improved with training.

Driving with Dementia

Alzheimer's Association
(www.alz.org/care/alzheimers-dementia -and-driving.asp)
Offers advice on talking with your loved one about their driving, as well as provides links to driving counseling support for caregivers.

National Institute on Aging
(https://www.nia.nih.gov/health/driving -safety-and-alzheimers-disease)
Intended for caregivers, this website from the NIA discusses safety, legal issues, and assessment for older drivers with Alzhei-mer disease or other forms of dementia.

Driver Rehabilitation

American Occupational Therapy Association
(https://www.aota.org/-/media/Corporate /Files/Practice/Aging/Driving/Spectrum -of-Driving-Services.pdf)
AOTA's comparison of different types of driving services and driver rehabilitation programs can help you determine what type of service your loved one needs.

To find a local provider:
- Call the occupational therapy depart-ments in local hospitals or rehabilitation centers.
- Locate an occupational therapist able to conduct driving assessment and loca-tions by zip code using the Find a Pro-vider tool available from AOTA (https:// www.aota.org/Practice/Productive -Aging/Driving.aspx).
- Search the online directory of the Asso-ciation for Driver Rehabilitation Special-ists to locate a provider (https://www .aded.net/search/custom.asp?id=1984).
- Check your local chapter of the Alzhei-mer's Association for lists of area driving evaluation programs (https://www.alz .org/help-support/caregiving/safety /dementia-driving).

Identifying Local Transportation Services

National Association of Area Agencies on Aging
(www.n4a.org/about-n4a)
The National Association of Area Agencies on Aging is a leading aging issues resource that provides specific regional services.

National Volunteer Transportation Center
(https://ctaa.org/national-volunteer-transportation-center/)
This organization provides training for volunteer drivers as well as connects drivers with older adults who need transportation.

Rides in Sight
(https://www.ridesinsight.org/)
A national nonprofit transportation system supported by Independent Transportation Network America, Rides in Sight is dedicated to helping find transportation alternatives. This service is membership-based; people 60 and older and visually impaired adults are eligible to join.

Driver's License Renewal

American Automobile Association
(https://exchange.aaa.com/safety/senior-driver-safety-mobility/senior-licensing-policies-practices)
AAA's Senior Licensing Laws website provides information on licensing policies and practices for older drivers.

Insurance Institute for Highway Safety
(http://www.iihs.org/iihs/topics/t/older-drivers)
An overview of older drivers and how their ability to drive changes over time is provided at this website.

State Departments of Motor Vehicles
Contact your state's DMV for information on driver's license renewal requirements.

BIBLIOGRAPHY

American Geriatrics Society. *Clinician's Guide to Assessing and Counseling Older Drivers*, 4th ed. New York: American Geriatrics Society, 2019.

Classen, S., O. Shechtman, and K. D. Awadzi. "Traffic Violations versus Driving Errors of Older Adults: Informing Clinical Practice." *American Journal of Occupational Therapy* 64, no. 2 (2010): 233–41.

Harkey, D. L., H. Huang, and C. V. Zegeer. *Accident Analysis of Older Drivers on Freeways*. Working Paper FHWA-RD-96-035. Washington, DC: Federal Highway Administration, August 1996.

Insurance Institute for Highway Safety. "Fatality Facts 2019: Older People." Posted March 2021. https://www.iihs.org/iihs/topics/t/older-drivers/fatalityfacts/older-people.

Iverson, D. J., G. S. Gronseth, M. A. Reger, et al. "Practice Parameter Update: Evaluation and Management of Driving Risk in Dementia. Report of the Quality Standards Subcommittee of the American Academy of Neurology." *Neurology* 74, no. 16 (2010): 1316–24.

CHAPTER 20

Who Will Speak for Me?

This chapter builds on the discussion in chapter 4.

Your decisions are yours to make until you are no longer able to. If you're extremely ill or living with dementia, there will need to be someone available to speak for you. This should be someone you trust and who knows your health care priorities.

What should I consider when deciding who should speak for me? Do I need a lawyer to make this official?

A *health care proxy* (in some states this is called a *medical power of attorney* or a *durable power of attorney for health care*) is a legal document in which you can appoint someone to make medical decisions for you if ever you are unable to make them for yourself. No lawyer is needed. The proxy only goes into effect if you are in a condition that prevents you from making the decision yourself. Choose someone who knows you well and who you trust to carry out your choices. Filling out the paperwork is important, but more important is making sure this person is aware of your preferences for care. It is extraordinarily hard for someone to stand in and make medical decisions for some-

one else. Being able to "hear their voice" based on conversations you have had in the past can really make a difference. Most health care proxy documents include a back-up proxy in case your first choice is unavailable. Forms to name a health care proxy can be downloaded online and may even be available in your doctor's office. These forms take only a few minutes to complete. Once you appoint a proxy, you will need to have your form signed by two witnesses, and then make sure the proxy and your medical provider have an actual copy. Note that a regular "durable power of attorney" is more for financial and other legal matters (such as accessing a bank account) and does not typically cover health care decisions.

What should I discuss with my proxy?

No one can identify all the possible medical decisions that might need to be made in future situations. Most discussions begin with feelings about emergency and end-of-life care, often what you've seen someone else go through and whether or not that's what you would want. There are several excellent "prompts" that can help you consider different situations and then discuss them with your proxy (see the

Resources section at the end of this chapter). A lot of your choices will come back to values, so if you completed a health care priority form (discussed in chapters 4 and 17), review this with your proxy.

You can also complete an advance directive, like a living will. A *living will* is a document that specifies the types of medical treatments you would or would not want if you found yourself in a serious medical situation and were unable to let your preferences be known. You can describe the situations under which you would want to attempt to prolong life or to withdraw care. Living wills usually address things like dialysis, artificial nutrition and hydration, mechanical ventilation, CPR (cardiopulmonary resuscitation), and your preferences as they relate to pain control, symptom management, and comfort care at the end of life. Many living wills also address organ donation in the case of death. Living wills are legal documents that vary from state to state and usually require an attorney and/or a notary for preparation.

Having a health care proxy is in many ways more powerful than having documents that state your choices about health care, like a living will. It is impossible to predict the nuances in medical decision-making that occur during serious medical illness, so it can be hard to translate the wishes you expressed in a living will to a situation you could not have predicted would occur. A proxy can be more flexible and respond to an emergent situation. Many people have both a living will and a health care proxy; in these cases, the health care proxy makes decisions as informed by the living will but is still able to act on unanticipated questions that may come up.

What if I don't designate a health care proxy? Who would make decisions for me?

When a patient without a proxy doesn't have the capacity to make a decision, a surrogate can be designated by the state. Each state has its own ranked list of potential surrogates, and the highest-ranked surrogate who agrees is given the authority. Below is an example of a typical order in which surrogates are assigned.

1. Previously existing court-appointed guardian
2. Patient's spouse
3. Patient's adult child (if there are more than one, typically a majority of the "reasonably available" children)
4. Patient's parent
5. Patient's domestic partner (if unmarried, in some states)
6. Adult sibling
7. Grandparent
8. Adult grandchild
9. Adult aunt/uncle
10. Adult niece/nephew
11. Close friend of the patient (in selected states)
12. Attending physician (in selected states) for those who have no family members or other surrogates to speak on their behalf, in consultation with a second physician and/or the health care institution's ethics committee.

Why wouldn't I want CPR? On TV, almost everyone comes back to life quickly without harm.

CPR is used to revive people found to be pulseless and nonresponsive. Older adults with multiple medical conditions are unlikely to have a good outcome from CPR. Most people, including doctors, overestimate survival and underestimate disability for CPR recipients. On television, CPR is effective more than 75 percent of the time, compared to 10 percent in real life. Those 80 and over have a 2 percent chance of living to hospital discharge, and many of these people have severe new neurological and functional deficits as a result of the resuscitation attempt. Other adverse outcomes include rib and sternal fractures from the chest compression, and if mouth-to-mouth resuscitation or a bag valve mask is used, swelling of the belly, which can lead to vomiting and aspiration.

If my health care proxy is conflicted about letting me die, could they agree to CPR or mechanical ventilation even though I've said I wouldn't want these? Is there anything I can do to make it more likely that my wishes are followed?

Your proxy could make that decision. One of the hardest things about being a proxy is to make a decision for someone based on what they wanted, rather than what you want. Completing a *DNR (Do Not Resuscitate)* and *POLST (Physician Orders for Life-Sustaining Treatment)* order provides more assurance that your wishes will be followed. These are actual medical orders that are signed by your physician.

A Do Not Resuscitate order means just that—if I die, do not try to bring me back to life with CPR, electrical shocks, or medications. When I discuss DNR orders with patients, I often explain that this order addresses the last moments of life, when the heart has stopped beating or when you can no longer breathe on your own. A DNR order does not mean do not treat. This is a common misconception. Infections, breathing problems, dehydration, and the like should be treated unless your proxy says that's not what you would want. DNR orders in the hospital differ than those for when you're at home. If you are in the hospital, you can ask your doctor to enter this order if you would not want CPR or mechanical ventilation if your heart stopped or if you stopped breathing. Most hospitals will require a new order each time you are admitted to the hospital. An out-of-hospital DNR can be used in the home. It needs to be signed by the doctor, can be obtained through your doctor's office, and you must have a copy of it to show emergency personnel for it to be honored. In the event of an emergency at home, emergency medical technicians are required to try to revive patients if they don't see an out-of-hospital DNR or a POLST. Therefore I tell my patients to keep this document somewhere where it is easy to find, like on the refrigerator or on the kitchen table.

People with a serious medical illness and a limited prognosis should consider a POLST (also called a *MOLST*, Medical Order for Life-Sustaining Treatment; *MOST*, Medical Orders on Scope of Treatment; *POST*, Physician's Orders on Scope of Treatment; or *TPOPP*, Transportable Physician Orders for Patient Preferences, depending on the state). A POLST is a document that addresses your wishes at the end of life and includes things like whether or not you want to go to the hospital if you suffer a serious or potentially life-ending event, as well as your preferences for CPR, mechanical ventilation, and artificial nutrition and hydration. These POLST medical orders are typically summarized on a highly visible, standardized form that is legal and valid across medical settings, such as in a hospital, rehabilitation center, or nursing home. Many POLST forms also leave room for you to list your specific goals for your medical care. POLST forms differ from state to state and are not available in every state. You can refer to www.polst.org to learn more.

These are life-and-death situations we're talking about. What if my proxy or surrogate isn't able to make a decision when the time comes?

It's stressful to make decisions about starting, withholding, or withdrawing life-sustaining therapies. It's a doctor's job to provide recommendations and provide support for the person making decisions. Let your proxy know that it is fine to ask for the provider's judgment to help in making decisions after providing input on what you would have wanted.

A *time-limited trial of therapy* can be useful if you don't know how someone is going to respond to a treatment, the prognosis is not clear, or if there is uncertainty about a patient's wishes. It is defined as "an agreement between clinicians and a patient/family to use certain medical therapies over a defined period to see if the patient improves or deteriorates according to agreed-on clinical outcomes." For example, a severely ill woman with chronic obstructive pulmonary disease (COPD) may require antibiotics and a ventilator to be able to survive a pneumonia. But if she loses muscle strength while on the ventilator, she may need the machine to help her breathe even after the pneumonia is cured. A time-limited trial of antibiotics while on the ventilator gives patients a certain number of days to see if the pneumonia improves and they can start to breathe on their own. If the patient deteriorates, the antibiotics and ventilator can be withdrawn, and goals shifted more purely to comfort and palliation.

What is the role of hospice and palliative care?

Bea has been in the hospital three times in the last eight months because of complications from her lung cancer treatment. She is having trouble breathing and is in a lot of pain, and now she can no longer do the things that are important to her. Bea thinks she wants to continue with the cancer treatment, but at the same time, she wonders if she will be able to manage, both physically and emotionally, if these symptoms continue. Her doctor suggested she meet with the palliative care team while in the hospital.

Palliative care is specialized medical care that focuses on relief from symptoms and the stress of living with a serious illness. It includes early identification, assessment, and treatment of pain and other problems—physical, psychosocial, and spiritual—for both the patient and the caregivers (see the Resources section at the end of this chapter). Palliative care is provided by a trained multidisciplinary team of doctors, nurses, and other specialists who will work with your other doctors to provide additional support. Palliative care is appropriate at any age and at any stage of a serious illness and can be provided along with curative care. Most hospitals now have palliative care services available to inpatients, and many have outpatient options as well.

Palliative care is often confused with hospice care. While both can provide comfort during serious medical illness, they are not the same thing. Palliative care can be provided from the time of diagnosis or at any time during the course of a serious illness.

Hospice care typically provides comfort care after most disease-directed treatments have stopped. Patients are eligible if they have a terminal diagnosis with a life expectancy of six months or less. Medicare A covers the services of the hospice team, the cost of durable medical equipment, and medications. The patient lives at home or in a long-term care facility and may be admitted to an inpatient facility to have intractable pain or other symptoms treated. Some geographical areas have live-in hospices, but they are not the norm. Medicare will only pay for hospitalizations for people enrolled in hospice if the person has uncontrollable symptoms, not for further treatment of the primary illness.

RESOURCES

General

My Health Priorities
(https://myhealthpriorities.org/)
This online, self-directed tool helps users identify their health priorities.

Organ Donation
(https://www.organdonor.gov/)
This website of the Health Resources and Services Administration provides information about the organ donation process and registration.

POLST
(www.polst.org)
Information on the Physician Orders for Life-Sustaining Treatment form.

Vial of Life
(https://www.vialoflife.com/area/#/)
Completing this form from the Vial of Life Project provides emergency personnel

access to medical information important in getting you the proper medical treatment.

Easy-to-Use Resources for Completing Advance Directive Documents

American Bar Association. "Tool Kit for Health Care Advance Planning." November 11, 2020. https://www.americanbar.org /groups/law_aging/resources/health_care _decision_making/consumer_s_toolkit_for _health_care_advance_planning/.
This resource doesn't create advance directives, but it has conversation scripts and resources for decision-making and communication when creating advance directives.

Five Wishes
(https://agingwithdignity.org/programs /five-wishes/)
The Five Wishes form from Aging with Dignity is the most popular advance directive in the United States.

National Hospice and Palliative Care Organization
(https://www.nhpco.org/advancedirective)
Download information on completing advance directives in your state.

Our Care Wishes
(https://www.ourcarewishes.org)
This free service from Penn Medicine allows you to create and share advance directives with loved ones and caregivers.

PREPARE for Your Care
(prepareforyourcare.org)
This is a free step-by-step program with video stories to help you complete an advance directive form, putting your wishes in writing. It includes information on how to discuss these with your doctor. It is available in Spanish, English, and some Chinese dialects.

BIBLIOGRAPHY

Quill, Timothy E., and Robert Holloway. "Time-Limited Trials Near the End of Life." *JAMA* 306, no. 13 (2011): 1483–84.

Sudore, R. L., et al. "Engaging Diverse English- and Spanish-Speaking Older Adults in Advance Care Planning: The PREPARE Randomized Clinical Trial." *JAMA Internal Medicine* 178, no. 12 (2018): 1616–25.

Acknowledgments

It took a village (and a pandemic) to get this book to you. This book exists only because of the belief and hard work of many, starting with Marsha Melnick, Susan Meyer, Gloria Loomis, Rachel Trusheim, and Joseph Eckenrode who understood, contrary to many others, that we'll all age if we're lucky, and that there's a need for a book to help guide us through this new stage of life. Drs. Claire Davenport and Jessi Israel wrote parts of specific chapters, Dr. Sharon See, Jennifer Chen, and Angel Liu helped with the research for the medication tables. The American Geriatrics Society (AGS) and Belvoir Media were generous in allowing use of some of their content, particularly on driving and from our newsletter, Focus on Healthy Aging.

I am indebted to Martha Ackelsberg, Ora Chaikin, Jessi Israel, Kenneth Karpel, Judith Plaskow, and Donna Moran Simpson for reviewing drafts of the entire manuscript, and to friends and colleagues who reviewed individual chapters, including Sheila Barton, Mary DeBare, Miguel Escalon, Fran Grossman, Greg Hinrichsen, Steve Kaplan, Gary Kennedy, Bruce Leipzig, Staci Leisman, Gloria Loomis, Marsha Melnick, Susan Meyer, Adrienne Ormond, Ira Rosenbloom, Karen Sauvigne, Sharon See, Brijen Shah, Mara Schonberg, Rachel Trusheim, and Mary Tinetti.

I would particularly like to thank my editor at Johns Hopkins University Press, Joe Rusko, and to thank Peter Rabins for connecting us.

For over 25 years I've been lucky to be part of the team that is the Brookdale Department of Geriatrics and Palliative Medicine at the Icahn School of Medicine at Mount Sinai. My patients and their lives provided the impetus for me to write this book, and I am deeply grateful to them for allowing me to be part of their lives. It is my sincere hope that the shared wisdom within this book will allow many others to benefit from what we have all experienced and learned together.

Personal Emergency Response Systems

What Is a Personal Emergency Response System (PERS), and How Does It Work?

Most PERSs incorporate a base unit and a "panic button" that typically is worn either as a pendant or bracelet (some systems also offer a wall button). If you fall, you press the button to activate the base unit. Some base units have automatic fall detectors which may cost extra. PERS can operate by landline or cellular network. Another option is a mobile Global Positioning System (GPS) for use when you are on the go. With these devices, the panic button uses the cellular network for communication between you and the response center, and GPS satellite technology to locate you. Don't worry that if you set off the device, emergency services will break down the door. When you sign up, you can tell the company where to find an extra door key, or have a lockbox installed outside your home and put a spare key in it.

What Options Do I Need to Consider?

You will need to decide whether to get a monitored or unmonitored system. With the monitored option, you pay a monthly fee, and the unit connects to an emergency response center with staff who will dispatch emergency services or contact a family member or neighbor if you need assistance. An unmonitored unit doesn't contact a live person—instead, it cycles through preprogrammed phone numbers of your choice until somebody answers, and then plays a prerecorded message requesting help. There is an upfront cost for the base unit and panic button for unmonitored systems, but there is no monthly fee.

Other things to look for include no installation or activation fees, a free trial period so that you can see how well the system works for you, and the freedom to cancel the service at any time without penalties. For landlines and cell phones, ask about the range for the panic button, the base unit's battery life, and whether there is a low-battery warning signal. If you're considering a monitored system, make sure it's staffed 24 hours a day, that calls are answered promptly by a person, and that the operators have received adequate training, preferably similar to that for 911 dispatchers.

Perhaps the most important thing to keep in mind when considering a PERS is that you must be wearing the device in order for it to be useful. If the PERS is on a table or hanging on the wall, you won't be able to trigger it if you have a fall or a medical emergency.

Assistive Devices

Canes

Canes can help you walk if you have arthritis or pain, especially of a knee or hip, mild balance problems, peripheral neuropathy, or if you have an injury to one foot or leg. Canes improve walking by reducing weight-bearing on the affected leg and improving support when that joint is in the air during walking. It improves balance by increasing the signals that sensors in the hand send to the brain about the location of the cane and the ground, and where these are in relation to the person.

Your cane needs to be the right length to maximize stability. The length should be the distance from the wrist to the ground when you're standing erect with your elbow bent about 20–30 degrees. Pistol-grip canes have more support than rounded ones. The more points the cane has that are on the ground, the greater the stability; however, four-point (or quad) canes are heavier and may be awkward and challenging to use correctly. Canes should be held in the hand opposite the affected leg. All canes must have a nonskid rubber tip.

Walkers

A walker may be necessary when a cane doesn't provide enough support, if your balance is off, if both legs are weak, or if you feel weak in general. The best type of walker for you depends on your gait, strength, and cognitive and cardio-

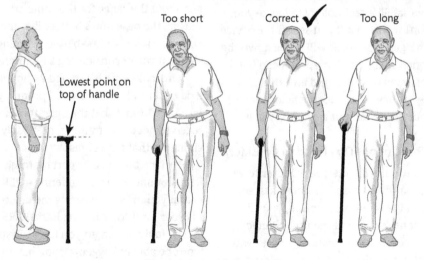

Too short   Correct ✔   Too long

Lowest point on top of handle

What length should my cane be?

pulmonary abilities. Walkers must be adjusted similarly to canes (see above) so one stays upright and doesn't need to lean forward to reach the walker. Walkers cannot be used on stairs.

Wheelchairs and Scooters

Wheelchairs and scooters should be used if someone cannot safely ambulate with a cane or walker. A wheelchair must be fitted according to body build, weight, disability, and prognosis. Incorrect fit can result in poor posture, joint deformity, reduced mobility, pressure injury, circulatory compromise, and discomfort. Home modifications may be necessary to accommodate the use of a walker or scooter at home.

TABLE A.1
Types of Walkers

	Standard	Front-Wheeled	Rolling Four-Wheeled
How they work	Needs to be picked up to move forward.	Doesn't need to be picked up, so it uses less energy. Gait is smoother, coordinated, and faster. Brakes engage when the walker is leaned on.	Able to move faster by decreasing energy expenditure. Can lean on the device and sit to rest when fatigued. Has hand brakes that can be locked when transferring to a chair or bed.
Who benefits	Those with good upper extremity strength and the ability to learn necessary coordination.	Those with Parkinson's disease, hip fracture, and mild deconditioning.	Those with cardiopulmonary disease and severe deconditioning.
Use in those with cognitive impairment	May not be able to learn necessary coordination.	More likely to be used correctly than standard walker.	Because the brakes are hand brakes and require the ability to remember how and when to use them, these may not be appropriate.
Advantages and disadvantages		Must have nonskid tips on the back legs. Tennis balls cut and placed on the rubber tips can help aid movement on carpeted surfaces.	Less stable than standard. User needs to have good balance and reaction times to use the brakes safely and be able to turn around safely to sit. Good for walking outside because of large wheels.

TABLE A.2
Types of Wheelchairs and Scooters

	Manual	Power	Scooter
How they work	Needs to be self-propelled or pushed.	Has controls (usually a joystick) that can be modified, so use of the upper extremities is not needed.	Operated with tiller and handlebar.
Who benefits	Those who are able to use their arms and have the strength and cardiovascular capacity to move themselves.	Those with bilateral arm weakness, diminished cardiopulmonary capacity, or other neurologic disorders that limit capacity to self-propel a manual wheelchair.	Similar to power wheelchair, except one must be able to operate it with the upper extremities. May be more acceptable to older adults than a power wheelchair.
Use in those with cognitive impairment	Depends on degree of impairment; may need a caregiver to propel.	Need mental alertness and cognitive ability to operate safely.	Need mental alertness and cognitive ability to operate safely.
Advantages and disadvantages	In one study, 61% of the older adults reported having difficulty with manual wheelchair propulsion. Easy to transport. Often used in nursing homes and by caregivers for ease of mobility.	Medicare will only cover for in-home use. Has a height-adjusted foot platform that can flip up when not in use.	Medicare will only cover for in-home use. Motorized scooters offer less trunk support than motorized wheelchairs. May require home and car modifications. Three-wheel scooter better for taller people; four-wheel scooter has a broader wheelbase to ensure even weight distribution for stability.

Sources: Modified from G. M. Harper, W. L Lyons, and J. F. Potter, MD, eds., *Geriatrics Review Syllabus*, 10th ed. (Albany, NY: Fry Publications, 2019), tables 35.2 and 35.3; Panel on Prevention of Falls in Older Persons, American Geriatrics Society, and British Geriatrics Society, "Summary of the Updated American Geriatrics Society / British Geriatrics Society Clinical Practice Guideline for Prevention of Falls in Older Persons," *Journal of the American Geriatrics Society* 59: (2011): 148–57.

Getting Ready to Meet with Your Doctor

Physicians are often taught that 80 percent of diagnoses can be made based on the history provided by the patient. To get the correct diagnosis, you need to be the best observer you can. This appendix contains pre-visit checklists for chapters 6–16 (except chapter 12). You should complete the relevant checklists and bring them to your evaluation. You may need to closely observe your symptoms for a few days before you can accurately do this. These checklists will help your provider make the right diagnoses.

There are also some general instructions you should follow for each visit:

- Bring the checklist with you to the visit.

- Bring all medications you take; include prescription drugs, over-the-counter medications, and the supplements and vitamins you get from the health food or drug store.

- Show the provider your medication bottles, and be honest about whether you take any recreational drugs.

- Make sure you have time alone with the medical provider if there are private issues you wish to discuss, or if you don't want family observing the physical examination or testing.

- Make plans before you leave the office for how you will get the test results.

- Make a follow-up appointment to discuss all the findings, possible diagnoses, and your response to treatment.

Chapter 6. Mind Matters

1. Provide some specific examples of the situations and behaviors that are concerning to you or your loved ones.

_____

_____

_____

2. Check all of the following that you are having difficulty with:
   - ☐ concentrating
   - ☐ learning and remembering new things
   - ☐ finding the right word
   - ☐ paying bills
   - ☐ organizing or managing your medications
   - ☐ driving
   - ☐ problem-solving
   - ☐ decision-making
   - ☐ getting lost in familiar places
   - ☐ other concerns: _____

3. If you checked any of the above, when did these concerns start, and are they progressing?

   _____

   _____

4. Are any of these interfering with your ability to keep appointments, make plans, and communicate, or are loved ones questioning whether you can live on your own?   Yes   No

5. Complete the following:

   - ☐ Do you have a history of anxiety, depression, or other psychological illness?   Yes   No

   - ☐ Are you are having significant pain?   Yes   No

   - ☐ Have there been changes in your medications or their doses recently?   Yes   No

     If so, which ones? _____

   - ☐ Are you taking any dietary supplements?   Yes   No

     Which ones? _____

   - ☐ Do you exercise regularly?   Yes   No

     What do you do? _____

   - ☐ Are you a current or former smoker?   Yes   No

     How many years did you smoke? _____

   - ☐ How much alcohol do you currently drink? _____

     Were you ever a heavy drinker?   Yes   No

☐ Do you use "recreational" drugs?   Yes   No

Have you ever overused these?   Yes   No

☐ Has anyone in your family had depression, anxiety, strokes,
heart attacks, dementia, panic attacks, or thyroid problems?   Yes   No

If so, who? _____

Make sure to review your medications with your provider.

Chapter 7. Energy Cycles

1. Provide some specific examples of the activities or situations that cause you to
feel that you have low energy or exercise intolerance (reduced ability to be active
or exercise at the level expected for your age and condition).

_____

_____

_____

2. When was the last time your energy or exercise tolerance felt normal?

_____

Circle your answers

3. Are you concerned about low energy, exercise intolerance, or both?

4. Do you feel this way periodically, such as every day or once a week, at a particular
time of day, or mainly when you do certain activities?

5. Has this gotten worse over time?   Yes   No

If you have *exercise intolerance*, complete the following:

☐ How far can you go before you need to stop (number of blocks, stairs)?
What were you previously able to do, and when?

_____

_____

☐ Check all of the following that happen to you when you're walking or exercising:
  ○ shortness of breath
  ○ palpitations (fast heart rate or awareness of heart beating)
  ○ leg pain
  ○ light-headedness or dizziness
  ○ chest pain or pressure
  ○ feeling of faintness
  ○ early feelings of exhaustion

☐ How long does it take for you to feel better after you stop doing the activity?

_____

☐ If you develop pain or pressure, describe exactly where it is. What does it feel like? (Examples: burning, heavy weight, stabbing, numbness, pins and needles.) Does it go anywhere or just stay where it starts?

_____

_____

_____

If you have *low energy*, complete the following:

☐ Describe how you spend your day.

_____

_____

☐ Are there days that you have more energy?   Yes   No

  If so, is there anything that you think contributes to this?

_____

☐ Has the amount of time you spend in bed or sleeping increased?   Yes   No
☐ Do you feel exhausted most days of the week?   Yes   No
☐ Has your walking speed slowed dramatically?   Yes   No

Nutrition history

☐ Have you unintentionally gained or lost weight over
  the past year?   Yes   No

  If so, how much? _____

☐ What do you eat on a usual day?

Breakfast _____

Lunch _____

Dinner _____

Snacks _____

☐ On a usual day, how many cups or glasses of fluid do you drink? _____

Check if you have any of the following conditions:

☐ Diabetes   ☐ Parkinson's disease

☐ Stroke   ☐ Cognitive impairment

☐ Neuropathy   ☐ COPD

☐ Severe arthritis   ☐ Heart Disease

Check if you currently have any of the following symptoms:

☐ Fevers or sweats

☐ Muscle weakness or rigidity

☐ Headaches

☐ Sleep problems (insomnia, daytime sleepiness, snoring)

☐ Severe pain

Have you had recent changes in any of the following?

☐ Desire or motivation to be active, involved?	Yes	No
☐ Mood (are you feeling sad, irritable, anxious?)	Yes	No
☐ Stress level (any recent upsetting or stressful events?	Yes	No

☐ Have you had a recent illness?   Yes   No

If yes, describe: _____

☐ Have there been changes in your medications
or their doses recently?   Yes   No

If so, which ones? _____

☐ Are you taking any dietary supplements?   Yes   No

Which ones? _____

☐ Do you exercise regularly?   Yes   No

What do you do? _____

☐ Are you a current or former smoker?   Yes   No

How many years did you smoke? _____

☐ How much alcohol do you currently drink? _____

Were you ever a heavy drinker?   Yes   No

☐ Do you use "recreational" drugs?   Yes   No

Have you ever overused these?   Yes   No

☐ Has anyone in your family had depression, anxiety, strokes,
heart attacks, panic attacks, or thyroid problems?   Yes   No

If so, who? _____

Make sure to review your medications with your provider.

Chapter 8. Ups and Downs

1. Provide some specific examples of the situations and behaviors that are concerning you.

   _____

   _____

2. Check any of the following that you felt over the past two weeks:*
   ☐ little interest or pleasure in doing things?
   ☐ nervous, anxious, or on edge?
   ☐ down, depressed, or hopeless?
   ☐ unable to stop or control worrying?
   ☐ tense or having trouble relaxing?
   ☐ worrying too much about different things?
   ☐ restless?
   ☐ easily annoyed or irritable?
   ☐ feeling afraid, as if something awful might happen?

   Comments: _____

   _____

*These items are from the Patient Health Questionnaire-2 Item and the General Anxiety Disorder-7 Item (see the bibliography at the end of chapter 8).

3. Are you concerned about your memory? If **yes**, check whether you are having difficulty with any of the following, and note when the concern started and whether it has progressed:

☐ concentrating
☐ learning and remembering new things
☐ finding the right word
☐ paying bills
☐ other concerns: _____

☐ organizing your medications
☐ driving
☐ problem-solving
☐ decision-making
☐ getting lost in familiar places

Comments: _____

_____

Complete the following:

☐ Do you have a history of anxiety, depression, or other psychological illness?	Yes	No
☐ Are you are having significant pain?	Yes	No
☐ Have there been changes in your medications or their doses recently?	Yes	No
If so, which ones? _____		
☐ Are you taking any dietary supplements?	Yes	No
Which ones? _____		
☐ Do you exercise regularly?	Yes	No
What do you do? _____		
☐ Are you a current or former smoker?	Yes	No
How many years did you smoke? _____		
☐ How much alcohol do you currently drink? _____		
Were you ever a heavy drinker?	Yes	No
☐ Do you use "recreational" drugs?	Yes	No
Have you ever overused these?	Yes	No
☐ Has anyone in your family had depression, anxiety, strokes, heart attacks, dementia, panic attacks, or thyroid problems?	Yes	No
If so, who? _____		

Make sure to review your medications with your provider.

Chapter 9. Balancing Acts

Circle your answers:

Are you afraid that you will fall?	Yes	No
Are you able to get up from a chair without difficulty?	Yes	No
Do you need help getting in and out of the tub or shower?	Yes	No

Do you use any of the following devices for mobility?

Cane	Yes	No
Walker	Yes	No
Wheelchair	Yes	No
Other (specify) _____		

Do any of the following limit the distance you can walk?

Pain	Yes	No
Shortness of Breath	Yes	No
Fatigue	Yes	No
Balance	Yes	No
Other (specify) _____		

Have you had a fall in the last year? If yes, complete the following.* Yes   No

How many falls did you have in the last year? _____

Date the last fall occurred? _____

What were the circumstances of the fall? _____

_____

Check all that occurred with or after the fall:
- ☐ Loss of consciousness
- ☐ Tripped/stumbled over something
- ☐ Lightheadedness, dizziness
- ☐ Rapid or irregular heartbeat
- ☐ I was on the ground or unable to get up for over five minutes
- ☐ I needed assistance to get up

Check if you have any of the following conditions:
- ☐ Diabetes
- ☐ Stroke
- ☐ Neuropathy

*Questions about falls from Reuben et al. (2003); see the Resources section at the end of chapter 9.

- ☐ Severe arthritis
- ☐ Parkinson's disease
- ☐ Cognitive impairment/memory problems
- ☐ Glaucoma
- ☐ Cataracts
- ☐ Severe pain
- ☐ Depression

Complete the following:

☐ Have there been changes in your medications
or their doses recently?   Yes   No

If so, which ones? _____

☐ Are you taking any dietary supplements?   Yes   No

Which ones? _____

☐ When was your last eye examination? _____

☐ Do you exercise regularly?   Yes   No

What do you do? _____

☐ Have you recently had physical therapy, and if so, when?   Yes   No

_____

☐ Are you a current or former smoker?   Yes   No

How many years did you smoke? _____

☐ How much alcohol do you currently drink? _____

Were you ever a heavy drinker?   Yes   No

☐ Do you use "recreational" drugs?   Yes   No

Have you ever overused these?   Yes   No

☐ Has anyone in your family had a neurological condition,
hip fracture, thyroid problems, or osteoporosis?   Yes   No

If so, who? _____

Make sure to review your medications with your provider.

Chapter 10. Sleep Cycles

Complete a sleep log for one or two weeks (see table 10.4).

Answer the following questions:

1. Check all of the following that concern you about your sleep
   - ☐ Difficulty falling asleep
   - ☐ Difficulty staying asleep
   - ☐ Getting up several times a night
   - ☐ Sleepy and wanting to go to bed early in the evening
   - ☐ Not sleepy until very late
   - ☐ Vivid dreams or nightmares
   - ☐ Other: _____

2. Circle your answer(s): Do you snore, breathe irregularly, stop breathing, or kick during the night? (Ask your bed partner.)

3. When did the concerns in questions 1 and 2 start? Have they progressed?

   _____

4. Check all of the following that happen at night or during sleep:
   - ☐ Pain
     Where? _____
   - ☐ Numbness and tingling
     Where? _____
   - ☐ Coughing
   - ☐ Shortness of breath
   - ☐ Leg cramping
   - ☐ Heartburn
   - ☐ Need to use the bathroom three or more times a night
   - ☐ Uncontrollable urge to move your legs
   - ☐ Excessive sweating
   - ☐ Feelings of stress
   - ☐ Other: _____

5. What do you do when you can't sleep? Do you stay in bed? Read, watch TV, use the computer, eat? Other?

   _____

   _____

Complete the following:

☐ Have there been changes in your medications
  or their doses recently?   Yes   No

  If so, which ones? _____

☐ Are you taking any dietary supplements?   Yes   No

  Which ones? _____

☐ Do you have a history of anxiety, depression,
  or other psychological illness?   Yes   No

☐ Are you currently under increased stress?   Yes   No

☐ Do you exercise regularly?   Yes   No

  What time of day? _____

☐ Are you a current or former smoker?   Yes   No

  How many years did you smoke? _____

☐ How much alcohol do you currently drink? _____

  Were you ever a heavy drinker?   Yes   No

☐ Do you use "recreational" drugs?   Yes   No

  Have you ever overused these?   Yes   No

☐ Has anyone in your family had sleep apnea, restless legs
  syndrome, depression, anxiety disorder, thyroid problems? Yes   No

  If so, who? _____

Make sure to review your medications with your provider.

Chapter 11. Urine Trouble

1. Provide some specific examples of the problems you are having and how they
   are affecting your life and activities.

   _____

   _____

   _____

2. Check all that apply:
   - ☐ It feels as if my bladder doesn't completely empty.
   - ☐ I feel strong urges to urinate but rarely leak.
   - ☐ I need to get up several times every night to urinate.
   - ☐ In general, I'm urinating much more often.
   - ☐ My stream doesn't start right away or is weak.
   - ☐ I need to strain to get my stream started.

3. Do you have accidents where you leak or lose urine?   Yes   No

   If yes:

   - ☐ Do you usually lose large or small amounts of urine?   Large   Small

   - ☐ How many pads or pull-ups do you use each day? _____

   - ☐ Using the figure on page 188, what type(s) of incontinence do you likely have?

   _____

   - ☐ If you have both urge and stress symptoms, which bothers you the most?

   _____

3 If you were to spend the rest of your life with your urinary condition just the
   way it is now, how would you feel about that?* (check one)
   - ☐ Delighted   ☐ Mostly dissatisfied
   - ☐ Pleased   ☐ Unhappy
   - ☐ Mostly satisfied   ☐ Terrible
   - ☐ Mixed

Check if you have any of the following conditions:
   - ☐ Diabetes   ☐ Cataracts
   - ☐ Stroke   ☐ Severe pain
   - ☐ Neuropathy   ☐ Depression or anxiety
   - ☐ Severe arthritis   ☐ Thyroid disease
   - ☐ Parkinson's disease   ☐ Leg swelling
   - ☐ Cognitive impairment/memory ☐ Cancer
     problems   ☐ Constipation

*Modified from the International Prostate Symptom Score (IPPS); M. J. Barry, F. J. Fowler, M. P.
O'Leary, et al., "The American Urological Association Symptom Index for Benign Prostatic
Hyperplasia," *Journal of Urology* 148 (1992): 1549–57.

Complete the following:

- ☐ Have there been changes in your medications
  or their doses recently?   Yes   No

  If so, which ones? _____

- ☐ Are you taking any dietary supplements?   Yes   No

  Which ones? _____

- ☐ Do you have a history of pelvic cancer, surgery, or radiation?   Yes   No

- ☐ For women, how many pregnancies and deliveries have you had?

  _____

- ☐ For men and women, do you do pelvic floor exercises
  (also called Kegels)?   Yes   No

- ☐ Do you exercise regularly?   Yes   No

  What types of exercises? _____

- ☐ Are you currently under increased stress?   Yes   No

- ☐ Are you a current or former smoker?   Yes   No

  How many years did you smoke? _____

- ☐ How much caffeine to you drink each day (include coffee, tea, soda, etc.)?

  _____

- ☐ How much alcohol do you currently drink? _____

  Were you ever a heavy drinker?   Yes   No

- ☐ Do you use "recreational" drugs?   Yes   No

  Have you ever overused these?   Yes   No

- ☐ Has anyone in your family had diabetes, sleep apnea,
  depression, anxiety disorder, thyroid problems?   Yes   No

  If so, who? _____

Make sure to review your medications with your provider.

Many people have pain in more than one place in their body. For this visit, decide which one(s) you want evaluated, mark the figure below to show the location of the pain(s), and complete the following.

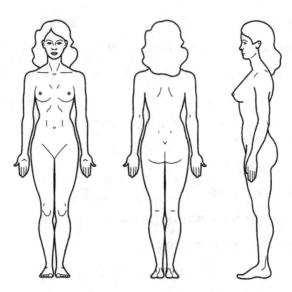

You can help your health care provider by identifying where you are experiencing pain in your body. Adobe Stock

☐ Being as specific as you can, where is the pain? If it moves, where does it go? Is it always there, or does it go away at times?

_____

_____

☐ What were you doing when the pain began? When did it start? Is this the first time you've had a pain like this?

_____

_____

☐ Do you have nausea, constipation, sweating, fever, or any other symptoms with the pain? Does it awaken you from sleep?

_____

_____

☐ Check what the pain feels like:
  ○ An ache
  ○ Pressure
  ○ Burning
  ○ Pins and needles
  ○ Stabbing
  ○ Other: _____

☐ What makes the pain better? What makes it worse? What medications and treatments have you tried to alleviate the pain? Did any work?

_____

_____

☐ How bad is the pain on a scale of 0 to 10, with 0 being no pain and 10 being the worst pain ever? _____

Complete the following:

☐ Have there been changes in your medications or their doses recently?   Yes   No
  If so, which ones? _____

☐ Are you taking any dietary supplements?   Yes   No
  Which ones? _____

☐ Are you currently under increased stress?   Yes   No

☐ Do you exercise regularly?   Yes   No
  What types of exercise? _____

☐ Are you a current or former smoker?   Yes   No
  How many years did you smoke? _____

☐ How much alcohol do you currently drink? _____
  Were you ever a heavy drinker?   Yes   No

☐ Do you use "recreational" drugs?   Yes   No
  Have you ever overused these?   Yes   No

Make sure to review your medications with your provider.

Provide some specific examples of the problems you are having and how they are affecting your life and activities.

_____

_____

_____

The next sections cover specifics of (1) abdominal pain and heartburn, (2) bowel concerns, including (3) constipation and (4) diarrhea, and (5) difficulty swallowing.

1. Complete the following if you have *abdominal pain or heartburn*:

   ☐ Being as specific as you can, where is the pain? If it moves, where does it go? Is it always there, or does it go away at times?

   _____

   _____

   _____

   ☐ When did you first have this pain? What were you doing when the pain began?

   _____

   _____

   _____

   ☐ Check what the pain feels like:
      ○ An ache
      ○ Pressure
      ○ Burning
      ○ Pins and needles
      ○ Stabbing or a knife
      ○ Cramping
      ○ Other _____

   ☐ Do you have nausea, vomiting, diarrhea, constipation, sweating, fever, bloating, gas, or any other symptoms with the pain? Does it awaken you from sleep?

   _____

   _____

   _____

☐ What makes the pain better? What makes it worse? What positions, medications and treatments have you tried to alleviate the pain? Did any work?

_____

_____

☐ How bad is the pain on a scale of 0 to 10, with 0 being no pain and 10 being the worst pain ever? _____

2. Complete the following if you're having *bowel concerns*, including *constipation* or *diarrhea*:

☐ When did this problem start? _____

☐ How often do you have bowel movements? _____

☐ Do you have pain when you move your bowels?   Yes   No

☐ Do you have pain anywhere other than the belly and/or rectum?   Yes   No

If yes, where? _____

☐ Referring to the Bristol stool chart below, what type of stool do you have?

_____

Bristol Stool Chart			
Type 1	Separate hard lumps	Type 5	Soft blobs with clear-cut edges
Type 2	Lumpy and sausage like	Type 6	Mushy consistency with ragged edges
Type 3	Sausage shape with cracks in the surface	Type 7	Liquid consistency with no solid pieces
Type 4	Like a smooth, soft sausage or snake		

Classifying stool by shape and consistency. Adapted from the Bristol scale

☐ Do your stools float in the toilet? Are they bloody or tarry? (circle answers)

☐ Do you use artificial sweetener regularly?   Yes   No

☐ Are there any foods or beverages that make abdominal problems worse? Better? What are they?

_____

_____

☐ Are you having new difficulty urinating?   Yes   No

☐ How much fiber do you eat (cereals, vegetables)? _____

_____

☐ How many glasses of liquids are you drinking daily? _____

☐ How much coffee do you drink daily? _____

☐ How much exercise do you get daily, and what kind? _____

_____

3. If you're *constipated*, complete the following:

    ☐ Are there certain positions that make it easier for you to have a bowel movement? What are they?

     _____

    ☐ Do you feel that you're unable to totally evacuate your rectum?   Yes   No

    ☐ Are you taking any laxatives or special foods to help with the constipation? If yes, what are they?

     _____

4. If you're having *diarrhea*, check if any of the following apply to you:
    ☐ Diarrhea at night
    ☐ Leaking stool, gas, or mucus (circle which one)
    ☐ Recent travel abroad
    ☐ Taking medications or special diet to help. If so, what?

     _____

5. If you are having *difficulty swallowing*, complete the following:

    ☐ When did this start? How often does it happen? _____

     _____

    ☐ Is the difficulty mainly when swallowing solids or liquids? (circle answer)

    ☐ Do you cough or choke when eating and drinking?   Yes   No

    ☐ Does your voice sound wet after eating or drinking?   Yes   No

    ☐ Do you have pain when you swallow?   Yes   No

     If yes, where is the pain? Back of throat? Chest? Other _____

☐ Does food reflux (backflow) into your mouth?	Yes	No
☐ Do you have a sour taste in your mouth after eating?	Yes	No

Complete the following:

☐ Have there been changes in your medications
or their doses recently?   Yes   No

If so, which ones? _____

☐ Are you taking any dietary supplements?   Yes   No

Which ones? _____

☐ Are you currently under increased stress?   Yes   No

☐ Do you have a neurological disease, diabetes, cancer, or have
had any abdominal or gynecologic surgery or radiation?   Yes   No

If yes, where? _____

☐ Are you a current or former smoker?   Yes   No

How many years did you smoke? _____

☐ How much alcohol do you currently drink? _____

Were you ever a heavy drinker?   Yes   No

☐ Do you use "recreational" drugs?   Yes   No

Have you ever overused these?   Yes   No

☐ Has anyone in your family had thyroid problems, inflammatory
bowel disease, GERD, or cancer?   Yes   No

If yes to cancer, what type? _____

Make sure to review your medications with your provider.

Chapter 15. Weighing In

Which of the following do you want to discuss at your visit?
- ☐ Being overweight or losing weight
- ☐ Being underweight or gaining weight
- ☐ Recent weight loss
- ☐ Other: _____

Check your answers to the following three questions:*

1. My appetite is:
   - □ very poor
   - □ poor
   - □ average
   - □ good
   - □ very good

2. When I eat:
   - □ I feel full after eating only a few mouthfuls
   - □ I feel full after eating about a third of a meal
   - □ I feel full after eating over half a meal
   - □ I feel full after eating most of the meal
   - □ I hardly ever feel full

3. Normally I eat:
   - □ less than one meal a day
   - □ one meal a day
   - □ two meals a day
   - □ three meals a day
   - □ more than three meals a day

Provide examples of typical meals for you:

Breakfast (or first meal) _____

Lunch (or second meal) _____

Dinner (or third meal) _____

Snacks (or additional meals) _____

Complete the following:

□ During the 24 hours of the day, how much time do you spend:

Sitting _____

Walking _____

Exercising (other than walking) _____

Sleeping _____

*Questions from the Council of Nutrition Appetite Questionnaire; M. G. Wilson, D. R. Thomas, L. Z. Rubenstein, et al., "Appetite Assessment: Simple Appetite Questionnaire Predicts Weight Loss in Community-Dwelling Adults and Nursing Home Residents," *American Journal of Clinical Nutrition* 82, no. 5 (2005): 1074–81.

☐ What do you consider your "typical" adult weight? _____

☐ When was the last time you weighed this amount? _____

☐ How much weight have you gained or lost over the last six months to a year?

_____

Check if you have any of the following:
☐ Difficulty swallowing
☐ Difficulty chewing
☐ Constipation
☐ Diarrhea
☐ Excessive volume when you urinate
☐ Severe pain. If yes, where? _____

☐ Light-headedness when you stand
☐ Depression, stress, or anxiety
☐ Swelling of legs, scrotum, or abdomen
☐ Shortness of breath or exhaustion with walking

Complete the following:

☐ Have there been changes in your medications or their doses recently?   Yes   No

If so, which ones? _____

☐ Are you taking any dietary supplements?   Yes   No

Which ones? _____

☐ Are you currently under increased stress or feeling depressed?   Yes   No

☐ Do you exercise regularly?   Yes   No

What types of exercise? _____

☐ Are you a current or former smoker?   Yes   No

How many years did you smoke? _____

☐ How much alcohol do you currently drink? _____

Were you ever a heavy drinker?   Yes   No

☐ Do you use "recreational" drugs?   Yes   No

Have you ever overused these?   Yes   No

☐ Has anyone in your family had thyroid problems, diabetes, or cancer?   Yes   No

If cancer, what kind? _____

Make sure to review your medications with your provider.

Chapter 16. Sex Talk

Which of the following do you want to address at the visit? Check all that apply.

☐ My sexual or gender orientation

☐ Practicing safe sex

☐ Little desire or interest in having sex

☐ Little pleasure from sex

☐ Difficulty getting aroused. Possible reasons (please check)
  ○ I feel unattractive
  ○ I'm not feeling excited after usual thoughts or fantasies
  ○ I'm not feeling excited after genital stimulation
  ○ My erection is inadequate
    ○ If yes, do you have sleep-associated erections?   Yes   No

☐ Inability to have an orgasm
  ○ With a partner
  ○ With self-stimulation
  ○ Multiple times as I did previously
  ○ As soon after the first orgasm as I did previously

☐ Pain during sex
  ○ During manual stimulation
  ○ During intercourse itself
  ○ In certain positions, or unable to find comfortable position

☐ Other concerns: _____

For each concern that you marked down:

☐ Provide some specific examples of the problems you are having and how they are affecting your life and activities.

_____

_____

_____

☐ When did this concern start? Was it suddenly or gradually?

_____

_____

☐ How often are you having this problem (these problems)?

_____

☐ Do you have a spouse or other romantic, intimate, or sexual partner? If yes, answer the following (if not, see below):

○ How long have you been together? _____

○ In general, how often have you had sex? _____

○ Was sex ever an issue in the past? _____

○ When was the last time you had sex with this person? _____

○ Describe the quality of your relationship. Do you think this could be interfering with your sex life?

_____

○ Is your partner in good health?   Yes   No

○ Do either of you have other sexual partners?   Yes   No

○ Do you self-stimulate? _____

○ Are your spouse or other partners male, female, both, or transgender?

_____

☐ If you don't have a regular partner:

○ How often do you self-stimulate? _____

○ How often do you try to have sex with another person? _____

○ When was the last time you had sex with another person? _____

○ Are your sexual partners male, female, both, or transgender?

_____

Complete the following:

☐ Have there been changes in your medications
or their doses recently?   Yes   No

If so, which ones? _____

☐ Are you taking any dietary supplements?   Yes   No

Which ones? _____

☐ Are you currently under increased stress or feeling depressed?   Yes   No

☐ Do you exercise regularly?   Yes   No

   What types of exercise? _____

☐ Are you a current or former smoker?   Yes   No

   How many years did you smoke? _____

☐ How much alcohol do you currently drink? _____

   Were you ever a heavy drinker?   Yes   No

☐ Do you use "recreational" drugs?   Yes   No

   Have you ever overused these?   Yes   No

☐ Do you or your partner have heart disease, high blood pressure,
   high cholesterol, diabetes, peripheral artery disease, Parkinson's disease,
   multiple sclerosis, or severe pain? (Circle answers and note Me/Partner.)

☐ Have you or your partner had a mastectomy, hysterectomy, prostate surgery,
   history of pelvic injury, surgery, radiation, or spinal injury or surgery?
   (Circle answers and note Me/Partner.)

☐ Has anyone in your family had thyroid problems, diabetes, or heart disease?

Make sure to review your medications with your provider.

Index

Page numbers in **boldface** refer to illustrations, boxes, and tables.

Index

anorgasmia, **323–24**, 324–25

antacids, **271, 278**

antiarrhythmics, **208, 221, 249, 275, 296, 304**

antibiotics, **82, 126, 210, 222, 251, 278–79, 297, 307**

anticholinergics: drugs to avoid, 29, **29–30**; drugs to use with caution, **31**; side effects, **125, 186, 208, 210, 277, 306**

anticonvulsants, **82, 125, 152, 209, 222, 245, 247, 249, 276, 297, 305, 323**

antidepressants: concerns for older adults, **247**; drugs to avoid, **30**; drugs to use with caution, **31**; indications and mechanism of action, **245**; side effects, **81, 105, 114, 125, 152, 171, 185, 209, 221, 249, 276, 305,** 323, **323**; withdrawal symptoms, **83**

antidiarrheals, **82, 152**

antidiuretic hormone (ADH), **181–82**

anti-dizziness medications: drugs to use with caution, **31**; side effects, **81, 105, 152, 276**

antiestrogens, **209**

antifungals, **222, 251, 279, 297**

antihistamines: drugs to avoid, **29–30**; side effects, **82, 126, 153, 186, 210, 221, 278, 307**

antihypertensives, **249, 296**

antimalarials, **210, 222**

antimetabolites, **297**

antimicrobials, **222, 251, 278–79, 297, 307**

anti-Parkinsonian medications: drugs to avoid, **30**; side effects, **82, 114, 125, 152, 171, 250, 276, 277, 305–6**

antipsychotics: drugs to avoid, **30**; drugs to use with caution, **31**; side effects, **82, 105, 125, 151, 171, 185, 210, 276, 305, 323**

antiseizure medications. *See* anticonvulsants

antispasmodics: drugs to avoid, **30**; side effects, **82, 105, 126, 152, 278, 306**

anti-thyroid medications, **306**

anti-tuberculosis medications, **210, 251, 279, 297**

antivirals, **279, 307**

anxiety, 77; drugs that cause or are associated with, **124–27**; disorders, **118**, 123–24

anxiolytics: drugs to avoid, **30**; side effects, **81, 105, 114, 125, 151, 171–72, 185, 222, 323**

appetite, **292**, 298

aripiprazole (Abilify), **31**

aromatase inhibitors, **153, 252**

arthritis, 253, 258. *See also* osteoarthritis

artificial tears, 204

ascorbic acid (vitamin C), **279**

aspiration, **264**, 274

aspirin, **31, 58,** 60–61, **221**

assisted living, 344

assistive devices, ix, 140–41, 156, 238, 258, 366, 366–68

asthma, **162**

atenolol (Tenormin), **28, 104, 151, 208, 275**

atorvastatin (Lipitor), **104, 170, 208, 221, 249, 275, 304, 323**

atropine, **105, 152, 306**

atropine/diphenoxylate (Lomotil), **82,** 152

attitude toward aging, 3–12

audiobooks, 204–5

audiograms, **215**

autoimmune medications, **251**

avanafil (Spedra), 325

azithromycin (Zithromax), **307**

back pain, 150, **154,** 248, 255

baclofen (Lioresal), **30**

bacteriuria, asymptomatic, 179

balance and falls, 134, **135, 136–37, 140,** 141; adapting to your new normal, 143–50; advice for loved ones, 156; age-related changes, 138–43, **139–40**; conditions that can worsen, 150; drugs that cause falls, 150, **151–53;** emergency fall plan, 144; evaluation of, 155–56; fear of falling, 142; getting ready to meet your doctor about, 376–77; physical therapy for, 146; predisposing and precipitating factors, **18;** prevention of falls, 50, 142–46, 157; resources, 157; risk factors, **18,** 142; risky behavior, 144; specialists for, 155, **155;** symptoms that need prompt medical attention, 150

balance exercises, 99, 145–46

barbiturates, **30, 82**

bariatric surgery, 287

Barrett's esophagus, 274

Baruch, Bernard, 4

beclomethasone (Qvar), **306**

bed rest, 103

Beers criteria, 29

behavior(s). *See* mood and behavior

behavioral health professionals, 130

behavioral therapy, 131, 188, 189, 193, 241

benign prostatic hyperplasia (BPH), **182, 183,** 187, 193, 196; alpha-blockers for, **186, 211, 222, 278, 324**

benzodiazepines, 29, 124; side effects, **114, 209, 221, 249, 276, 305;** withdrawal symptoms, **83**

benztropine (Cogentin), **30, 82, 125, 277, 306**

deconditioning, 103

decongestants, **126**, **153**, **172**, **186**, **210**, 297

deliberate practice, 116

delirium, 78–79

dementia, 69, 70, **72**, 80; advice for loved ones, 86, 87–88, 257; behaviors that suggest, 86–87; driving with, 354; drugs for, **172**, **306**; earliest signs, 83; incontinence with, 198; risk factors, 76; sleep disorders with, 173; types of, **84**. *See also* Alzheimer disease; cognitive abilities

denosumab (Prolia, Xgeva), **297**

dentures, 301–2

depression, 80, 103, **113**; anhedonia, 122–23; drugs that cause, 122, **124–27**; major depressive disorder (MDD), **117–18**, 122, 123; and sex, 323; subsyndromal, **118**, 122, 123. *See also* antidepressants; mood and behavior

desipramine (Norpramin), **31**, **81**, **125**, 323

desloratadine (Clarinex), **82**

DEXA (dual energy X-ray absorptiometry), **64**

dexamethasone (Decadron), **82**, **126**, **153**, **170**, **186**, **209**, **222**, **250**, **297**, **306**

dexamphetamine (Dexedrine, Zenzedi), **125**, **172**, **305**

diabetes, 194; drugs for, **125**, **152**, **186**, **222**, **250**, **277**, **297**, **306–7**; drugs to avoid, **30**; prevention of, 66; screening for, **58**, 58–59, 66; treatment of, 59

diarrhea, 267, 273–74, 282–83; drugs that cause, **275–79**

diastole, **94**

diastolic BP, **94**

diazepam (Valium), **30**, **105**, **125**, **151**, **171**, **221**, **323**

dicyclomine (Bentyl), **30**, **82**, **105**, **126**, **152**, **278**, **306**

didanosine/ddI (Videx), **251**, **279**, **307**

dietary changes: foods that cause gas, 272–73; healthy diet, 217; Mediterranean diet, 270, 300; resources, 284, 310; suggestions for, 299–301; ways to increase energy, 97; ways to increase fiber intake, 269

dietary supplements, 32, 36–37, 298

difficult decisions, 331–34, 360–61

digestion, **262–63**, 283. *See also* gastrointestinal problems

digoxin (Lanoxin), **208**, **275**, **296**, **304**

diltiazem (Cardizem), **104**, **151**, **185**, **275**, **304**

dimenhydrinate (Dramamine), **31**, **81**, **105**, **152**, **276**

diphenhydramine (Benadryl): concerns for older adults, **246**; side effects, 29, **82**, **126**, **153**, 165, 169, **172**, **186**, **210**, 278, **307**

diphtheria, 55–56

disc herniation, **235**, 255

disequilibrium, 150

disinhibition, 115

diuretics, **81**, **104**, **124**, **151**, **170**, **185**, 191, 195, **208**, **221**, **249**, **275**, **296**, **304**, **323**

diverticulitis, 280–81

diverticulosis, **265**, 280

dizziness, 150; anti-dizziness medications, **31**, **81**, **105**, **152**, **276**; drugs that cause, **151–53**. *See also* balance and falls

docetaxel (Taxotere, Docefrez), **252**

doctors: choosing, 8; getting ready to meet, 369–92. *See also* health care providers; specialists

dolasetron (Anzemet), **278**

donepezil (Aricept), **114**, **152**, **172**, **186**, **249**, **276**, **306**

Do Not Resuscitate (DNR) orders, 358–59

dopamine agonists, **125**, **152**, **250**, **277**, **306**

double voiding, 184–87

dowager's hump, **139**

doxazosin (Cardura), **105**, **185**, **208**, **275**, **304**, **324**

doxepin (Silenor, Sinequan), **30**, **81**, **105**, **185**

doxycycline (Periostat, Vibramycin), **222**, **251**, **279**

doxylamine (Unisom, Nytol Maximum Strength), **29**, 165

DPP-4 inhibitors, **250**, **277**, **307**

driving, 50, 201–2, 347–55, **351**; adapting to your new normal, 349–52; advice for loved ones, 352–53; age-related changes, 347–49; evaluation of, 350–51, 353–54; resources, 353–55

droperidol, **172**

drug levels, **24**, **25**

drug side effects: cognitive changes, 79–80, **81–82**; depression, anxiety, and mania, 122, **124–27**; eye symptoms and disease, **208–11**; falls, muscle weakness, dizziness, and bone loss, 150, **151–53**; GI symptoms, 268, **275–79**; hearing loss and tinnitus, 220, **221–22**; joint pain, muscle pain and cramps, and peripheral neuropathy, **249–52**; low energy or exercise intolerance, 103, **104–5**; nutrient deficiencies, **296–97**, 303; sexual impairment, **323–24**; sleep disturbances, 167, **170–72**; urinary incontinence, **185–86**,

fluids, 184, 269
fluoroquinolones, **82**, **126**, **153**, 210, 251, 278, **307**
fluorouracil (Adrucil), **297**
fluoxetine (Prozac), **105**, **171**, **276**, 305
fluphenazine (Prolixin), **151**
flu shots, **51**, 52, **53**, 54–55
fluticasone (ArmonAir), **250**
FODMAPs (fermentable oligosaccharides, disaccharides, monosaccharides, and polyols), 272–73
food: intake, **292**, 302; lists, 284; preparation, 303; resources, 310–11
foot abnormalities or pain, 150, **155**
footwear, 144
formoterol (Perforomist), **250**, **277**
fractures, 50, 147, 255
frailty, 92, **96**
free recall, **71–72**
frontotemporal dementia (FTD), **84**
functional incontinence, **188**, 193–94
furosemide (Lasix), **81**, **104**, 151, **170**, **185**, 208, **221**, 249, 275, **296**, **304**, 323

gabapentin (Neurontin), **81**, **104**, 124, 151, 185, 221, 245, 276, 305, 323
gait: problems, **155**; speed, **135**, 138
galantamine (Razadyne), **152**, **186**, **222**, 249, **276**, **306**
gallbladder disease, 280
gallstones, **265**, 266–67
gamma-aminobutyric acid (GABA), **305**
gastrocolic reflex, 268
gastrointestinal (GI) medications, **82**, **105**, **126**, 152–53, 210, 251, 278, **297**, **306**
gastrointestinal (GI) problems, 260–85; adapting to your new normal, 267–73; advice for loved ones, 283–84; age-related changes, 260–67, **264–66**; conditions that mimic or worsen, 274–83; drugs that cause, **275–79**; evaluation for, 283; getting ready to meet your doctor about, 384–87; resources, 284; specialists for, 283; symptoms that need prompt medical attention, 273–74. *See also specific problems*
gastrointestinal (GI) system, **261**
gender identity, 318
generalized anxiety disorder (GAD), **118**, 123. *See also* anxiety
gentamicin, **222**, **297**
GERD (gastroesophageal reflux disease), **162**, **264**, 266, 270, 274; drugs for, **271–72**; drugs

that cause or worsen, 270, **275–79**. *See also* gastrointestinal problems
geriatric health care providers, 21. *See also* health care providers
geriatric medical information, 21–22
Geriatrics 5M's, 19–20
geriatric syndromes, 17–19, 179
giant cell arteritis (GCA), 248, 253
glaucoma, **206**, 206, **208–11**; medications, **308**
glimepiride (Amaryl), **125**, **306**
glipizide (Glucotrol), **105**, **125**, 152, **170**, **306**
GLP-1 agonists, **277**, **307**
glucose, 59
glyburide (Diabeta, Glynase, Micronase), **30**, **105**, **125**, 152, **170**, 211, **306**
Goldilocks approach, **26**, 26–33
gonadotropin-releasing hormone agonists, **126**
goserelin (Zoladex), **126**
gout, 253
GPS (Global Positioning System), 365
grief, 115, 122
group therapy, 121

H_2 blockers: for GERD, **271**; side effects, **82**, **126**, **153**, 210, 278, **297**, **306**
hair cells, **214**
hallucinations, visual, 121
haloperidol (Haldol), **31**, **82**, 151, 171, **185**, 323
headaches, 248
head trauma, 77
health care, 38–46; advice for loved ones, 45–46; resources, 46. *See also* medical care
health care providers, 21, 43–45. *See also* primary care provider; specialists
health care proxy (HCP), 45, 356–59
health goals, 40–43, **44**, 45
health information resources, 284
health management, 40
health priorities, 39–45, **44**, 101, 360
hearing, 212–24, **213–15**, 215–16, 223; adapting to your new normal, 217–19; advice for loved ones, 220–23; age-related changes, 199, 212–16, **216**, 348; aids, 73, 218–19; conditions that mimic or worsen, 219–20; drugs associated with changes in, 220, **221–22**; measurement of, **215**; resources, 223–24; symptoms that need prompt medical attention, 219
heart: failure, **162**; health, 76, 320
heartburn, **162**, 266, **275–79**. *See also* GERD

lean body mass (LBM), **288**, **295**
learning new things, 69–70, **71**, 74
leg cramps, **163**, 255
leg pain, **154**, 255
leg swelling, 194, 195
lesbian, gay, bisexual, trangender, or queer (LGBTQ) people, 318
letrozole (Femara), **153**, **252**
leucovorin, **297**
leukotriene receptor antagonists, **126**
leuprolide (Lupron), **126**
levetiracetam (Keppra), **82**, **125**, **152**, **249**, **276**
levocetirizine dihydrochloride (Xyzal), **82**
levodopa/carbidopa (Sinemet), **82**, **114**, **125**, **171**
levofloxacin (Levaquin), **82**, **126**, **153**, **210**, **251**, **278**, **307**
levothyroxine (Synthroid), **28**, **170**, **186**, **306**
Lewy body dementia (LBD), **84**
libido, **313**, **323–24**
lidocaine, 243–44
lidoderm, **246**
life expectancy, 5
life review, 119
ligaments, **230**, **234**
lightheadedness, 150
light sensitivity, **208–11**
limbic system, **112**, **113**
linagliptin (Tradjenta), **307**
liothyronine (Cytomel), **170**
lisdexamfetamine (Vyvanse), **125**, **305**
lisinopril (Prinivil, Zestril), **104**, **151**, **170**, **185**, **275**, **304**
lithium (Eskalith, Lithobid), **171**
local services, 345–46, 355
local support, 335–37
local transportation services, 355
lockjaw (tetanus), 55–56
long-term care (LTC) insurance, 338
long-term memory, **73**, **74**
loratadine (Claritin), **82**, **210**
lorazepam (Ativan), 29, **30**, **81**, **83**, **114**, **125**, **171**, **221**, **323**
losartan (Cozaar), **104**, **151**, **275**, **304**
loved ones, xi
low-density lipoprotein (LDL), 59–60
low energy, 106–7; drugs that cause, 103, **104–5**
lower esophageal sphincter (LES), **262–63**
low vision, 204
lumbar stenosis, **154**, **155**, 254, 255
lung cancer screening, **62**, 63

macronutrients, **289**, **290**
macular degeneration, 204–5; age-related, **206**, 207; medications associated with, **210**
magnesium antacids, **278**
magnesium deficiency, **296**, **297**
magnetic gait, **84**
magnetic resonance imaging (MRI), 121
major depressive disorder (MDD), **117**, **118**, 122, 123
malabsorption, 282–83
mammography, **62**
mania: behaviors, 121–22; drugs that cause, **124–27**
marijuana, medical, **246**, **247**
massage, therapeutic, 241, 258
mattresses, 238
measles, **53**
mechanical ventilation, 358–59
meclizine (Antivert, Bonine), **31**, **81**, **105**, **126**, **152**, **210**, **276**, **278**, **307**
median nerve, **232**
Medicaid, 338, 340, 346
medical care, 13–22. *See also* health care
medical information resources, 21–22, 284
medical power of attorney, 356
Medicare, 146, 338; annual wellness visits (AWVs), 51–52; Part D, **35**; Welcome to Medicare visits, 51
medications, 19, 23–37, **24**, **25**; adverse effects, 14–15, 23–24, **24**, 32; advice for loved ones, 33; Beers criteria, 29; costs, **35**, 37; deprescribing, 36; dosage, 33; drugs to avoid or use with caution, **29–30**; Goldilocks approach to, **26**, 26–33; higher-risk, 29, **29–31**; newly approved, 32; over-the-counter (OTC), 23, **34**; personal lists, 27, **28**, **34**; pill esophagitis, 267–68; polypharmacy, 26–27; prescribing cascade, 24; resources, 36–37; reviewing, **51**, 145, 268; tips for taking, **34–35**; underdosing, 27–29; withdrawal symptoms, 80, **83**, 167, 248, 274. *See also* drug side effects
meditation, **112**, 120–21, 132
Mediterranean diet, 270, 300
medroxyprogesterone, **306**
meglitinide analogs, **250**, **277**, **307**
melatonin, **81**, 166
memory, 69–70, **70**, **72**, **73–74**; cued recall, **72**; free recall, **71–72**; resources, 88; strategies to help, 73–77. *See also* cognitive abilities
meningitis, 55
metabolic equivalents (METs), **93**, **95**

metabolism, **288–89**
metaxalone (Skelaxin), **81**, **104**, **125**, **275**
metformin (Glucophage, Glumetza), **152**, **277**, **297**, **307**
methimazole (Tapazole), **306**
methocarbamol (Robaxin), **30**, **104**, **151**, **185**, **246**
methyldopa, **104**, **124**, **304**
methylphenidate (Ritalin, Concerta), **125**, **151**, **172**, **305**
methylprednisolone (Solu-Medrol), **82**, **126**, **153**, **170**, **186**, **209**, **222**, **250**, **277**, **297**, **306**
metoclopramide (Reglan), **126**, **153**
metolazone (Zaroxolyn), **81**, **104**, **208**, **249**, **275**, **296**, **304**, **323**
metoprolol (Lopressor, Toprol), **81**, **104**, **124**, **151**, **170**, **221**, **275**, **304**, **323**
metronidazole (Flagyl), **251**, **307**
micronutrients, **289–91**, **295–96**
microscopic colitis (MC), 282
miglitol (Glyset), **277**, **307**
mild cognitive impairment (MCI), 83
mindfulness-based stress reduction (MBSR), **112**, 131
mindfulness meditation, 120–21
mineral supplements, **279**
ministrokes, **84**
minocycline, **251**, **279**
mirabegron (Myrbetriq), **153**, 192, **251**
mirtazapine (Remeron), **81**, **152**, **209**, **276**, **305**, 323
mixed dementia, 80, **84**
mobility, 19, 134, **135**, 156, 157; conditions that can worsen, 150; evaluation of, 155–56; physical therapy for, 146; specialists for, 155, **155**
modafinil (Provigil), **125**, **151**, **172**, **305**
montelukast (Singulair), **126**
mood and behavior, 110–33; adapting to your new normal, 119–21; advice for loved ones, 128–29; age-related changes, 17, 114–16, **117–18**; biology of, **111**; brain areas involved in, **113**; conditions that mimic or worsen, 122–24; evaluation of, 127–28; getting ready to meet your doctor about, 374–75; resources, 130–32; symptoms that need prompt medical attention, 121–22
morning stiffness, 236
morphine: **245**; side effects, **81**, **104**, **125**, **151**, **185**, **245**, **249**, **275**, **304**; withdrawal symptoms, **83**
moving homes, 335–36, 341

moxifloxacin (Avelox), **251**, **278**
multi-complexity, 19–20
multicomponent approaches, 132
multitasking, 70, **72**
muscle: mass, **95**, **294**, 302; relaxation, 241; spasms, 252; sprains, 252; strains, 253; strength, **295**, 302; weakness, **151–53**
muscle pain, 252–53; drugs that cause, 249–52; heat for, 239
muscle relaxants: concerns for older adults, 247; drugs to avoid, **30**; indications and mechanism of action, 246; side effects, **81**, **104**, **125**, **151**, **185**, **275**
musculoskeletal system, **135**; adapting to your new normal, 237–38; age-related changes, **233–35**; anatomy of, **228–30**
music therapy, 241

nadolol (Corgard), **170**
naproxen (Aleve, Naprosyn), 24, **31**, **81**, **104**, **151**, **185**, **208**, **221**, **245**, **275**, **304**
naps, 161
nateglinide (Starlix), **250**
National Institutes of Health (NIH), 16
nausea and/or vomiting, **275–79**
nebulizers, 42
neomycin, **297**
nerve pain, 236–37, 254–55
neurodegenerative disorders, **114**, **118**
neurological diseases, 150
neurological drugs, **125**, **151–52**, **171–72**, **185–86**, **209–10**, **221–22**, **249**, **276**, **305**, **323**
neurotransmitters, **112–13**, **114**
new opportunities, 10
nicardipine (Cardene), **221**
nicotine, **308**
nifedipine (Procardia), **151**, **170**, **185**
nighttime urination, **162**. See also nocturia
nitrates, **275**, **304**
nitrofurantoin (Macrodantin), **251**
nitroglycerin (Nitrostat), **275**, **304**
nizatidine (Axid), **82**, **126**, **210**, **271**, **297**, **306**
nocturia, 179, **181–82**, 194–95
nonsteroidal anti-inflammatory drugs (NSAIDs), 24, 236; concerns for older adults, 247; drugs to avoid, **30**; drugs to use with caution, **31**; indications and mechanism of action, 245; side effects, **81**, **104**, **151**, **185**, **208**, **221**, **264–65**, **275**, **304**; topical, 243
normal aging, ix, 13–26; balance and falls, 138–43, **139–40**; cognitive abilities, 69–70, **71–72**; energy, 91–92, **95**; GI problems,

260–67, **264–66**; hearing, 212–16; mood and behavior, 114–16, **117–18**; musculoskeletal, **233–35**; pain, **233**; sex, 312–18, **316–17**; sleep cycle, 158–61, **160**; urination, 179–83, **181–82**; vision, 200–202, **203**; weight, 286–99, **292–97**

normal pressure hydrocephalus (NPH), **84**

nortriptyline (Pamelor), **31**, **81**, **125**, **221**, **245**, **276**, **305**

numbness and tingling (pins and needles), **163**

nursing home care, 344

nutrition, 50, **289–91**, **295–96**; conditions that mimic or worsen problems, 303; drugs that cause deficiencies, **296–97**, 303

nutritional supplements, **279**, 298

obesity, 92, 286–87, **288**

obesity paradox, **293**

obstructive sleep apnea (OSA), 167–68, **169**

Occam's Razor, 17

occupational therapy (OT), 238, 241–42

ofloxacin (Floxin), **278**

olanzapine (Zyprexa), **30**, **105**, **151**, **185**, **305**, **323**

old age, 4–8

older adults, 14–19

olmesartan (Benicar), **275**

omeprazole (Prilosec), **28**, **82**, **105**, **153**, **251**, **271**, **306**

onabotulinumtoxin A (Botox), **252**

ondansetron (Zofran), **153**, **278**

online dating, 321–22

opioids: concerns for older adults, **247**; indications and mechanism of action, **245**; side effects, **81**, **104**, **125**, **151**, **185**, **249**, **275**, **304**; withdrawal symptoms, **83**

oral health, **51**, 303

oral pain medications, 244

orgasm, **313**, **316**

Osler, Sir William, 38

osteoarthritis (OA), 232, **233–34**, 236; hip, **154**, 253–55; knee and hip, 148, **154**, **155**, 255; specialists for, **155**; spinal, **234–35**, 255. *See also* pain

osteonecrosis of the jaw, 147

osteopathic manipulative treatment (OMT), 242

osteophytes, 236

osteoporosis, **64**, 143, 146–47; drugs, **222**, **297**

overactive bladder, 194

overflow fecal incontinence, 281

overflow incontinence, **188**, 192–93

over-the-counter (OTC) medications, 23, **34**; artificial tears, 204; side effects, 79–80, 268

overweight, 92, 189, 286–87, **288**

oxaliplatin (Eloxatin), **297**

oxybutynin (Ditropan), **31**, **82**, **126**, **153**, **186**, **251**, **278**

oxycodone (Percocet), **81**, **83**, **104**, **151**, **185**, **227**, **245**, **249**, **275**, **304**

oxymetazoline (Afrin, Dristan), **126**, **153**, **172**, **186**

paclitaxel (Taxol), **252**

pain: abdominal, 280–81; aches and pains, 225–59; acute, 225, **226**; advice for loved ones, 256–57; back, 150, **154**, 248, 255; biology of, **225–26**; chronic, **226**; common conditions, 252–55; conditions that mimic or worsen, 150, 248–53; evaluation of, 256; foot, 150; getting ready to meet your doctor about, 382–83; inflammatory, **227**; leg, 255; management, 239–47, 258; muscle, 252–54; nerve, 254–55; neuropathic, **227**, 236–37; nociceptive, **226–27**; persistent, 225, **226**, 239; prevention of, 237–38; radicular, **235**, 254; referred, **227**; resources, 258; severity, **233**; during sex, 319–20; somatic, **226**; symptoms that need prompt medical attention, 150, 248; types of, **226–27**; visceral, **226–27**

pain medications, 147–48, **227**, 236, 242–44, **245–46**; precautions for older adults, **246–47**; sensitivity to, **233**; side effects, **104**, **124–25**, **151**, **185**, **208**, **221**, **249**, **275**, **304–5**, **323**

palliative care, 359–61

pantoprazole (Protonix), **105**, **126**, **153**, **251**, **271**, **278**, **297**, **306**

pap smears, 61, **62**

paradox of positive aging, 114–15, **117**

Parkinsonism, **151**

Parkinson's disease (PD), **84**, **114**, **118**

paroxetine (Paxil), **31**, **81**, **83**, **105**, **171**, **305**, **323**

Patient Priorities Care Initiative (PPCI), 39, 45, 46

pelvic floor muscle exercises, **190**

penicillin, **307**

peptic ulcers, **264–65**, 280

periodic limb movements during sleep (PLMS), 169, **169**

peripheral nervous system (PNS), **231–32**

peripheral neuropathy, 149–50, **249–52**, 254

perphenazine (Trilafon), **125**

personal amplifiers, 218

personal care aides, 338, **339–40**, 340

personal emergency response systems (PERSs), 365

personality changes, 115, **117**, 121–22

pertussis (whooping cough), 55–56

phenobarbital, **30**, **82**, **297**

phenylephrine (SudafedPE), **126**, **153**, **172**, **186**, **210**, **297**

phenytoin (Dilantin), **82**, **152**, **249**, **276**, **297**, **305**, **323**

phosphodiesterase inhibitors, 325

physical activity, 99–100, 108

physical therapy (PT), 100, **139**, 146, 241–42

Physician Orders for Life-Sustaining Treatment (POLST), 358–60

physiological changes, 14–15

physiologic reserves, 14

pill esophageal injury, 280

pill esophagitis, 267–68

pinched nerves, 254

pins and needles (numbness and tingling), **163**

pioglitazone (Actos), **152**, **170**, **186**, **250**, **306**

piroxicam (Feldene), **208**

platinum, **252**, **297**

pneumococcal conjugate vaccine (PCV), **53**, 55

pneumococcal polysaccharide vaccine (PPSV23), **53**, 55

pneumonia, **53**, 55

polymyalgia rheumatica (PMR), 236, 253

polypharmacy, 26–27

positive aging, 114–15, **117**

postherpetic neuralgia (PHN), 56

postprandial hypotension, 141, 149

postural hypotension, 141, 148–49

posture, 138, **139**, 146, 238

potassium, **295–96**; deficiency, **296–97**; supplements, **279**

pramipexole (Mirapex), **82**, **125**, **152**, **171**, **250**, **277**, **306**

pramlintide (SymlinPen), **250**

pravastatin (Pravachol), **104**, **170**, **249**, **323**

prazosin (Minipress), **275**, **304**

prediabetes, 59, 66

prednisone, **82**, **126**, **153**, **170**, **186**, **209**, 222, **246**, **250**, **277**, **297**, **306**

pregabalin (Lyrica), **81**, **104**, **151**, **185**, **245**, **305**, **323**

prehabilitation, 148

presbycusis, 212–13, **216**

presbyopia, ix, 203

prescription drugs. *See* medications

prevention, 47–66, **48–49**; advice for loved ones, 64–65; of constipation, 268; of falls, 142–43, 145–46, 157; of injury, 143; osteoporosis, 146–47; resources, 65–66; urge suppression, **191**

primary care provider (PCP), 38. *See also* health care providers

primidone (Mysoline), **82**, **297**, **323**

problem-solving therapy, 130

procainamide, **249**

prochlorperazine maleate (Compazine), **31**, **276**

progesterone, **277**

progestins, **306**

prokinetics, **126**

promethazine hydrochloride (Phenergan), **221**

propantheline, **30**, **82**, **105**, **126**, **152**, **278**, **306**

propranolol (Inderal), **81**, **124**, **170**, **275**, **304**, **323**

proprioception, **136**

propylthiouracil, **306**

prostate: cancer screening, **48**, **62**, 63; enlargement, **182**, 183; shrinkers, **324**

prostate-specific antigen (PSA) screening, **48**, **62**

prostatitis, 196

protein, **289**, **295**; recommended daily amount, **295**, 299, 302; recommended dietary intake, 299–300, 302; ways to increase energy, 97, 99

proton pump inhibitors (PPIs): for GERD, 271–72; side effects, **82**, **105**, **126**, **153**, **251**, **278**, **297**, **306**

protriptyline (Vivactil), **171**

pseudoephedrine (Sudafed), **126**, **153**, **172**, **186**, **210**, **297**

psychoeducational skills-building, 132

psychological drugs. *See* psychotropic drugs

psychotherapy, 121, 130–32

psychotropic drugs, **125**, **151–52**, **171–72**, **185–86**, **209–10**, **221–22**, **249**, **276**, **305**, **323**

pulmonary drugs, **126**, **171**, **210**, **250**, **277**, **297**, **306**

pulmonary rehabilitation, 41, 100

quetiapine (Seroquel), **31**, **82**, **105**, **151**, **185**, **305**, **323**

quinapril (Accupril), **124**

taxanes, 252
temazepam (Restoril), **81**, **83**, 165, **209**, **249**, **276**, **305**
temperature extremes, 50
tendons, **230**, **234**
tenofovirDF (Viread), **153**
terazosin (Hytrin), **105**, **185**, **186**, **211**, **222**, **275**, **278**, **304**, **324**
terbutaline, **171**, **250**, **277**
testosterone: levels, 102, **317**; replacement, 102, 315
tetanus, diphtheria, and pertussis, **53**, 55–56
tetracyclines, **251**, **278**, **279**, **307**
theophylline, **126**, **171**, **277**
therapeutic massage, 241
therapists, behavioral health, 130
thiazolidinediones, **152**, **186**, **250**, **306**–7
thioridazine (Mellaril), **30**, **82**, **125**, **185**, **210**, **323**
thyroid drugs, **170**, **306**
time-limited trials, 359
time management, 101
timolol, **221**
tinnitus, 219, **221**–22
tiotropium (Spiriva), **210**
tizanidine (Zanaflex), **246**
tobramycin, **297**
toileting, 184
tolazamide, **125**
tolbutamide (Orinase), **125**, **222**, **306**
tolcapone (Tasmar), **152**, **172**, **250**, **276**, **305**
tolteradine (Detrol), **31**, **82**, **126**, **153**, **186**, **251**, **278**
topical pain medications, 243–44
topiramate (Topamax, Qudexy XR), **125**, **209**, **221**, **305**, **323**
torsemide (Demadex), **249**
total energy expenditure, **288**
touch hunger, **117**, 129
tramadol (Ultram), **81**, **83**, **104**, **125**, **151**, **185**, **249**, **275**, **304**
transcutaneous electrical nerve stimulation (TENS), 241
transportation services, 351–52, 355
trauma, 14–15
trazodone (Desyrel), **81**, **152**, **209**, **276**
trial of therapy, time-limited, 359
triamterene-hydrochlorothiazide (Dyazide), **81**, **151**, **249**, **275**, **323**
triazolam (Halcion), **81**, **83**, **125**, **185**, **209**, **249**, **276**, **305**
tricyclic antidepressants (TCAs): indications

and mechanism of action, **245**; side effects, **81**, **105**, **125**, **152**, **185**, **209**, 323, **323**
trifluoperazine (Stelazine), **210**
trihexyphenidyl (Artane), **30**, **82**, **125**, **277**, **306**
triptans, **208**

ulcers, **263**, **264–65**, 280
underweight, **288**, **293**, 298
uninhibited bladder contractions (UBCs), **181**, 189, **191**
universal adaptations to prevent falls, 144–46
upper esophageal sphincter (UES), **262**
urge incontinence, **188**, 189–92, 194
urge suppression, **191**
urinary incontinence, 41–42, 179, **181**; with dementia, 198; medications and, **185–86**, 188, 191; new-onset, 183; treatments for, 187–89; types of, **188**. *See also* urination
urinary medications, **153**, **185–86**, **211**, **251**, **278**, **324**
urinary retention, 281
urinary system, **180**
urinary tract infections (UTIs), 179, **181**
urination, 179–98, **180**; adapting to your new normal, 183–95; advice for loved ones, 197; age-related changes, 179–83, **181–82**; conditions that mimic or worsen, 195–96; double voiding, 184–87; evaluation of, 196–97; getting ready to meet your doctor about, 379–81; nocturia, 179, **181–82**, 194–95; symptoms that need prompt medical attention, 195; ways to avoid problems, 183–84
US Preventive Services Task Force (USPSTF), **49**

vaccines, 52–57
vaginal atrophy, 196
valproic acid (Depakene, Depakote, Divalproex), **82**, **152**, **221**, **249**, **276**, **305**, **323**
valsartan (Diovan), **275**
vancomycin (Vancocin), **222**
vardenafil (Levitra, Staxyn), **209**, 325
vascular dementia (VD), **84**
venlafaxine (Effexor), **81**, **83**, **105**, **114**, **152**, **171**, **185**, **221**, **245**, **276**, **323**
verapamil (Calan), **104**, **185**, **275**, **304**
vertebra, **231**
vertebral compression fractures, 255
vertigo, 150, **155**
vestibular system, **136–37**
vilazodone (Viibryd), 323

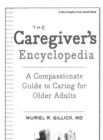
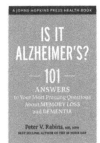
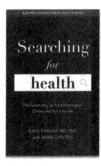
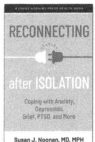
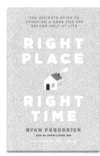
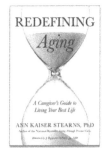

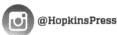
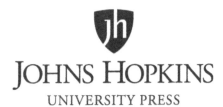